INTERVENTIONAL CARDIOLOGY

Edited by **Ibrahim Akin**

Interventional Cardiology
http://dx.doi.org/10.5772/65543
Edited by Ibrahim Akin

Contributors

Rodrigo Estévez-Loureiro, Mario Castaño, Tomas Benito-Gonzalez, Javier Gualis, Armando Perez De Prado, Felipe Fernandez Vazquez, Stefan Baumann, Hussien Heshmat, Mahmoud Elmahdy, Mohamad Abdelmeguid, Yassir Mohamed Helmy El Haddad, Tobias Becher, Frederik Eder, Christian Fastner, Michael Behnes, Dirk Loßnitzer, Christina Dösch, Martin Borggrefe, Uzair Ansari, Ibrahim El-Battrawy, Gregor Leibundgut, Matthias Kaspar, Abdul Wahab Hritani, Suhail Allaqaband, M. Fuad Jan, Mustafa Yildiz, Ibrahim Akin, Dogac Oksen, Takashi Murashita, Vladimir Ganyukov, Roman Sergeevich Tarasov, Hamidreza Sanati

Published by InTech

Janeza Trdine 9, 51000 Rijeka, Croatia

Publishing Process Manager Martina Blecic
Technical Editor SPi Global
Cover InTech Design team

First published July, 2017
Printed in Croatia
Legal deposit, Croatia: National and University Library in Zagreb

Additional hard copies can be obtained from orders@intechopen.com

Interventional Cardiology, Edited by Ibrahim Akin
p. cm.
Print ISBN 978-953-51-3293-6
Online ISBN 978-953-51-3294-3

For EU product safety concerns:
IN TECH d.o.o., Prolaz Marije Krucifikse Kozulić 3, 51000 Rijeka, Croatia,
info@intechopen.com or visit our website at intechopen.com.

Meet the editor

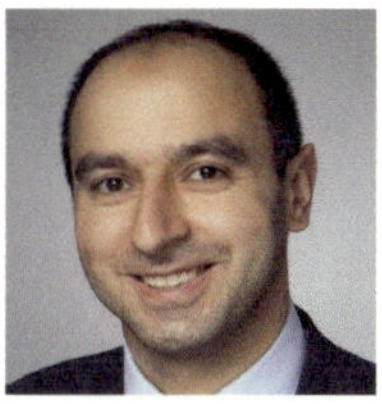

Professor Akin graduated from the University of Medicine in Hannover in 2004 and completed his clinical training in catheterization laboratory in Chemnitz, University Hospital of Rostock, and the Heart Center at Bad Segeberg. He has specialized in the field of interventional cardiology and has also extensive experience in cardiac device therapy, cardiac electrophysiology, and the treatment of structural heart disease. Professor Akin was nominated as chief of the cardiac catheterization laboratories at the University Hospital Mannheim in 2013, consolidating the interventional expertise in the treatment of coronary heart disease and structural heart disease in the region. He has maintained an active role in the practice of cardiac electrophysiology and implantation of cardiac devices and, in 2015, was promoted to the additional position of deputy chief of cardiology. His clinical research is primarily relegated to the field of invasive cardiology, with special interests in coronary stent technology, left atrial appendage interventions, modern cardiac device therapies, as well as treatment of patients suffering from cardiac arrest and ion-channel diseases.

Contents

Preface

The practice of interventional cardiology has undergone a sea of change since its initiation in clinical routine by Andreas Gruentzig in the 1970s. The continuing stream of innovation addressing the treatment of occlusive coronary artery disease, which began with the use of bare-metal stents 30 years ago, was followed by the era of the drug-eluting stents 10 years later. The recent advent of bioresorbable scaffolds, improved coronary imaging modalities with IVUS and OCT, as well as optimized supportive treatment has established interventional therapies as standard procedures for management of coronary artery disease. Additionally, several interventional therapeutic strategies have become increasingly relevant in the treatment of structural heart disease. The complexity of all these modern interventions, enabled by the availability of vastly improved noninvasive and invasive methods, demands optimal planning and a detailed discussion in an interdisciplinary heart team.

The chapters in this textbook outline and describe the essential branches of interventional cardiology. It offers an insight into the differential plans of treatment for patients suffering from an acute coronary syndrome, detailing the increased role of the cath lab as well as highlighting the role of an established 24-hour on-call treatment protocol and a dedicated myocardial infarction support network. These components are necessary prerequisites for the design of an optimal cardiac management structure. The concomitant development of modern antithrombotic therapies and stents has also contributed to the improved long-term outcomes that we witness today. Additionally, the treatment of acute cardiac disease has been supported by the use of mechanical circulatory support systems and is especially relevant in high-risk procedures and cardiogenic shock. There is also mention in this book of technical advancements in treatments for chronic total coronary occlusions, which offer patients effective alternative therapies in comparison to the conservative options routinely adopted earlier. The high success rates at the hands of trained interventionalists have led to the widespread practice of these reperfusion procedures. While discussing interventions in structural heart disease, special emphasis has been laid on mitral valve repair, thus extrapolating the treatment options for heart failure. Finally, a chapter has also been dedicated to recent data emphasizing the significance of interventional thromboembolic prophylaxis and the importance of a conceptual heart team in the management of a patient.

This book attempts to offer a unique perspective to the practice of interventional cardiology, and we hope that the information outlined in these chapters would be extremely useful in the daily clinical scenario.

Professor Ibrahim Akin
Chief of Interventional Cardiology and Cardiovascular Research
Deputy Chief of Internal Medicine
Medical Faculty Mannheim
University of Heidelberg, Germany

Section 1

Coronary Intervention

Chapter 1

Radial Access in Primary PCI for Acute Myocardial Infarction

Hussien Heshmat, Yassir El haddad,
Mahmoud Farouk and Mohamed Abdel Meguid

Additional information is available at the end of the chapter

http://dx.doi.org/10.5772/intechopen.69131

Abstract

Transradial approach (TRA) is now considered the standard of care in many centers for elective and primary percutaneous coronary intervention (PCI). The use of the radial approach in ST-segment elevation myocardial infarction (STEMI) patients has been associated with a significant reduction in major adverse cardiac events. However, it is still unclear if the side of radial access (right vs. left) has impact on safety and effectiveness of TRA in primary PCI. So this chapter was conducted to summarize the benefits of transradial access over transfemoral access based on the most recent studies and to compare between using either right radial or left radial as an access for transradial procedure.

Keywords: primary PCI, left radial access, right radial approach, AMI

1. Introduction

Primary percutaneous coronary intervention (PPCI) angioplasty saves life and improves outcomes in patients with acute ST-segment elevation myocardial infarction (STEMI). The vascular access in this life-threatening situation has an impact on mortality and morbidity. In this chapter, we will discuss the preferred vascular access in PPCI; radial vs. femoral and review the studies that compared right radial vs. left radial in acute myocardial infarction.

2. Vascular access in acute myocardial infarction; radial or femoral

There is ongoing debate about which of the two commonly used primary percutaneous coronary intervention (PCI) methods, the traditional femoral artery access, or the radial artery access should physicians use. Some physicians support use of the femoral artery method because of concerns on the adequacy of support with the radial route. The claim is that femoral approach can provide stronger support for more complex procedures that require bulkier hardware; kissing balloons, crush techniques, and rotablation. However, most PPCI procedures do not entail densely calcific lesions or complex bifurcations. Most of the trials show that using radial access is feasible in the PPCI procedure and compared with femoral access; can provide a bleeding and mortality advantage.

ST-segment elevation myocardial infarction (STEMI) patients treated with primary percutaneous coronary intervention (PPCI) are likely to benefit from the bleeding reduction by using the radial approach as these patients have more risk for access site bleeding and bleeding-related complications as in primary percutaneous intervention we use aggressive antiplatelet and antithrombotic therapies [1]. Using the radial approach may allow higher doses of anticoagulants to be used for further ischemic reduction with minimal bleeding incidence in comparison with using the femoral approach [2]. In addition, the use of the radial approach in STEMI patients has been associated with a significant reduction in major adverse cardiac events (MACE) during follow-up [3].

3. Trials that compared radial and femoral access in primary PCI

We summarize the most important trials that compared radial and femoral access in primary PCI (**Table 1**).

These trials strongly suggest benefits from the radial approach in terms of reduction of bleeding and possible mortality. There still remain some concerns on the longer door to balloon times with the radial approach.

Study name	Year	Study design	No. of patients (TRI vs. TFI)	Endpoints Results (TRI vs. TFI) P value	Comments (other outcomes)
TEMPURA [4]	2003	Prospective randomized study	77 vs. 72	MACE 5.2 vs. 8.4% $P = 0.444$	Characteristics of coronary intervention were similar in both groups except total procedure time, which was significantly shorter in the TRI group.
RADIAL-AMI [5]	2005	Multicenter pilot trial	25 vs. 25	Procedure time 32 vs. 28 min $P = 0.04$	Despite longer procedure time, Contrast use or fluoroscopy time shows no significant difference.

Study name	Year	Study design	No. of patients (TRI vs. TFI)	Endpoints Results (TRI vs. TFI) P value	Comments (other outcomes)
FARMI [6]	2007	Prospective randomized study	57 vs. 57	Bleeding complications 2 vs. 11 *P* value significant	Coronary angiography duration shorter in TRI than TFI group, but PCI duration was the same.
Li et al. [7]	2007	Prospective randomized study	184 vs. 186	Significantly less Bleeding complications with TRI 2 vs.7	Time procedure is same in TRI and TFI group.
Yan et al. [8]	2008	Prospective randomized study	57 vs. 46	Local complications 1.8 vs. 13.1% $P < 0.05$	All procedure data and MACE show no significant difference between the two groups.
RADIAMI [9]	2009	Prospective randomized study	50 vs. 50	Different procedure data $P > 0.05$ insignificant.	Time to ambulation in TRI group was significantly shorter then in TFI group ($p = 0.003$).
Gan et al. [10]	2009	Prospective randomized study	90 vs. 105	Different procedure data were similar.	Puncture-related complications were lower in the TRI group than the TFI group ($P < 0.05$).
Hou et al. [11]	2010	Prospective randomized study	100 vs. 100	Different procedure data $P > 0.05$ insignificant.	Vascular complications and total hospital stay were lower in TRI group than TFI group ($p < 0.01$).
RADIAMI II [12]	2011	Prospective randomized study	49 vs. 59	Different procedure data using star closure device.	D2B is longer in TRI group than TFA group ($p = 0.009$), but MACE and bleeding complications were the same.
RIFLE-STEACS [13]	2012	Multicenter randomized parallel group study	500 vs. 501	30-day NACEs 13.6 vs. 21% $P = 0.003$.	Lower cardiac mortality ($p = 0.020$), bleeding ($p = 0.026$), and hospital stay ($p = 0.03$) in TRI group.
RIVAL [14]	2012	Multicenter randomized parallel group study	3507 vs. 3514	Complications at 30 days.	Large hematoma and Pseudo aneurysm needing closure in TFI group more than TRI ($p <$ 0.0001, $p = 0.006$).
STEMI-RADIAL [15]	2012	Prospective randomized study	348 vs. 359	Complications at 30 days, 1.4 vs. 7.2%, $P =$ 0.0001.	Contrast utilization were significantly reduced in TRI than TFI ($p = 0.01$). Mortality shows no difference between two groups.
Ocean race [16]	2014	Prospective randomized study	52 vs. 51	Quality of life.	Radial access is associated with significantly fewer problems with mobility and self-care and better psychological outcome after PCI.

Study name	Year	Study design	No. of patients (TRI vs. TFI)	Endpoints Results (TRI vs. TFI) P value	Comments (other outcomes)
Kasem et al [17]	2014	Retrospective study	150 vs. 63	D2B and contrast volume.	TRI is not associated with prolonged door to balloon time or excess contrast utilization. Also TRI is associated with lower mortality, less need for invasive hemodynamic support and fewer local complications.
ALKK PCI registry [18]	2015	Prospective observational study	2530 vs. 15,270	Complications, bleeding and mortality 1.8 vs. 5.1% $P < 0.001$.	TRI group show higher procedural success rate and lower vascular access complications and mortality.
Warren J. c. et al. [19]	2015	Multicenter prospectively collected study	2947 patients	Door to balloon time 30 vs. 27 min. $P < 0.001$.	Time to first balloon longer with TRI group than with TFI, but no difference mortality and reinfarction rates between TRI and TFI.
Haq et al. [20]	2015	Retrospective data	45 vs. 47	Demographic and procedure data insignificant except D2B.	D2B is longer in TRI group than TFA group ($p = 0.021$).
MATRIX [21]	2015	A Randomized, multicenter study	4197 vs. 4207	MACE at 30 days 8.8 vs. 10.3% $P = 0.0307$	NARC and BARC higher in TFI than TRI group ($p = 0.0092$, $p = 0.013$) and all-cause mortality ($p = 0.045$).
Graham et al. [22]	2016	Prospective randomized study	338 vs. 1553	30-day major bleeding 3.7 vs. 1.2% $P = 0.18$ insignificant.	30-day death and reinfarction show no significant statistically difference between two groups ($p = 0.11$, $p = 0.56$).
Kołtowski et al [23]	2016	Prospective randomized study	52 vs. 51	The cost between the two access points 3060 vs. 3374 EUR was insignificant.	The indirect costs were lower in the radial group. Introduction of radial access as the default approach in all centers may significantly reduce the overall financial burden from a social perspective.
Lee et al. [24]	2016	Prospective randomized study	336 vs. 1609	procedural success, complications, mortality and MACE TRI < TFI. significant better in TRI group	In octogenarians, TRI was more effective than the TFI approach in PPCI.

Study name	Year	Study design	No. of patients (TRI vs. TFI)	Endpoints Results (TRI vs. TFI) P value	Comments (other outcomes)
Kilic et al. [25]	2017	Prospective registry	1310 vs. 2270	30-day all-cause mortality 1.7 vs. 4.6% $p < 0.001$.	Radial access is associated with improved outcome in patients with an acute coronary syndrome.

TRI, transradial intervention; TFI, transfemoral intervention; D2B, door to balloon; MACE, major adverse cardiac events; NARC, net adverse clinical events; BARC, Bleeding Academic Research Consortium.

Table 1. Trials of (TRI) vs. (TFI) in acute myocardial infarction.

4. Right vs. left radial artery access

Transradial cardiac catheterization can be performed either by using right or left radial access. But the catheterization laboratory setup, patient preparation, and overall techniques are different from using right radial access to left radial access. The transradial operator should be proficient with both right and left radial accesses. The modern cardiac catheterization laboratory and its support staff should also be proficient to handle these differences efficiently in order to maximize the advantages gained by using either right or left radial in transradial procedures.

5. Historical aspects

Transradial catheterization was started by using the left radial artery as an access for the procedure. The original description of transradial catheterization was introduced by Lucien Campeau in 1989. Campeau successfully completed a coronary angiography by utilization of left radial artery as an access for the transradial procedure. Campeau prepared the left wrist in hyperextension position to facilitate the puncturing of the radial artery. Campeau completed the procedure by using 18-gage needle, 5-Fr sheath, and 5-Fr catheters [26]. The right radial approach was utilized by Ferdinand Kiemeneij in the first description of transradial PCI in 1993. Ferdinand Kiemeneij successfully completed a percutaneous coronary intervention by the utilization of right radial artery as an access for the transradial procedure. Kiemeneij completed the procedure by using 22-gage access needles, 6-Fr sheath, and 6-Fr guiding catheters [27].

Since 1993, the right radial approach became the preferable vascular access by the majority of transradial operators. The disruption of the traditional laboratory setup and the relocation of the operator in the left radial approach to the left side of the patient, on the contrary, the right radial approach is more familiar as the femoral approach in the catheter and equipment manipulation from the right side by both the operator and the support staff. However, the left radial artery access has advantages over the right radial approach in lower incidence of vascular anomalies less than right radial and using the left radial approach mimetic the femoral approach regarding the manipulation of the catheters and support of guiding catheters. **Table 2** summarizes the differences and similarities between right and left transradial accesses based on the most recent studies [28].

	Right radial access	Left radial access
Acceptability	More popular	Less popular (if indicated only)
Preparation and setup	More standardized	Less standardized (disrupt traditional setup)
Comfort for the operator	More comfortable	Less comfortable
Learning curve	Longer	Shorter
Catheter manipulation	More challenging (similar with experts)	Better control
Radiation dose	Similar (longer with trainees)	Similar (shorter with trainees)
Efficacy and safety	Similar	Similar

Table 2. Comparison between right and left radial access [28].

6. Preprocedural assessment

The choice of right radial vs. left radial is decided by the transradial operator and patient-related factors. Transradial operator may choose the left radial in special conditions as in requiring cannulation of the LIMA or in a presence of a contraindication for using the right radial access. The left radial approach may be preferred in specific patients who have a higher risk for right radial artery (RRA) touristy like in female gender, short stature, low body weights, and elderly.

6.1. Right radial access

The patient is positioned supine on the table in the same manner as the transfemoral route. An arm board extension is attached to the right-hand side of the table. Arm boards are available in different shapes and designs. Perhaps best suited for this purpose may be the trapezoid-shaped fiberglass board, with the narrow end tucked under the mattress at shoulder level and the broad area at the wrist.

The patient should be prepared with the wrist exposed, the forearm placed in the supine position and the hand gently taped in position, with the wrist hyper extended and supinated. A pulse oximetry probe is placed on the right index finger or thumb to allow for continuous monitoring of the circulation to the hand throughout the procedure. After the wrist has been appropriately prepared, it will be examined for the radial artery. Infiltrate local anesthetic subcutaneously at least 2 cm proximal to the radial styloid process (in the region where the radial artery pulse is best appreciated) to form a small wheal. The skin is sterilized with an alcohol-based skin preparation. The groin should also be prepared for access in the event of a failed radial artery insertion. The angiography drape is applied so as to expose the wrist in an area where the radial artery pulse will be palpable.

Radial artery puncture can be done using open needle technique (anterior wall puncture) or trans-fixation technique (posterior wall puncture). After the artery has been successfully punctured, introduce the guide wire through the cannula. Once the guide wire has been smoothly advanced through the device, remove the cannula while leaving the guide wire in place. Introduce the sheath (with the dilator inserted) over the guide wire into the radial artery. A small superficial skin incision may be made where the guide wire enters through the skin to facilitate smooth passage of the sheath and to prevent radial artery spasm.

After the sheath is fully advanced, the guide wire and the dilator assembly may be removed. After the removal of the dilator, the sidearm may be used for administration of compatible medications as antispasmodic agents (e.g., verapamil 2.5–5 mg diluted in blood, nitrates 100–200 mic) through the sheath via the sidearm. And anticoagulants (e.g., heparin 5000 U) may be administered either via the sheath or IV, depending on the procedure performed.

6.2. Left radial access

There are more variations in catheterization laboratory setup, patient preparation, and equipment setup with the left radial compared to the right radial approach. Some operators prefer to perform the left radial procedure from the left side of the patient. In this case, the patient is positioned, prepped, and draped in a similar fashion as that of right radial access, only the arm board is attached to the left side of the table, and the equipment is arranged as a mirror image of the right-sided approach.

The patient is positioned supine on the table in the typical manner as the transfemoral route. A pulse oximeter probe is placed on the left index finger or thumb to allow continuous monitoring throughout the procedure. The operator achieves vascular access either from left side of the patient or from the right side of the patient, as if performing a left femoral artery puncture. After needle puncture and sheath insertion in a typical manner as right radial approach, the left forearm is pronated and adducted, such that the left wrist rests close to the right inguinal area. The operator then performs the catheterization procedure on the right side of the patient with a general setup that closely resembles the transfemoral approach.

7. Trials of right vs. left radial elective PCI

In previously published studies, comparing RRA with left radial artery (LRA) in elective PCI, it has been shown that both approaches are safe, have similar success rates, volume of contrast agent, and similar rate of crossover to different approach [29–32]. On the other hand, controversy between these researches regarding number of catheters used, Fluoroscopy time, and radiation exposure in LRA compared to RRA was obvious. Dominici et al. [29] and Kado et al. [32]

have shown a reduction in fluoroscopy time and number of catheters used in LRA compared to RRA, while Freixa et al. [31] and the "transradial approach (left vs. right) and procedural times during percutaneous coronary procedures (TALENT) study" demonstrated similar procedure and fluoroscopy time between both approaches when performed by well-trained operators [30]. Moreover, decreased radiation exposure with LRA was detected by Kado et al. [32] which is not concordant with the results of sub-study of the "TALENT" trial, which demonstrated no differences in radiation dose between the two approaches [33]. Recently, several studies have shown that the LRA might be associated with shorter procedural time and lower cerebrovascular complications when compared with the RRA in elective PCI [29, 34, 35].

8. Right vs. left radial access in acute myocardial infarction

Data from published studies addressing the best transradial approach (TRA) (right vs. left) in the setting of primary PCI are scarce, while data in the setting of elective PCI are controversial. Although the right radial artery (RRA) approach is usually the first point of access, tortuosity within the brachial and subclavian arteries may result in more radiation exposure, lengthy procedure, or even procedural failure [34, 36, 37]. Alternatively, the left radial artery (LRA) approach, although unflavored and less extensively studied, may offer an advantage from the point-of-view of vascular anatomy [29, 33].

Since delay in the reperfusion, time is considered the main cause of mortality in STEMI patients [38, 39], it is essential to decrease the reperfusion time when undergoing primary PCI. As the choice of transradial access site over the femoral approach is preferred in patients with STEMI because of less bleeding complications, it remains undetermined whether RRA or LRA provides a shorter procedural time in STEMI patients undergoing primary PCI. Up to date, only a few researches have compared the access side (right vs. left) during primary PCI [40–42].

We did a retrospective study on 400 consecutive patients presenting to our hospital with STEMI. Primary PCIs were performed for 202 patients using the right radial approach and 198 using the left radial approach. Results show that there was no significant difference in demographics and clinical characteristics for patients included in both groups with mean age 57 ± 12.8 years, with male predominance (77.2%). There was no significant difference between the right radial and left radial regarding success rate (97.5 for RRA vs. 98.4% for LRA; $P = 0.77$), contrast amount used (151.2 ± 12.4 ml for the RRA vs. 150.8 ± 19.6 ml for the LRA; $P = 0.41$), fluoroscopy time (FT) (13.2 ± 4.3 min for the RRA vs. 12.8 ± 3.5 min for the LRA), needle-to-balloon time (18.2 ± 2.8 min vs. 17.8 ± 6.5 min for RRA & LRA respectively, $P = 0.12$), number of catheters, postprocedure vascular complications, in-hospital reinfarction, and stroke/transient ischemic attack (TIA) or death. We concluded that both right radial access and left radial access are safe and effective in primary PCI, as both approaches have a high success rate and comparable needle-to-balloon time [40].

A recent retrospective study done on 135 patients compared LRA vs. RRA in STEMI patients. Primary PCIs were performed for 85 patients using the right radial approach and 50 using the left radial approach. Results show that there was no significant difference in room procedural times, success rates, and comparable safety. But the authors attributed these results to the choice of LRA in patients known to be at risk for RRA failure (old age, female gender, lower body weight, and lower BMI). As in the patients of the LRA group, there were more females (40 vs. 20%, $P = 0.02$), significantly older (69.7 ± 14.8 vs. 60.0 ± 12.5 years, $P < 0.0001$), lower body weights (78.0 ± 16.3 vs. 95.1 ± 26.8 kg, $P \leq 0.0158$), shorter stature (169.3 ± 10.8 vs. 173.9 ± 10.3 cm, $P = 0.02$), and lower BMI (27.2 ± 5.1 vs. 31.2 ± 7.7 kg m^{-2}, $P \leq 0.01$) [41].

A recent prospective study on 200 STEMI Chinese patients compared LRA vs. RRA. Primary PCIs were performed for 100 patients using the right radial approach and 100 using the left radial approach. Results show that there were no significant differences in the demographics and clinical characteristics for patients included in both groups. There was no significant difference between the right radial and left radial regarding procedural success rate (98 for left vs. 94% for right; $P = 0.28$). But there was significant difference between the right radial and left radial regarding needle-to-balloon time (16.0 ± 4.8 LRA vs. 18.0 ± 6.5 min RRA; $P = 0.02$), fluoroscopy time (7.4 ± 3.4 LRA vs. 8.8 ± 3.5 min RRA; $P = 0.01$), and CAK dose area product (51.9 ± 30.4 vs. 65.3 ± 49.1 Gy cm^2; $P = 0.04$). Fu and colleagues attributed these results to the anatomical advantage of LRA, which allows for quicker and easier delivery of a PCI device, such as a balloon or aspiration catheter. They also mentioned that all operators participating in this study had been well trained to perform the left radial PCI procedure before the study [42].

Another recent prospective study on 206 patients with acute myocardial infarctions who required emergency percutaneous coronary intervention and were divided into the following two groups: a group that underwent percutaneous coronary intervention through the left radial artery and other group that underwent percutaneous coronary intervention through the femoral artery. The times required for angiographic catheter and guiding catheter placements, the success rate of the procedure, and the incidence of vascular complications in the two groups were observed. Results show that there was no significant difference in catheter placement time or the ultimate success rate of the procedure between the two groups. However, the left radial artery group showed a significantly lower incidence of vascular complications than the femoral artery group ($P < 0.05$) [43].

9. Conclusion

The choice of TRA access site (right vs. left) in primary PCI depends on the experience of performing operator and demographics of treated population. With well-trained operators in both approaches, no significant difference in safety or effectiveness of either approach can be detected, as demonstrated in our study and by the "TALENT" study (senior group) in elective PCI and Larsen et al. in primary PCI [30, 41]. On the other hand, LRA shows better outcomes (compared to RRA) with less trained operators or those trained mainly on LRA, as demonstrated by the results of "TALENT" study (the fellow group) and by Fu et al. [30, 42].

Populations characterized by short stature or low BMI (e.g., Chinese population in Fu et al.) [42] showed better outcomes with LRA in primary PCI. On the other hand, Saito et al. [44] revealed lower success rates via LRA in Japanese patients, which were due to a higher reported frequency of left subclavian arteries originating too distally and/or tortuosity not permitting catheter advancement to the aortic root.

Similarity between RRA and LRA in safety and effectiveness gives more space for TRA in primary PCI, as more patients can achieve rapid and successful revascularization (similar to TFA) but with the added safety margin that TRA provides.

Author details

Hussien Heshmat*, Yassir El haddad, Mahmoud Farouk and Mohamed Abdel Meguid

*Address all correspondence to: hheshmat@kasralainy.edu.eg

Cardiology Department, Faculty of Medicine, Cairo University, Cairo, Egypt

References

[1] Mehta SR, et al. Effects of radial versus femoral artery access in patients with acute coronary syndromes with or without ST-segment elevation. Journal of the American College of Cardiology. 2012;**60**(24):2490-2499

[2] Rao SV, et al. The transradial approach to percutaneous coronary intervention: Historical perspective, current concepts, and future directions. Journal of the American College of Cardiology. 2010;**55**(20):2187-2195

[3] Arzamendi D, et al. Effect on bleeding, time to revascularization, and one-year clinical outcomes of the radial approach during primary percutaneous coronary intervention in patients with ST-segment elevation myocardial infarction. The American journal of cardiology. 2010;**106**(2):148-154

[4] Saito S, et al. Comparative study on transradial approach vs. transfemoral approach in primary stent implantation for patients with acute myocardial infarction: results of the test for myocardial infarction by prospective unicenter randomization for access sites (TEMPURA) trial. Catheterization and Cardiovascular Interventions. 2003;**59**(1):26-33.

[5] Cantor WJ, et al. Radial versus femoral access for emergent percutaneous coronary intervention with adjunct glycoprotein IIb/IIIa inhibition in acute myocardial infarction—the RADIAL-AMI pilot randomized trial. American Heart Journal. 2005;**150**(3):543-549

[6] Brasselet C, et al. Randomised comparison of femoral versus radial approach for percutaneous coronary intervention using abciximab in acute myocardial infarction: Results of the FARMI trial. Heart. 2007;**93**(12):1556-1561

[7] Wei-min L. et al, Safety and feasibility of emergent percutaneous coronary intervention with the transradial access in patients with acute myocardial infarction. Chinese Medical Journal. 2007;**120**(7):598-600

[8] Yan Z-x, et al. Safety and feasibility of transradial approach for primary percutaneous coronary intervention in elderly patients with acute myocardial infarction. Chinese Medical Journal. 2008;**121**(9):782-786

[9] Chodór P, et al. RADIal versus femoral approach for percutaneous coronary interventions in patients with acute myocardial infarction (RADIAMI): A prospective, randomized, single-center clinical trial. Cardiology Journal. 2009;**16**(4):332-340

[10] Gan L, et al. Effectiveness and feasibility of transradial approaches for primary percutaneous coronary intervention in patients with acute myocardial infarction. Journal of Nanjing Medical University. 2009;**23**(4):270-274

[11] Hou L, et al. Comparative study on transradial versus transfemoral approach for primary percutaneous coronary intervention in Chinese patients with acute myocardial infarction. Saudi Medical Journal. 2010;**31**(2):158-162

[12] Chodór P, et al. Radial vs femoral approach with StarClose clip placement for primary percutaneous coronary intervention in patients with ST-elevation myocardial infarction. RADIAMI II: A prospective, randomised, single centre trial. Kardiologia Polska. 2010;**69**(8):763-771

[13] Romagnoli E, et al. Radial versus femoral randomized investigation in ST-segment elevation acute coronary syndrome: The RIFLE-STEACS (Radial Versus Femoral Randomized Investigation in ST-Elevation Acute Coronary Syndrome) study. Journal of the American College of Cardiology. 2012;**60**(24):2481-2489

[14] Jolly SS, et al. Radial versus femoral access for coronary angiography and intervention in patients with acute coronary syndromes (RIVAL): A randomised, parallel group, multicentre trial. The Lancet. 2011;**377**(9775):1409-1420

[15] Bernat I, et al. STEMI-RADIAL: A prospective, randomized trial of radial vs. femoral access in patients with ST-segment elevation myocardial infarction. In: Transcatheter Cardiovascular Therapeutics (TCT) Scientific Symposium. 2012

[16] Koltowski L, et al. Quality of life in patients with ST-segment elevation myocardial infarction undergoing percutaneous coronary intervention—radial versus femoral access (from the OCEAN RACE Trial). The American Journal of Cardiology. 2014;**114**(4):516-521

[17] Kasem H, Elteby I, Dashti R, Aljarallah MA. Radial versus femoral access in a newly initiated primary PCI service. European Heart Journal Acute Cardiovascular Care. 2014;**3**(2):44

[18] Bauer T, et al. Use and outcome of radial versus femoral approach for primary PCI in patients with acute ST elevation myocardial infarction without cardiogenic shock: Results from the ALKK PCI registry. Catheterization and Cardiovascular Interventions. 2015;**86**(S1):S8-S14

[19] Cantor WJ, et al. Reperfusion times for radial versus femoral access in patients with ST-Elevation myocardial unfarction undergoing primary percutaneous coronary intervention. Circulation. Cardiovascular Interventions. 2015;**8**(5):e002097

[20] Haq M, et al. Transradial versus transfemoral approach for primary percutaneous coronary intervention–single centre experience over a period of two years. University Heart Journal. 2017;**11**(2):56-62

[21] Valgimigli M, et al. Radial versus femoral access in patients with acute coronary syndromes undergoing invasive management: A randomised multicentre trial. The Lancet. 2015;**385**(9986):2465-2476

[22] Graham JJ, et al. Radial versus femoral access for percutaneous coronary intervention in ST-elevation myocardial infarction patients treated with fibrinolysis: Results from the randomized routine early invasive clinical trials. Cardiovascular Revascularization Medicine. 2016;**17**(5):295-301

[23] Kołtowski Ł, et al. Cost-effectiveness of radial vs. femoral approach in primary percutaneous coronary intervention in STEMI–Randomized, control trial. Hellenic Journal of Cardiology. 2016;**57**(3):198-202

[24] Lee HW, Cha KS, Ahn J, Choi JC, Oh JH, Choi JH, Lee HC, Yun E, Jang HY, Choi JH, Hong TJ. Comparison of transradial and transfemoral coronary intervention in octogenarians with acute myocardial infarction. International Journal of Cardiology. 2016;**202**:419-424

[25] Kilic S, et al. Effects of radial versus femoral artery access in patients with acute myocardial infarction: A large centre prospective registry. Netherlands Heart Journal. 2017;**25**(1):33-39

[26] Campeau L. Percutaneous radial artery approach for coronary angiography. Catheterization and Cardiovascular Diagnosis. 1989;**16**(1):3-7

[27] Kiemeneij F, Laarman GJ. Percutaneous transradial artery approach for coronary stent implantation. Catheterization and Cardiovascular Diagnosis. 1993;**30**(2):173-178

[28] Shah RM, et al. Comparison of transradial coronary procedures via right radial versus left radial artery approach: A meta-analysis. Catheterization and Cardiovascular Interventions. 2016;**88**(7):1027-1033

[29] Dominici M, et al. Left radial versus right radial approach for coronary artery catheterization: A prospective comparison. Journal of Interventional Cardiology. 2012;**25**(2):203-209

[30] Kanei Y, et al. Randomized comparison of transradial coronary angiography via right or left radial artery approaches. The American Journal of Cardiology. 2011;**107**(2):195-197

[31] Freixa X, et al. Right versus left transradial approach for coronary catheterization in octogenarian patients. Catheterization and Cardiovascular Interventions. 2012;**80**(2):267-272

[32] Kado H, et al. Operator radiation exposure and physical discomfort during a right versus left radial approach for coronary interventions. JACC: Cardiovascular Interventions. 2014;**7**(7):810-816

[33] Sciahbasi A, et al. Transradial approach (left vs right) and procedural times during percutaneous coronary procedures: TALENT study. American Heart Journal. 2011;**161**(1): 172-179

[34] Norgaz T, Gorgulu S, Dagdelen S. A randomized study comparing the effectiveness of right and left radial approach for coronary angiography. Catheterization and Cardiovascular Interventions. 2012;**80**(2):260-264

[35] Pristipino C, et al. Prospective registry of vascular access in interventions in lazio region study group. Major improvement of percutaneous cardiovascular procedure outcomes with radial artery catheterisation: Results from the PREVAIL study. Heart. 2009;**95**(6):476-482

[36] Lo TS, et al. Radial artery anomaly and its influence on transradial coronary procedural outcome. Heart. 2009;**95**(5):410-415

[37] Kawashima O, et al. Effectiveness of right or left radial approach for coronary angiography. Catheterization and Cardiovascular Interventions. 2004;**61**(3):333-337

[38] Luca GD, et al. Time delay to treatment and mortality in primary angioplasty for acute myocardial infarction. Circulation. 2004;**109**(10):1223-1225

[39] Cannon CP, et al. Relationship of symptom-onset-to-balloon time and door-to-balloon time with mortality in patients undergoing angioplasty for acute myocardial infarction. JAMA. 2000;**283**(22):2941-2947

[40] Elmahdy MF, ElMaghawry M, Hassan M, Kassem HH, Said K, Elfaramawy AA. Comparison of safety and effectiveness between right versus left radial arterial access in primary percutaneous coronary intervention for acute ST segment elevation myocardial infarction. Heart, Lung and Circulation. 2017;**26**(1):35-40

[41] Larsen P, et al. Comparison of procedural times, success rates, and safety between left versus right radial arterial access in primary percutaneous coronary intervention for acute ST-segment elevation myocardial infarction. Catheterization and Cardiovascular Interventions. 2011;**78**(1):38-44

[42] Fu Q, et al. Randomized comparative study of left versus right radial approach in the setting of primary percutaneous coronary intervention for ST-elevation myocardial infarction. Clinical Interventions in Aging. 2015;**10**:1003

[43] Qi G, et al. Emergency percutaneous coronary intervention through the left radial artery is associated with less vascular complications than emergency percutaneous coronary intervention through the femoral artery. Clinics. 2017;**72**(1):1-4

[44] Saito S, et al. Transradial coronary intervention in Japanese patients. Catheterization and Cardiovascular Interventions. 1999;**46**(1):37-41

Chapter 2

Current Concept of Revascularization in STEMI Patients with Multivessel Coronary Artery Disease: Evidence Base and Our Own Randomized Trial Results

Vladimir I. Ganyukov and Roman S. Tarasov

Additional information is available at the end of the chapter

http://dx.doi.org/10.5772/67884

Abstract

The use of personalized approach for the optimal revascularization strategy in patients with ST-segment elevation myocardial infarction (STEMI) and multivessel coronary artery disease (MVCAD) is based on complete revascularization by using latest generation drug-eluting stents, with the choice between multivessel primary stenting and staged stenting strategy. The chapter includes theoretical rationale, original single-center study, an original calculator for choosing optimal revascularization strategy, and a clinical case example.

Keywords: ST-segment elevation myocardial infarction, multivessel stenting, personalized approach, calculator

1. Introduction

The current guidelines recommend culprit vessel revascularization as a standard treatment option in primary percutaneous coronary intervention (PPCI) [1–6]. Nevertheless, patients with ST-segment elevation myocardial infarction (STEMI) and multivessel coronary artery disease (MVCAD) constitute up to 50% of all STEMI cases [7, 8]. As known, MVCAD is associated with an adverse short- and long-term outcome after STEMI [9–11]. The definition and criteria of MVCAD, timing for nonculprit vessel revascularization, and a number of other tactical issues are actively discussed in the recent literature [5, 6]. There are three established PCI approaches for treatment of MVCAD and STEMI: (1) PPCI of infarct-related artery (IRA) only (culprit vessel revascularization only, CO) with percutaneous coronary intervention (PCI) of noninfarct-related artery based on findings ischemia (spontaneous or during noninvasive stress-testing); (2) multivessel primary stenting (MPS): IRA is opened with the further dilatation of other significantly narrowed arteries during the same PPCI procedure; (3) multivessel staged stenting (MSS): the IRA only is treated during the first PPCI procedure with subsequent complete revascularization during the second intervention. In this chapter, we justify the use of personalized approach for the optimal revascularization strategy in patients with STEMI and MVCAD using the latest generation of drug-eluting stents (DES) with choosing MPS or MSS according to our original calculator. The chapter includes theoretical rationale, original single-center study, an original calculator for choosing optimal revascularization strategy, and a clinical case example.

2. The evolution of treatment strategies and guidelines for revascularization in patients with STEMI and MVCAD. The current evidence base. What do we know?

Earlier results of trials comparing MPS and CO approaches were controversial [12–19], probably due to the heterogeneity of patient samples, variable endpoints, distinct inclusion criteria and different study protocols. European and American Cardiology Societies for 2010–2013 [1–3] recommended limiting PPCI to the vessel with a culprit stenosis with the exception of cardiogenic shock and persistent ischemia after PCI. Moreover, performance of PPCI in a noninfarct artery was considered harmful [2].

However, randomized controlled trial (RCT) results [20–23] demonstrated usefulness and safety of multivessel stenting in patients with STEMI and MVCAD, both with MPS and MSS approaches. The current guidelines were updated by this data [4–6].

MPS approach was tested in two randomized controlled trials: PRAMI (Preventive Angioplasty in Acute Myocardial Infarction) [20] and CvLPRIT (Complete Versus Culprit-Lesion Only Primary PCI) [21]. In PRAMI trial, combined endpoint defined as cardiac death, nonfatal recurrent myocardial infarction (MI), or refractory angina at mean follow-up of 23 months occurred in 21 (9%) patients treated with MPS approach compared to 53 (22%) patients treated with CO approach (hazard ratio (HR): 0.35; 95% confidence interval (CI): 0.21–0.58) [20]. Authors concluded that MPS approach significantly reduces the risk of adverse cardiovascular events, as compared to PCI limited to IRA [20]. In the CvLPRIT trial, authors showed that major adverse cardiac events (MACE) including all-cause mortality, recurrent MI, heart failure, and ischemic-driven revascularization at 12 months follow-up occurred in 15 (10%) patients treated with MPS approach compared to 31 (21%) patients treated with CO approach (HR: 0.45; 95% CI: 0.24–0.84) [21]. In concordance with the PRAMI trial, researchers concluded that complete revascularization is beneficial for patients with STEMI and MVCAD in comparison with CO approach [21].

The MSS approach was also tested in two randomized controlled trials: DANAMI 3 PRIMULTI (Third Danish Study of Optimal Acute Treatment of Patients With ST-segment Elevation Myocardial Infarction) [22] and PRAGUE-13 (Primary Angioplasty in Patients Transferred From General

Community Hospital to Specialized PTCA Units With or Without Emergency Thrombolysis) [23]. In the DANAMI 3 PRIMULTI trial, the MSS approach was based on the fractional flow reserve (FFR) value ≤ 0.80. Combined endpoint, defined as recurrent MI, all-cause mortality, and ischemia-driven revascularization at 27 months follow-up occurred in 40 (13%) patients treated with MSS approach and in 68 (22%) patients treated with CO approach (HR: 0.56; 95% CI: 0.38–0.83) [22]. Therefore, the MSS approach in patients with STEMI and MVCAD reduced the risk of adverse outcomes [22]. However, PRAGUE-13 trial did not find significant differences between MSS and CO approaches (frequencies of primary composite endpoint including all-cause mortality, recurrent MI, or stroke at 38 months follow-up were 13.9% vs. 16.0%, respectively) [23].

All these findings provided the possibility for endorsement (class IIb) of MPS and MSS strategies to patients with STEMI and MVCAD by European and American Cardiology Societies since 2014 [4] and 2015 [5], respectively. Moreover, in 2016, the American Cardiology Society accepted appropriate use criteria for coronary revascularization in patients with acute coronary syndrome considering revascularization of arteries with nonculprit stenosis at initial procedure or during the initial hospitalization [6]. According to these criteria, (1) stable patients immediately following PCI of culprit artery and one or more additional severe/intermediate (50–70%) stenoses may be defined as appropriate for MPS approach; (2) asymptomatic patients after successful treatment of culprit artery by PPCI and one or more additional severe/intermediate (50–70%) stenoses are appropriate for MSS approach if having ischemia on noninvasive testing/FFR ≤ 0.80; (3) asymptomatic patients after successful treatment of culprit artery by PPCI and one or more additional severe stenoses may be appropriate for MSS approach [6].

Hence, both MPS and MSS approaches have sufficient evidence base for being applied to patients with STEMI and MVCAD and are included in recent clinical guidelines. However, there is a number of unresolved issues such as stent choice, effect of residual SYNTAX score, timing of staged PCI, and the choice between two multivessel stenting approaches. Addressing these issues is crucially important for personalized treatment of STEMI and MVCAD.

3. Unresolved issues and prospects for revascularization in STEMI patients

3.1. Multivessel stenting versus staged revascularization with second-generation drug-eluting stents in ST-elevation myocardial infarction patients: results of randomized trial

3.1.1. Study population

The purpose of this open-label safety/efficacy randomized clinical trial (NCT01781715) is to determine outcomes of 136 consecutive patients with STEMI and multiple coronary artery disease (CAD) undergoing multivessel stenting in primary PCI or staged PCI with second-generation DES (Resolute Integrity™ Stent, Medtronic). Primary endpoints of this study were: (1) all death (cardiac and noncardiac), (2) any MI (STEMI and non-STEMI), (3) TVR. Secondary: (1) composite rate of all death, any MI and TVR, (2) stent thrombosis (ST).

We examined patients with STEMI and multivessel CAD undergoing primary PCI. Between October 2011 and October 2014 in our 24 h catheterization laboratory randomized 136 patients with multivessel CAD (defined as ≥70% diameter stenosis of two or more epicardial coronary arteries or their major branches by visual estimation with diameter ≥2.5mm). Inclusion criteria were (1) Subject must be at least 18 years of age; (2) Subject is able to verbally confirm understandings of risks and benefits of treatment of either multivessel stenting or staged PCI using the zotarolimus-eluting stent (Resolute Integrity™ Stent, Medtronic) and he or she or his or her legally authorized representative provides written informed consent prior to any study-related procedure; (3) Subject must have significant stenoses (≥70%) of two or more than two coronary arteries and requiring primary PCI for acute ST elevation myocardial infarction (STEMI) within 12 h; (4) Target lesions must be located in a native coronary artery with visually estimated diameter of less than 2.5 mm and more than 4.0 mm; (5) Target lesion(s) must be amenable for percutaneous coronary intervention.

Exclusion criteria were as follows: (1) Single lesions; (2) Acute heart failure Killip III-IV; (3) ≥50% left main stenosis; (4) Small vessels' diameter (<2.5mm); (5) The patient has a known hypersensitivity or contraindication to any of the following medications: heparin, aspirin, clopidogrel or ticagrelor, zotarolimus. Included were patients with the presence of prolonged (more than 30 min) chest pain, started less than 12 h before hospital arrival and ST elevation of at least 1 mm in two or more contiguous limb electrocardiographic leads or 2 mm in precordial leads.

Procedure success was defined as the achievement of an angiographic residual stenosis of less than 20% and a thrombolysis in myocardial infarction (TIMI) flow grade 3 after treatment of the lesions. Before the procedure patients were treated with loading doses of aspirin, clopidogrel or ticagrelor, unfractioned heparin. Post-PCI medical oral treatment included aspirin, statins, and clopidogrel or ticagrelor, which was recommended for 12 months in all cases after second-generation zotarolimus-eluting stent implantation. Signed informed consent for primary PCI and for the study was obtained from all patients before the procedure. Soon after every diagnostic angiography, the eligible patients were randomly allocated to two different strategies: 1. Multivessel stenting in primary PCI (MS primary): the IRA was opened followed by dilatation of other significantly narrowed arteries during the same procedure. 2. Multivessel stenting in staged revascularization (MS staged): the IRA only was treated during the primary intervention while the complete revascularization was planned in a second procedure (10.1 ± 5.1 days). The study protocol conforms to the ethical guidelines of the 1975 Declaration of Helsinki and was approved by the institution's human research committee.

3.1.2. Definitions and endpoints

Clinical and procedural data were collected by reviewing hospital records and angiographic runs stored in DICOM CDs. The primary endpoint of the study was the incidence of major adverse cardiac events (MACE) defined as cardiac or noncardiac death, reinfarction, and repeat coronary revascularization. For repeat revascularization we included all PCI or CABG occurring after the baseline procedure and justified by recurrent symptoms, reinfarction, or objective evidence of significant ischemia on provocative testing. In the staged group we classified as repeat revascularization only unplanned procedures. Follow-up was obtained by outpatient visits or phone interviews.

We estimated clinical and angiographic criteria of ST. The incidence of ST was assessed throughout the follow-up period, according to the conventional ARC (Academic Research Consortium) classification [24]. Clinical criteria consisted of acute onset of chest pain persisting for >15 min and/or accompanied by ST-segment elevation or depression of at least 1 mm in two contiguous leads in the distribution of the target vessel. All patients with the clinical suspicion of ST underwent immediate coronary angiography to confirm the diagnosis followed by PCI.

Angiographic criteria of stent thrombosis consisted of partial or complete occlusion within the previously implanted stent with evidence of fresh thrombus. Within the first 18 h after index MI, recurrent MI required recurrent symptoms of myocardial ischemia associated with recurrent ST-segment elevation or depression of at least 1 mm in two contiguous limb electrocardiographic leads or 2 mm in precordial leads lasting at least 30 min. After 18 h, recurrent MI was defined as appearance of new Q waves, new left bundle-branch block, and/or enzyme evidence (level of creatine kinase MB fraction and/or troponin) of MI.

3.1.3. Statistical analysis

Continuous variables are presented as mean ± SD, categorical variables as percentages. For the endpoint "death" patients were censored at death or December 2015 if alive. For MACE patients were censored at the date of first MACE or at the end of follow-up. Follow-up was 100% complete. We used Chi Squared and Mann Whitney "U" test for statistical analysis to compare clinical, demographic, angiographic, PCI characteristics, and outcomes in groups. All analyses were performed using STATISTICA 8.0 (StatSoft, Tulsa, OK, USA).

3.1.4. Results

3.1.4.1. Baseline characteristics

In general population the mean age was 59 ± 10.6 (31–88) years; 92 (67.2%) were men. The incidence of diabetes mellitus in study cohort was 22.1%. The MS primary group included 67 patients, and the MS staged group 69 patients. The elective procedure in the MS staged group was performed on average 10.1 ± 5.1 days after the primary PCI. We evaluated the results in two study groups (MS primary vs. MS staged).

Table 1 shows the baseline clinical and demographic characteristics in study groups. Patients of MS primary and MS staged group were comparable for all clinical and demographic characteristics. The majority of patients in both groups were male, had hypertension and acute heart failure Killip 1.

Table 2 shows the baseline angiographic characteristics and special features of PCI. Mean SYNTAX score in the groups did not exceed 19 points, which corresponds to an intermediate

Variables	MS primary (n = 67)		MS staged (n = 69)		P
	n	%	n	%	
Age, years	58.6 ± 10.2		59.1 ± 11.1		0.6
Male	48	71.6	43	62.3	0.3
LVEF, %		50.7 ± 9.2		51.8 ± 7.3	0.5
Hypertension	64	94	61	88.4	0.4
Diabetes mellitus	16	23.9	14	20.3	0.8
Peripheral artery disease	13	19.4	20	29	0.3
Previous MI	10	14.9	4	5.8	0.2
Previous stroke	0	0	2	2.9	0.5
Acute heart failure (Killip II)	10	14.9	8	11.6	0.8

Table 1. Patient clinical and demographic characteristics.

Variables	MS primary (n = 67)		MS staged (n = 69)		P
	n	%	n	%	
Three-vessel disease	32	47.8	31	44.9	0.9
SYNTAX score	19.1 ± 7.9		18.6 ± 7.1		0.9
SYNTAX score ≥23 points	18	26.9	16	23.2	0.8
Contrast medium, ml	325.8 ± 110.2		373 ± 154.5		0.06
Mean number of stents	2.6 ± 0.5		2.7 ± 0.6		0.7
Total mean stent length, mm	57.5 ± 13.4		58 ± 16.2		0.6
Mean stent diameter, mm	3.3 ± 0.4		3.3 ± 0.5		0.3

Table 2. Baseline angiographic characteristics and special features of procedures.

severity of coronary lesions. About half of the patients in each group had 3-vessel CAD. Total mean stent length in each group exceeded 57 mm. There were no statistically significant differences between angiographic characteristics in the groups.

3.1.4.2. Events

Follow-up was completed in 100% of patients. Over the 12-month observation, there were no significant differences in frequency of adverse cardiovascular events among groups. After a follow-up of 12 months, there was only one noncardiac death in MS staged group (colon cancer). At the same time, fatality outcomes in the groups did not exceed 3% (**Table 3**). Survival free of MI and re-PCI was 62 (92.5%) patients in MS primary group and 67 (97.1%) in MS staged group (p>0.05).

Variables	MS primary (n = 67)		MS staged (n = 69)		P
	n	%	n	%	
All death	2	3	2	2.9	0.9
of them within 30 days	2	100	1	50	–
Cardiac death	2	3	1	1.4	0.6
MI	5	7.5	2	2.9	0.6
of them within 30 days	1	20	2	100	–
TVR	2	3	1	1.4	0.6
of them within 30 days	0	0	0	0	–
Non-TVR	0	0	1	1.4	0.9
of them within 30 days	0	0	1	100	–
Combined endpoint (cardiac death + MI + TVR)	4	5.9	3	4.3	0.7
Stent thrombosis (on the number of patients)	4	5.9	2	2.9	0.7
of them within 30 days	1	25	2	100	–

Table 3. 12-month outcomes.

3.1.5. Discussion

The main finding of the present randomized study is that after a follow-up of 12 months, in STEMI patients with multiple coronary lesions treated with multivessel PCI (primary and staged (10.1 ± 5.1 days)) with second-generation DES (Resolute Integrity), revascularization had satisfactory outcomes in two different strategies of PCI despite the initial severity of patients, including a high frequency of occurrence of diabetes (22.1%) and the average length of the stented segment 57.8 ± 14.6 mm.

According to previous guidelines, PCI should be performed only in IRA, at least in patients without cardiogenic shock [25]. This recommendation was based on the hypothesis that single-vessel PCI has a more favorable benefit-to-risk ratio and better financial implications. Some studies suggest that the more conservative strategy of treating only the IRA could avoid complications arising from longer procedures, such as the larger use of contrast medium with a potentially increased risk of contrast-induced nephropathy, the increased administration of radiation, as well as the danger of ischemia in noninfarcted myocardial regions [15, 18].

There is no randomized data to definitely answer the issues about the specific scientific merits of any of the approaches (multivessel stenting in primary PCI or staged PCI) [26]. And there is no evidence base for second-generation DES in STEMI patients with multivessel CAD, but in recent years, with the development of new advanced devices the outcome of multivessel PCI has markedly improved [17, 19].

However, the results of recent randomized trials challenged these recommendations [1, 4, 27]. The approach to the choice of revascularization strategy in patients with STEMI and MVCAD was detailed in 2014 ESC/EACTS Guidelines on myocardial revascularization [4]. The basic position of the recommendations is that the primary percutaneous coronary intervention (PCI) should be limited to infarct-related artery (IRA) (excepting cardiogenic shock or persistent ischemia, IIa class, level of evidence B) [4]. However, in patients with ischemia in noninfarct area primary PCI should be also performed for nonculprit lesions up to one week after admission (evidence grade IIa, Level B). Moreover, it is possible to carry out revascularization of nonculprit lesions at the time of primary PCI (evidence IIb class, level B) [20]. These standards came with the publication of the data from a randomized trial describing the preventive importance of PCI in nonculprit lesions (PRAMI) [1]. Nevertheless, the PRAMI trial does not respond to a key question—in which cases do we need to perform MS?

To the best of our knowledge the present study is the first that estimates throughout a follow-up the multivessel stenting during primary PCI and multivessel staged (10.1 ± 5.1 days) PCI with second-generation DES in STEMI patients with multivessel disease. We found that aggressive approach (multivessel stenting at the time of primary PCI or staged PCI) in STEMI patients with Resolute Integrity stents is associated with low risk of MACE in 12-month follow-up period. It is clear when compared with the published data. Twelve-month incidence of MACE in STEMI patients with multivessel disease in general cohort (BMS and DES) is 23.9–28%, re-MI 1.6–8.8%, death 3.3–6.3%, ST 1.8–4.3% [12, 15, 18]. In our study, we observed 12-month MACE, re-MI, death, and ST in 5.1, 5.1, 2.9, and 4.4% of patients, respectively.

Indeed, the inflammatory reaction arising during acute coronary syndromes and responsible for plaque instability is not limited to the culprit lesion, but involves the entire coronary tree [28]. Our results suggest that the multivessel approach (primary and staged) with second-generation DES is safe and possibly less expensive than an incomplete approach by reducing the probability of further unplanned procedures. We suppose that multivessel revascularization could decrease the risks and discomfort for patients associated with new unscheduled procedures. This hypothesis was also confirmed in the PRAMI trial. In PRAMI trial it was shown that in patients with STEMI and multivessel coronary artery disease undergoing infarct artery PCI, preventive PCI in noninfarct coronary arteries with major stenoses significantly reduced the risk of adverse cardiovascular events, as compared with PCI limited to the infarct artery [20].

In two other randomized trials, investigators have specifically assessed the value of preventive PCI in patients with acute STEMI undergoing PCI in the infarct artery. In one study, 69 patients were randomly assigned (in a 3:1 ratio) to preventive PCI (52 patients) or no preventive PCI (17 patients) [29]. At 1 year, in the preventive-PCI group, there were nonsignificant reductions in the rates of repeat revascularization (17 and 35%, respectively) and cardiac death or myocardial infarction (4 and 6%, respectively). In the other trial, 214 patients were randomly assigned to one of three groups: no preventive PCI (84 patients), immediate preventive PCI (65 patients), and staged preventive PCI performed during a second procedure about 40 days later (65 patients) [17]. At 2.5 years, the rate of repeat revascularization was less frequent in the immediate—and staged—preventive-PCI groups combined, as compared with the group receiving no preventive PCI (11 and 33%, respectively), and there was a non-significant decrease in the rate of cardiac death (5 and 12%, respectively). The results of these studies are consistent with those of our study.

3.1.6. Conclusions

There is no doubt about the fact that the results of revascularization in STEMI patients with multivessel CAD may be improved by using the latest generation of DES (Resolute Integrity™ Stent, Medtronic). It is clear that further research in this area should be directed to the search criteria according to which it would be possible to choose a strategy of revascularization for PCI differentiated. Also important is to have an objective angiographic criteria indicating sufficient volume of revascularization performed in the hospital period with primary or staged multivessel stenting. In this context, in the next section of this chapter will be presented the relevant data of our own study—prognostic role of initial and residual SYNTAX score in STEMI patients after primary PCI.

4. Prognostic role of initial and residual SYNTAX score in patients with ST-segment elevation myocardial infarction after primary percutaneous coronary intervention

4.1. Methods

We recruited 327 consecutive patients and carried out a single-center registry study. The study was performed in accordance with the principles of Good Clinical Practice and the Declaration of Helsinki. The local ethical committee approved the study and all the participants provided written informed consent after receiving a full explanation of the study. Criteria of inclusion were (1) hospital admission within 12 h of STEMI onset requiring the performance of primary PCI; (2) MVCAD defined as hemodynamically significant (≥70%) stenosis of two or more coronary arteries; (3) technical ability to perform PCI. Criteria of exclusion were (1) acute heart failure Killip class III-IV (pulmonary edema and cardiogenic shock); (2) left main coronary artery stenosis ≥50%. Before PCI, all patients received a loading dose of acetylsalicylic acid (250–500 mg) and clopidogrel (600 mg). Successful PCI was defined as the reduction of stenosis to <20% and a TIMI flow grade 3. After the PCI, all the patients received aspirin, statins, and clopidogrel during 1 year of follow-up.

We first evaluated the prognostic value of initial SYNTAX score that was calculated before PCI. Patients were divided into two groups depending on the severity of coronary lesions: SYNTAX ≤ 22 points (n = 213) and SYNTAX ≥ 23 points (n = 114). We then evaluated residual SYNTAX score that was calculated after PCI. Likewise, patients were stratified into two groups: SYNTAX ≤ 8 points (n = 243) and SYNTAX ≥ 9 points (n = 74). The SYNTAX score was assessed using a calculator (http://www.rnoik.ru/files/syntax/index.html).

4.2. Results

4.2.1. Baseline characteristics

Table 4 demonstrates the baseline clinical and demographic characteristics in study groups. As shown, patients with severe coronary atherosclerosis (SYNTAX ≥ 23**)** were characterized by (1) older age; (2) decreased left ventricular ejection fraction (LVEF); (3) more frequent past medical history of MI; (4) more severe acute heart failure compared to those with SYNTAX ≤ 22.

Table 5 shows a comparison of clinical and demographic characteristics of patients after primary PCI. Patients with SYNTAX ≥ 9 were characterized by (1) older age; (2) higher prevalence of females; (3) decreased LVEF; (4) more frequent past medical history of MI and peripheral artery disease compared to those with SYNTAX ≤ 8.

Variables	Patients (n = 327)				P value
	Initial SYNTAX ≤ 22 (n = 213)		Initial SYNTAX ≥ 23 (n = 114)		
	n	%	n	%	
Age, years	59.1 ± 9.9		60.9 ± 10.6		0.08
Male gender	142	66.6	74	64.9	0.8
LVEF, %		52.5 ± 7.2		48.4 ± 8.8	0.000009
Arterial hypertension	188	88.3	103	90.3	0.7
Diabetes mellitus	47	22	20	17.5	0.4
Peripheral artery disease	56	26.3	33	28.9	0.7
Past medical history of MI	21	9.8	29	25.4	0.0001
Past medical history of stroke	8	3.7	3	2.6	0.8
Acute heart failure (Killip class II)	17	7.9	21	18.4	0.009

Table 4. Patient clinical and demographic features (initial SYNTAX score groups).

Variables	Patients (n = 317)				P value
	Residual SYNTAX ≤ 8 (n = 243)		Residual SYNTAX ≥ 9 (n = 74)		
	n	%	n	%	
Age, years	58.8 ± 9.9		63.1 ± 10.6		0.001
Male	76	31.3	34	55.9	0.03
LVEF, %		51.4 ± 7.6		49.2 ± 9.2	0.08
Hypertension	218	89.7	68	91.9	0.7
Diabetes mellitus	45	18.5	20	27	0.2
Peripheral artery disease	59	24.3	28	37.8	0.03
Previous MI	31	12.8	17	23	0.05
Acute heart failure (Killip II)	29	11.9	10	13.5	0.9

Table 5. Patient clinical and demographic features (residual SYNTAX score groups).

Analysis of the angiographic parameters and features of revascularization revealed a direct relationship between the initial SYNTAX ≥ 23 and residual SYNTAX ≥ 9 (**Table 3**). In comparison with residual SYNTAX ≤ 8 patients, those with SYNTAX ≥ 9 patients had (1) a higher prevalence of initial SYNTAX ≥ 23; (2) more frequent three-vessel disease; (3) more rare use of multivessel stenting strategy; (4) less percentage of successful PCI in IRA (**Table 6**).

4.2.2. Events

Within 1 year of follow-up, five deaths were reported in initial SYNTAX ≤ 22 group (**Table 7**). Four of them were due to MACE; the fifth was from cancer. Cases of cardiac death were due to (1) rupture of the myocardium on the second day after unsuccessful PCI of IRA; (2) stent thrombosis; (3) sudden cardiac arrest. We also observed seven nonfatal MI (**Table 4**). Three of them developed as a result of stent thrombosis, two as a result of destabilized nonculprit lesions, one as a complication of elective PCI, and one occurred 2 months after the

Variables	**Residual SYNTAX ≤ 8 (n = 243)**		**Residual SYNTAX ≥ 9 (n = 74)**		**P value**
	n	**%**	**n**	**%**	
Three-vessel disease	119	49	62	83.8	0.0001
Initial SYNTAX score	18.9 ± 7.7		26.8 ± 7.7		0.0000001
Procedure success	235	96.7	66	89.2	0.02
Multivessel stenting	80	32.9	7	9.5	0.0001
Staged PCI	163	67.1	67	90.5	0.0001
Mean time between PCI, days	80.1 ± 49.5		80.1 ± 46.4		0.9

Table 6. Baseline lesions and angiographic characteristics (residual SYNTAX score groups).

Variables	**Initial SYNTAX ≤ 22 (n = 213)**		**Initial SYNTAX ≥ 23 (n = 114)**		**P value**
	n	**%**	**n**	**%**	
Death from all causes	5	2.3	12	10.5	0.004
Cardiovascular death	4	1.9	11	9.6	0.003
Myocardial infarction	7	3.3	12	10.5	0.02
Repeated target vessel revascularization	10	4.7	9	7.9	0.4
Repeated nontarget vessel revascularization	2	0.9	2	1.8	0.9
Stent thrombosis	4	1.9	10	8.8	0.008
Combined endpoint*	10	4.7	12	10.5	0.008

*All death + MI + TVR.

Table 7. Outcomes after 1 year of follow-up (initial SYNTAX score groups).

index event. Six out of ten cases of repeated target vessel revascularization were caused by the development of in-stent restenosis (**Table 4**). Four other cases were associated with stent thrombosis. Twelve deaths were reported in patients with initial SYNTAX ≥ 23; eleven of them were caused by MACE while the twelfth was due to stroke (**Table 4**). Out of these, eleven deaths, five were the result of stent thrombosis, three were the result of an unsuccessful PCI and progressive acute heart failure, two patients died due to myocardial rupture, and the last case was associated with air embolism of the right coronary artery. Only one case of repeated target vessel revascularization out of nine was the result of in-stent restenosis, while the other eight were performed in patients with stent thrombosis (**Table 7**).

Initial SYNTAX score ≥ 23 was significantly associated with a higher risk of death from any cause, cardiac death, recurrent MI, stent thrombosis, and combined endpoint (**Table 8**).

There was a significantly higher frequency of death from any cause, recurrent MI, and repeated nontarget vessel revascularization among patients with residual SYNTAX ≥ 9 compared to those with residual SYNTAX ≤ 8 (**Table 9**).

Residual SYNTAX ≥ 9 successfully predicted MACE such as death, recurrent MI, and repeated nontarget vessel revascularization (**Table 10**).

Major adverse cardiovascular outcomes	**OR (95% CI)**
Death from any cause	4.9
Cardiac death	5.6
Recurrent myocardial infarction	3.5
Stent thrombosis	5.0
Combined endpoint	2.4

Table 8. Prognostic factors of MACE based on the initial SYNTAX score.

Variables	**Residual SYNTAX ≤ 8 (n = 243)**		**Residual SYNTAX ≥ 9 (n = 74)**		**P value**
	n	**%**	**n**	**%**	
Death	7	2.9	10	13.5	0.001
Myocardial infarction	10	4.1	8	10.8	0.05
Repeated target vessel revascularization	11	4.5	9	12.2	>0.05
Repeated nontarget vessel revascularization	6	2.5	7	9.5	0.02
Stent thrombosis	5	2.1	5	6.8	>0.05

Table 9. Outcomes after 1 year of follow-up (residual SYNTAX score groups).

Major adverse cardiovascular outcomes	OR (95% CI)
Death	3.4 (1.5–7.9)
Recurrent myocardial infarction	2.7 (1.2–6.1)
Repeated nontarget vessel revascularization	2.6 (1.2–5.5)

Table 10. Prognostic factors of MACE based on the residual SYNTAX score.

4.3. Discussion

The main objective of this study was to determine the value of initial and residual SYNTAX score for prediction of adverse revascularization outcomes in patients with STEMI and MVCAD. To the best of our knowledge, there is little evidence demonstrating the prognostic value of initial and residual SYNTAX score in STEMI patients who underwent primary PCI. Meanwhile, there is a need for objective criteria including the severity of coronary lesions, which could optimize the choice of revascularization strategy for these patients [30, 31].

Here we showed that initial SYNTAX ≥ 23 points can predict the development of MACE within 1 year of follow-up. Patients with SYNTAX ≥ 23 had significantly higher incidence of adverse outcomes such as death, MI, and stent thrombosis. However, residual SYNTAX score can be even more informative since it reflects the completeness of myocardial revascularization and risk of adverse events in the short- and long-term follow-up. Residual SYNTAX score ≥ 9 was significantly associated with an increased risk of death, recurrent MI, and repeated nontarget vessel revascularization. High residual SYNTAX score was more prevalent in groups with a predominance of female patients, three-vessel coronary disease, peripheral atherosclerosis, past medical history of MI, and reduced LVEF. It is known that these clinical and demographic indicators themselves have an adverse effect on long-term prognosis after MI [30, 31]. However, it cannot be excluded that adverse cardiovascular events are more dependent on revascularization completeness in the hospital period and, therefore, on residual SYNTAX score at the time of discharge from the hospital. It is important to note the direct association of the initial SYNTAX score ≥ 23 with residual SYNTAX score ≥ 9 points. We suggest that patients with initial severe coronary atherosclerosis are likely to retain a high residual SYNTAX at the end of hospitalization.

This highlights the need for complete revascularization in the early stages, including MS strategy (simultaneous and staged a tightly limited time interval between PCI), as well as a combination of primary PCI with subsequent coronary bypass surgery. Moreover, patients with high residual SYNTAX score may need more efficient schemes of anticoagulant and antiplatelet therapy with the use of modern drugs (bivalirudin, ticagrelor, prasugrel). Considering the desirability of multivessel PCI strategy targeting not only IRA but also nonculprit lesions in a limited time interval [4], we assume that the target value of residual SYNTAX score in STEMI patients to the end of in-hospital period is ≤ 8 points. This algorithm is particularly reasoning given a sufficiently high proportion of unsuccessful PCI in patients with severe initial and residual SYNTAX (10.8%).

4.4. Conclusions

Both initial and residual SYNTAX score can predict death from all causes and/or MACE in patients with STEMI and MVCAD. Patients with high initial SYNTAX score tend to have a high residual SYNTAX score. Therefore, the patients with high initial SYNTAX score require complete revascularization and efficient antiplatelet therapy. Probably, it is required to develop a model of differentiated selection of the optimal revascularization strategy for STEMI patients to reduce the residual SYNTAX score to the end of in-hospital period to ≤ 8 points using primary multivessel stenting or staged PCIs. These results may be useful for risk stratification in patients with STEMI and MVCAD. In this context, in the next section of this chapter will be presented the relevant data of our own study—personalized choice of optimal strategy revascularization in STEMI patients with MVCAD.

5. Personalized choice of optimal revascularization strategy in patients with STEMI and MVCAD

5.1. Methods and statistical analysis

Having recruited 327 consecutive patients, we carried out a single-center registry study. Criteria of inclusion were (1) hospital admission within 12 h of STEMI onset requiring the performance of PPCI; (2) MVCAD defined as hemodynamically significant (≥70%) stenosis of ≥ 2 coronary arteries; (3) technical ability to perform PPCI. Criteria of exclusion were (1) acute heart failure Killip class III-IV, i.e., pulmonary edema and cardiogenic shock; (2) left main coronary artery stenosis ≥ 50%. Before PPCI, all patients received a loading dose of acetylsalicylic acid (250–500 mg) and clopidogrel (600 mg). Successful PPCI was defined as the reduction of stenosis to < 20% and a TIMI flow grade 3. After the PCI, all the patients received aspirin, statins, and clopidogrel during 1 year of follow-up. Patients were divided into two groups: treated with MPS approach (n =91) and treated with MSS approach (n = 236). The second stage of PCI in those who were treated with MSS approach was carried out 3–6 months after PPCI. After 12 months of follow-up, both cardiac and noncardiac death, recurrent MI, and repeat coronary revascularization were defined as primary endpoints. Repeated revascularization was performed utilizing PCI after the baseline procedure due to the recurrent symptoms, recurrent MI, or significant ischemia at provocative testing. In patients treated with MSS approach, we defined only unplanned procedures as repeated revascularization. Follow-up was conducted by outpatient visits or phone interviews.

We collected the data on age, gender, acute heart failure (Killip class), left ventricular ejection fraction, SYNTAX score, peripheral atherosclerosis (PA), past medical history of myocardial infarction or stroke, arterial hypertension, diabetes mellitus, MVCAD, and use of drug-eluting stents.

Risk stratification models were obtained using stepwise logistic regression with the calculation of ROC curve and area under the curve (**Figures 1** and **2**).

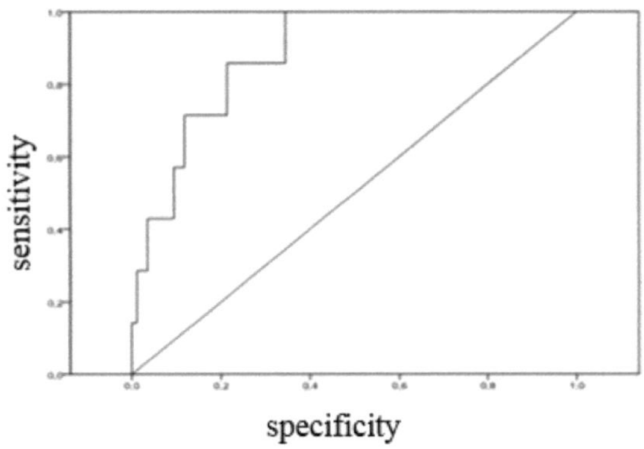

Figure 1. ROC curve of the model calculated for MPS strategy.

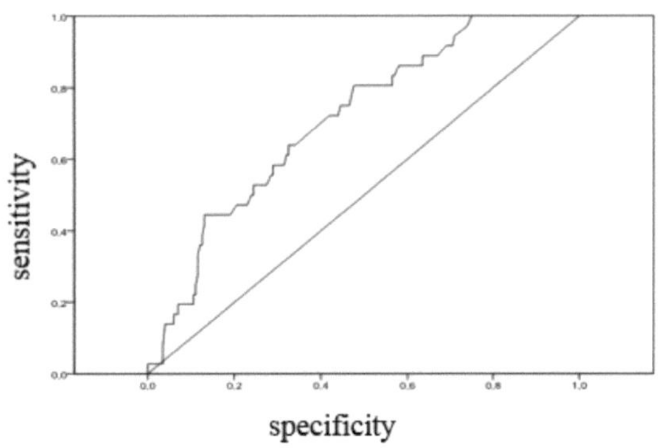

Figure 2. ROC curve of the model calculated for MSS strategy.

We further developed an original calculator for choosing the optimal stenting strategy (Microsoft Excel).

5.2. Results

5.2.1. Baseline characteristics

Patient groups did not have any significant differences in clinical or demographic characteristics (**Table 11**) as well as in angiographic features (**Table 12**) and characteristics of vascular access or implanted stents (**Table 13**).

Strikingly, there were no significant differences in outcomes between two revascularization strategies (**Table 14**).

Prognostic coefficients for each group of patients are presented in **Table 15**.

The values of prognostic coefficients were directly related to the risk of adverse outcome (**Table 15**). Past medical history of MI, severe coronary atherosclerosis (SYNTAX score ≥ 23), elderly age, and female gender showed significant predictive ability of an adverse outcome for patients treated with MPS, while past medical history of MI or stroke, PA, arterial hypertension, three-vessel disease, and the use of non-DES were the predictors of an adverse outcome in those treated using MSS approach. The following clinical case represents an example of utilizing interactive calculator for the selection of the optimal revascularization strategy in a patient with STEMI and MVCAD.

5.3. Clinical case: using a calculator for a personalized selection of the optimal revascularization strategy in a patient with STEMI and MVCAD

Female, 64 years old, was admitted to the hospital with STEMI. The time from onset of symptoms to hospital admission was 4 h. The patient had a number of cardiovascular risk factors: diabetes, hypertension, PA (two-sided stenosis of internal carotid arteries), and residual effects of stroke. ECG showed signs of ST-segment elevation in leads V1–V5 > 2 mm. Ejection fraction on echocardiography was 33%.

Variables	MPS (n = 91)		MSS (n = 236)		P
	n	%	n	%	
Age, years	59.2 ± 10.2		60.1 ± 10.2		0.6
Male gender	62	68.1	154	65.3	0.6
LVEF, %		51.1 ± 8.8		50.7 ± 7.8	0.97
Arterial hypertension	79	86.8	208	88.1	0.9
Diabetes mellitus	17	18.7	49	20.8	0.8
Peripheral artery disease	20	21.9	68	28.8	0.4
Past medical history of MI	9	9.9	40	16.9	0.3
Past medical history of stroke	0		12	5.1	0.5
Acute heart failure (Killip class II)	11	12.1	28	11.9	0.8

LVEF—left ventricular ejection fraction; MI—myocardial infarction.

Table 11. Patient clinical and demographic features.

Variables	MPS (n = 91)		MSS (n = 236)		P
	n	%	n	%	
Three-vessel disease	50	54.9	132	55.9	0.9
SYNTAX score	18.9 ± 7.5		21.5 ± 8.6		0.1
LAD-IRA	36	39.5	86	36.4	0.8
Cx-IRA	17	18.7	53	22.5	0.8
RCA-IRA	38	41.7	97	41.1	0.9

IRA—infarct-related artery; LAD—left anterior descending artery; Cx—circumflex artery; RCA—right coronary artery.

Table 12. Baseline angiographic characteristics.

Variables	MPS (n = 91)		MSS (n = 236)		P
	n	%	n		n
Femoral access	43\91	47.3	255\472	54.6	0.5
Radial access	46\91	50.5	212\472	45.4	0.6
Shoulder access	2\91	2.2	5\472	1	0.7
Successful PCI	84\91	92.3	444\472	94.1	0.9
Contrast medium, ml	328.2 ± 120.7		364.1 ± 165.5		0.07
The average number of stents implanted in IRA	1.3 ± 0,5		1.4 ± 0,6		0.7
DES in IRA	48	52.7	125	52.9	0.9
The average number of stents implanted in non-IRA	1.2 ± 0.5		1.4 ± 0.7		0.7
DES in non-IRA	41	45	116	49.2	0.7
The average length of IRA stented segment, mm	28.9 ± 12.6		29.3 ± 13.7		0.8
The average length of non-IRA stented segment, mm	24.2 ± 11.7		28.1 ± 15.4		0.5
The average diameter of IRA stent, mm	3.3 ± 0.4		3.4 ± 0.5		0.8
The average diameter of non-IRA stent, mm	3.2 ± 0.5		3.2 ± 0.4		0.9

Table 13. Characteristics of vascular access and implanted stents in patient groups.

According to angiography data, multiple coronary disease occurred: subtotal lesion of the proximal and distal segment of right coronary artery (RCA), thrombotic occlusion of the proximal segment of left anterior descending (LAD) artery with blood flow TIMI 0, subtotal bifurcation stenosis of circumflex (Cx) artery (**Figure 3**).

Variables	MPS (n = 91)		MSS (n = 236)		P
	n	%	n	%	n
Death from all causes	3	3.3	14	5.9	0.5
Cardiac death	3	3.3	12	5.1	0.7
MI	3	3.3	16	6.8	0.3
Target vessel revascularization	4	4.4	13	5.5	0.9
Nontarget vessel revascularization	0	0	4	1.7	0.5
Combined endpoint*	7	7.7	24	10.2	0.6
Stent thrombosis	3	3.3	11	4.7	0.8

*Combined endpoint—death, MI and unplanned revascularization (TVR and non-TVR).

Table 14. Outcomes after 1 year of follow-up.

Risk factor	Presence of risk factor	Prognostic coefficients for MPS	Prognostic coefficients for MSS
Elderly age	No	0.031	0.132
	Yes	0.192	0.195
Female	No	0.048	0.169
	Yes	0.138	0.134
Acute heart failure (Killip class)	1	0.079	0.144
	2	0.091	0.214
Peripheral atherosclerosis	No	0.071	0.132
	Yes	0.1	0.203
Past medical history of MI	No	0.049	0.1353
	Yes	0.3	0.25
Arterial hypertension	No	0.125	0.043
	Yes	0.072	0.165
Diabetes mellitus	No	0.068	0.15
	Yes	0.111	0.163
Past medical history of stroke	No	–	0.147
	Yes	–	0.273
Three-vessel disease	No	0.064	0.097
	Yes	0.091	0.189
SYNTAX score ≥23	No	0.045	0.150
	Yes	0.16	0.156
LVEF	(3) ≤40%	0.111	0.077
	(2) 41–49%	0.148	0.224
	(1) ≥50%	0.036	0.128
DES	No	0.075	0.182
	Yes	0.078	0.041

MI—myocardial infarction; LVEF—left ventricular ejection fraction; DES—drug-eluting stents.

Table 15. Prognostic factors of unfavorable outcome depending on the revascularization strategy.

Using our original calculator, we counted the probability of an adverse outcome for MPS and MSS strategies (**Figure 4**). As seen from **Figure 4**, MPS strategy was selected as favorable, while MSS strategy showed a poor prognosis for the patient.

Hence, the patient underwent multivessel stenting of LAD, Cx and RCA (five DES implanted in total) (**Figure 5**).

The patient's conditions were satisfactory. On the 14th day, the patient was discharged from the hospital. There was no angina but patient experienced chronic heart failure II-III functional

http://dx.doi.org/10.5772/67884

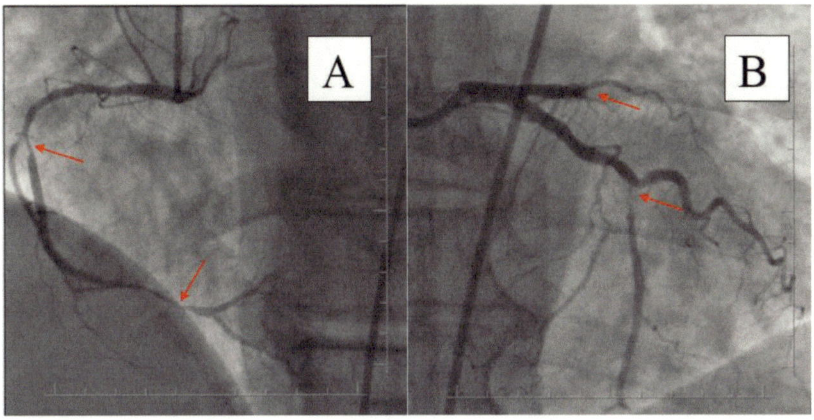

Figure 3. Angiography of the patient with STEMI and multiple coronary disease. A: Subtotal lesion of the proximal and distal segment of right coronary artery; B: Thrombotic occlusion of the proximal segment of left anterior descending artery and subtotal bifurcation stenosis of circumflex artery.

class (NYHA classification). Current diabetes and arterial hypertension were adequately controlled with proper medications. After 2 years, the patient underwent repeated coronary angiography. There were no stenoses of coronary arteries (**Figure 6**). According to echocardiography, LVEF was 45%, with a remained anterior wall hypokinesis.

Therefore, we successfully selected an optimal revascularization strategy. This restored the function of anterior myocardial wall, prevented destabilization of Cx and RCA stenosis, and provided a satisfactory quality of life.

5.4. Conclusions

Here we defined the risk factors of an adverse outcome and designed a calculator for the personalized choice of the optimal revascularization strategy for patients with STEMI and MVCAD.

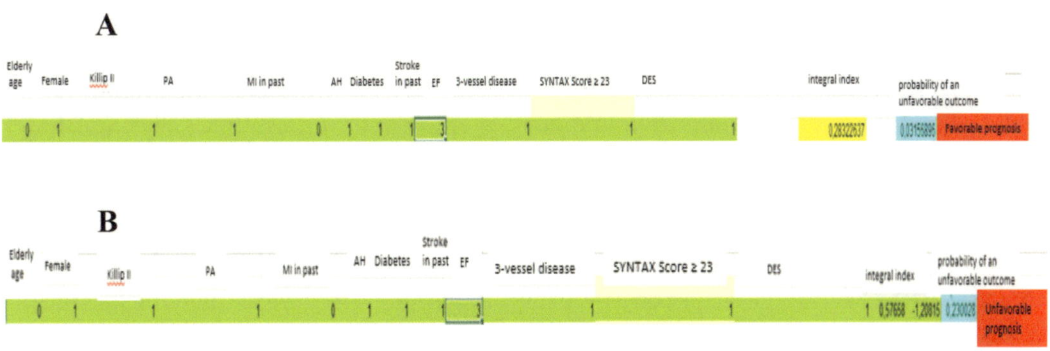

Figure 4. Using the model to calculate the probability of unfavorable prognosis for MPS (A) and MSS strategies (B); 1—presence of factor; 0—absence of factor; 3—LVEF ≤ 40%; PA—peripheral atherosclerosis; MI—myocardial infarction; AH—arterial hypertension; EF—ejection fraction; DES—drug-eluting stents.

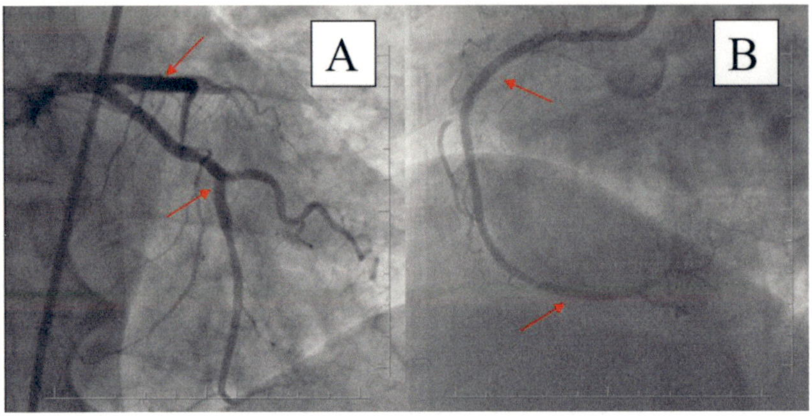

Figure 5. Angiography of the patient with STEMI after stenting. A—LAD and Cx; B—RCA.

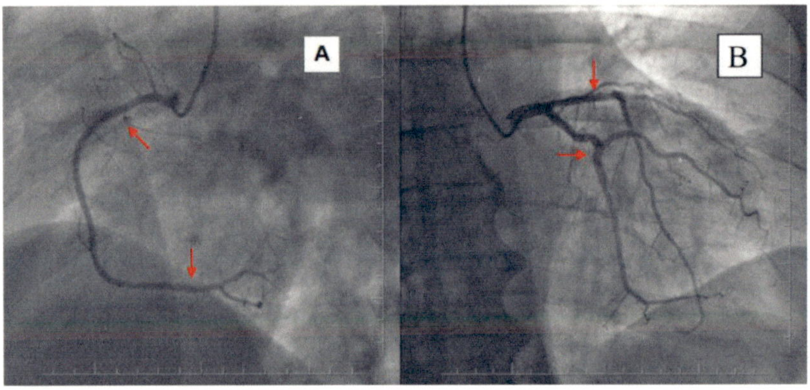

Figure 6. Angiography of the patient with STEMI 24 months after stenting A—RCA; B—LAD and Cx.

6. Conclusions

Around 50% of patients with STEMI have MVCAD that significantly worsens prognosis. There are three treatment approaches to these patients: culprit vessel intervention only, with ischemia-based PCI of non-IRA, MV stenting either at the time of PPCI or as a planned, staged procedure. Both MPS and MSS have evidence base and are approved by the current clinical guidelines. Treatment of culprit vessel only leads to worse outcomes. Complete revascularization, achievable through either MPS or MSS, is the key aim that was confirmed by our single-center registry study of initial and residual SYNTAX score. However, the choice between MPS and MSS is a crucially important issue. Here we defined the risk factors of adverse outcomes after either of these strategies and developed an original calculator for the choice of an optimal stenting strategy. Moreover, we carried out a randomized clinical trial and revealed that results of revascularization in patients with STEMI and MVCAD may be improved by using the latest generation DES such as Resolute Integrity™ Stent.

http://dx.doi.org/10.5772/67884

Hence, we justify the use of personalized approach for the optimal revascularization strategy in patients with STEMI and MVCAD using the latest generation of DES with choosing MPS or MSS according to our original calculator.

Author details

Vladimir I. Ganyukov[1]* and Roman S. Tarasov[2]

*Address all correspondence to: ganyukov@mail.ru

1 Laboratory of Interventional Cardiology, State Research Institute for Complex Issue of Cardiovascular Diseases, Kemerovo, Russia

2 Laboratory of Reconstructive Surgery, State Research Institute for Complex Issue of Cardiovascular Diseases, Kemerovo, Russia

References

[1] Wijns W, Kolh P, Danchin N, et al. Guidelines on myocardial revascularization: the task force on myocardial revascularization of the European Society of Cardiology (ESC) and the European Association for Cardio-Thoracic Surgery (EACTS). Eur Heart J. 2010;31(20):2501-2555.

[2] O'Gara PT, Kushner FG, Ascheim DD, et al. 2013 ACCF/AHA guideline for the management of ST-elevation myocardial infarction: executive summary: a report of the American College of Cardiology Foundation/American Heart Association Task Force on Practice Guidelines. Circulation. 2013;127:529-555.

[3] Steg PG, James SK, Atar D, et al. ESC guidelines for the management of acute myocardial infarction in patients presenting with ST-segment elevation. Eur Heart J. 2012;33:2569-2619.

[4] Windecker S, Kolh P, Alfonso F, et al. for the Task Force on Myocardial Revascularization of the European Society of Cardiology (ESC) and the European Association for Cardio-Thoracic Surgery (EACTS). 2014 ESC/EACTS guidelines on myocardial revascularization. Eur Heart J. 2014;35:2541-2619.

[5] Levine GN, O'Gara PT, Bates ER, et al. 2015 ACC/AHA/SCAI focused update on primary percutaneous coronary intervention for patients with ST-elevation myocardial infarction: an update of the 2011 ACCF/AHA/SCAI Guideline for Percutaneous Coronary Intervention and the 2013 ACCF/AHA Guideline for the Management of ST-Elevation Myocardial Infarction: a report of the American College of Cardiology/American Heart Association Task Force on clinical practice guidelines and the society for cardiovascular angiography and interventions. J Am Coll Cardiol. 2016;67:1235-1250.

[6] Patel MR, Calhoon JH, Dehmer GJ, et al. ACC/AATS/AHA/ASE/ASNC/SCAI/SCCT/STS 2016 appropriate use criteria for coronary revascularization in patients with acute coronary syndromes. http://dx.doi.org/10.1016/j.jacc.2016.10.034

[7] Cardarelli F, Bellasi A, Ou FS, et al. Combined impact of age and estimated glomerular filtration rate on in-hospital mortality after percutaneous coronary intervention for acute myocardial infarction (from the American College of Cardiology National Cardiovascular Data Registry). Am J Cardiol 2009;103:766-771.

[8] Park DW, Clare RM, Schulte PJ, et al. Extent, location, and clinical significance of non-infarct related coronary artery disease among patients with ST-elevation myocardial infarction. JAMA 2014;312:2019-2027.

[9] Parodi G, Mernisha G, Valenti R, et al. Five year outcome after primary coronary intervention for acute ST elevation myocardial infarction: results from a single centre experience. Heart. 2005;91:1541-1544.

[10] Muller DW, Topol EJ, Ellis SG, et al. Thrombolysis and angioplasty in myocardial infarction (TAMI) study group. Multivessel coronary artery disease: a key predictor of short-term prognosis after reperfusion therapy for acute myocardial infarction. Am Heart J. 1991;121:1042-1049.

[11] Sorajja P, Gersh BJ, Cox DA, et al. Impact of multivessel disease on reperfusion success and clinical outcomes in patients undergoing primary percutaneous coronary intervention for acute myocardial infarction. Eur Heart J. 2007;28:1709-1716.

[12] Hannan EL, Samadashvili Z, Walford G, et al. Culprit vessel percutaneous coronary intervention versus multivessel and staged percutaneous coronary intervention for ST-segment elevation myocardial infarction patients with multivessel disease. J Am Coll Cardiol Intervent. 2010;3:22-31.

[13] Toma M, Buller CE, Westerhout CM, et al. Nonculprit coronary artery percutaneous coronary intervention during acute ST-segment elevation myocardial infarction: insights from the APEX-AMI trial. Eur Heart J. 2010;31:1701-1707.

[14] Cavender MA, Milford-Beland S, Roe MT, et al. Prevalence, predictors, and in-hospital outcomes of non-infarct artery intervention during primary percutaneous coronary intervention for ST-segment elevation myocardial infarction (from the National Cardiovascular Data Registry). Am J Cardiol. 2009;104:507-513.

[15] Corpus RA, House JA, Marso SP, et al. Multivessel percutaneous coronary intervention in patients with multivessel disease and acute myocardial infarction. Am Heart J. 2004;148:493-500.

[16] Kornowski R, Mehran R, Dangas G, et al. Prognostic impact of staged versus "one-time" multivessel percutaneous intervention in acute myocardial infarction: analysis from the HORIZONS-AMI (harmonizing outcomes with revascularization and stents in acute myocardial infarction) trial. J Am Coll Cardiol. 2011;58: 704-711.

[17] Politi L, Sgura F, Rossi R, et al. A randomised trial of target-vessel versus multi-vessel revascularization in ST-elevation myocardial infarction: major adverse cardiac events during long-term follow-up. Heart. 2010;96:662-667.

[18] Roe MT, Cura FA, Joski PS, et al. Initial experience with multivessel percutaneous coronary intervention during mechanical reperfusion for acute myocardial infarction. Am J Cardiol. 2001;88:170-173, A6.

[19] Varani E, Balducelli M, Aquilina M, et al. Single or multivessel percutaneous coronary intervention in ST-elevation myocardial infarction patients. Catheter Cardiovasc Interv. 2008;72:927-933.

[20] Wald DS, Morris JK, Wald NJ, et al. Randomized trial of preventive angioplasty in myocardial infarction. N Engl J Med. 2013;369:1115-1123.

[21] Gershlick AH, Khan JN, Kelly DJ, et al. Randomized trial of complete versus lesion-only revascularization in patients undergoing primary percutaneous coronary intervention for STEMI and multivessel disease: the CvLPRIT trial. J Am Coll Cardiol. 2015;65:963-972.

[22] Engstrøm T, Kelbæk H, Helqvist S, et al. Complete re-vascularisation versus treatment of the culprit lesion only in patients with ST-segment elevation myocardial infarction and multivessel disease (DANAMI 3-PRIMULTI): an open-label, randomised controlled trial. Lancet. 2015;386:665-671.

[23] Hlinomaz O. Multivessel coronary disease diagnosed at the time of primary PCI for STEMI: complete revascularization versus conservative strategy: the PRAGUE 13 trial. Paper presented at EuroPCR, 19-22 May 2015, Paris, France.

[24] Cutlip DE, Windecker S, Mehran R, et al. Clinical endpoints in coronary stent trials: a case for standardized definitions. Circulation. 2007;115:2344-2351.

[25] Gabriel S, Stefan K, James, DA, et al. The task force on the management of ST-segment elevation acute myocardial infarction of the European Society of Cardiology (ESC). Eur Heart J. 2012. doi:10.1093/eurheartj/ehs215.

[26] Widimsky P, Holmes Jr David R. How to treat patients with ST-elevation acute myocardial infarction and multi-vessel disease? Eur Heart J. 2010. doi:10.1093/eurheartj/ehq410.

[27] Binder RK, Maier W, Luscher TF. Multi-vessel revascularization in ST-segment elevation myocardial infarction: where do we stand? Eur Heart J. 2016;37:217-220. doi:10.1093/eurheartj/ehv722.

[28] Goldstein JA, Demetriou D, Grines CL, et al. Multiple complex coronary plaques in patients with acute myocardial infarction. N Engl J Med. 2000;343:915-922.

[29] Di Mario C, Mara S, Flavio A, et al. Single vs multivessel treatment during primary angioplasty: results of the multicenter randomised HEpacoat for culprit or multivessel stenting for Acute Myocardial Infarction (HELP AMI) study. Int J Cardiovasc Intervent. 2004;6:128-133.

[30] Tarasov R, Ganyukov VI. Determination of optimal revascularization strategy in ST-segment elevation myocardial infarction patients with multivessel coronary disease with interactive calculator. Complex Issu Cardiovasc Dis. 2015;(4):42-52 (in Russ.). doi:10.17802/2306-1278-2015-4-42-52.

[31] Garg S, Sarno G, Serruys PW, et al. Prediction of 1-year clinical outcomes using the SYNTAX score in patients with acute ST-segment elevation myocardial infarction undergoing primary percutaneous coronary intervention. J Am Coll Cardiol Intervent. 2011;4(1):66-67.

Section 2

Chronic Total Occlusion

Chapter 3

Chronic Total Occlusions

Gregor Leibundgut and Mathias Kaspar

Additional information is available at the end of the chapter

http://dx.doi.org/10.5772/68067

Abstract

The following chapter provides a brief overview on the prevalence, clinical features, and histological findings in chronically occluded coronary arteries. The role of coronary collaterals and myocardial viability as well as left ventricular function for the evaluation of treatment strategies of chronic total occlusions (CTO) will be discussed. Imaging modalities such as computed tomography and intracoronary imaging are discussed for their significance in CTO assessment and intervention. Finally, important clinical and procedural aspects, latest interventional strategies and techniques, the armamentarium of dedicated tools for CTO interventions, as well as evidence from published trials and clinical research in the field will be presented.

Keywords: chronic total occlusions, coronary artery disease, percutaneous intervention

1. Introduction

A chronic total occlusion (CTO) of a coronary artery is defined as complete closure of the vessel lumen for at least 3 months (**Figure 1**). The true prevalence of CTOs in the general population is unknown and assumed to be around 15–20% [1–3] but varies widely (30–50%) in patients with significant coronary artery disease (CAD) [1–5].

Percutaneous coronary intervention (PCI) of CTOs is considered to be the most challenging procedure in interventional cardiology and is associated with higher periprocedural failure and complication rates. At this, the presence of a CTO influences treatment recommendations and is a strong predictor against PCI as a treatment strategy [5].

CTO PCI in specialized centers is currently performed with success rates greater than 80% and decreasing complication rates, suggesting a favorable risk/benefit ratio supporting its

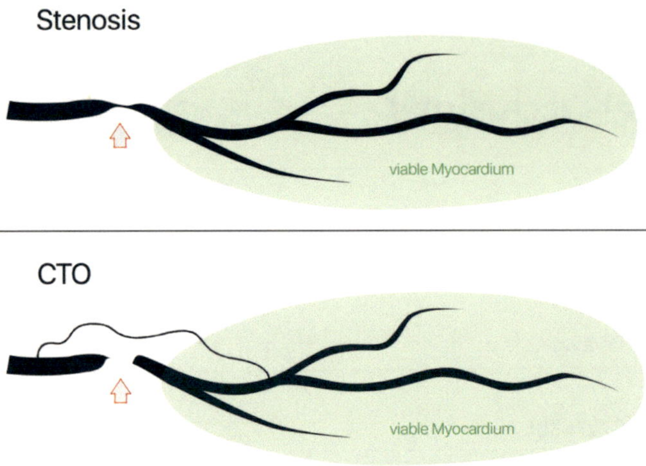

Figure 1. Stenosis versus chronic total occlusion.

increasing selection as a treatment option [6]. However, discrepant CTO PCI quantity and success rates exist among catheterization laboratories [1] and may be explained by individual skills among operators, lesion assessment, and the absence of consensual treatment strategies. Recently, CTO PCI has become more predictable as a consequence of dedicated tools, standardized procedural techniques, and continuous educational programs.

Contemporary PCI strategies with dedicated devices significantly improved procedural success, and the introduction of drug-eluting stents (DES) led to better long-term patency with preservation of left ventricular (LV) function. Still, there is little systematic evidence that post-procedural outcomes have relevantly changed, although much retrospective data suggest CTO PCI as favorable.

2. Basics of chronic total occlusions

2.1. Definition

A "true" total occlusion is defined as a coronary lesion with thrombolysis in myocardial infarction (TIMI) flow grade 0. In order to be classified as "chronic," the occlusion needs to be present for at least 3 months. It is difficult in clinical practice to determine the period of time for which a total occlusion has been present. The age of the occlusion is usually specified by detailed assessment of medical history and cardiovascular symptoms over the past 3 months [7–9]. Despite using contemporary criteria for CTO, Fefer et al. reported determined CTO duration in only 46% of cases, whereas another recent survey showed a known occlusion duration in 61% of CTO cases, with the undetermined duration of CTO as a predictor of procedural failure and major adverse cardiac events (MACE) [1, 10].

2.2. Prevalence and clinical features

In a recent report from the Canadian multicenter CTO registry, about 15% of patients without previous coronary artery bypass graft (CABG) surgery or known CAD and about 18% of patients with clinically significant CAD show at least one CTO on coronary angiogram [9]. In these registries, only 40% had a prior history of myocardial infarction (twice as high as without CTO), and more than 50% of CTO patients showed normal LV ejection fraction [11]. Furthermore, 64% of these patients underwent medical therapy, 26% were referred to CABG (with 88% successfully bypassing CTO), and only 10% underwent PCI of the CTO [1, 9]. In this study, only 5% of patients with a CTO were asymptomatic and it was in general difficult to attribute symptoms to the CTO in symptomatic multi-vessel disease (MVD) cases. Interestingly, recanalization of an occluded left anterior descending artery (LAD) rather than PCI of an occluded right coronary artery (RCA) results in greater increase of left ventricular function and more beneficial autonomic nervous system parameters with a potential antiarrhythmic effect [12].

Patients with CAD and CTO are mostly men, tend to be older, and usually have a higher cardiac risk profile. Interestingly, peripheral artery disease was found to be the strongest clinical predictor for the presence of a CTO [5]. In comparison to men, females with CTO tend to have less vessel disease, are usually older, have a higher frequency of hypertension and diabetes, and smoke less, but overall sex has no influence on CTO PCI failure [9, 13].

2.3. Spatial distribution of CTO

Few prospective surveys and a report from the National Heart, Lung, and Blood Institute (NHLBI) Dynamic Registry show CTO located in the RCA in over 50% of the cases [1, 14]. These figures are consistent with the Canadian multicenter CTO registry report, where, in most of the cases, CTO was found in the RCA (47%), 20% in the LAD, 16% in the left circumflex (LCX), and 17% in multiple locations [1, 9]. In a recent post-mortem analysis in CTO with and without CABG, CTO was most frequently located in the RCA (57.9%), followed by the LAD (22.1%) and LCX (20.0%), mainly located in the proximal segment (68.4%) of the vessel [15].

Garcia et al. examined the clinical and angiographic characteristics as well as clinical outcomes of >1300 consecutive CTO PCIs prospectively and retrospectively in multiple centers in the US. The study showed that proximal lesions were more common, and these patients had a higher prevalence of adverse comorbidities, mostly heart failure with reduced left ventricular ejection fraction (LVEF). Furthermore, proximal lesions had more adverse angiographic features (including proximal cap ambiguity, side branch at proximal cap, blunt or no stump, and moderate or severe calcification) but had more interventional collaterals and showed a higher angiographic complexity, resulting in longer and more complex procedures. The retrograde approach was used in half of the cases involving proximal CTO lesions and was successful in one-third of these cases. Surprisingly, procedural success and complication rates were similar to mid- and distal lesions [16].

3. Histopathology

Wang et al. demonstrated that acute coronary occlusions leading to segment elevation myocardial infarction (STEMI) seem to predominately occur in predictable spots within the proximal third of the coronary arteries and that for each 10 mm increase in distance from the ostium, the risk of an acute coronary occlusion significantly decreased by 13–30%, depending on the coronary vessel [17].

In contrast to this, sparse information exists concerning the genesis of CTO and its regional distribution in terms of recanalization. In some publications, soft plaque rupture during acute coronary syndrome (ACS) with rapid thrombotic occlusion followed by its organization is described as the main cause of CTO and only a few appear to derive from atheroma progression [18]. Furthermore, it seems that once thrombotic occlusion occurs the thrombus tends to disseminate retrograde from the site of occlusion to the proximal segments of the vessel with a major side branch [19]. It is known that due to increased chronic hypoxic induction of neovasculature, the affected vessel segment stays biologically active and shows a marked heterogeneity in compensatory angiogenesis with an unpredictable wide range of coronary collateral circulation [20].

3.1. Collaterals and microchannels in CTO

Successful guidewire crossing may be facilitated by the presence of intravascular microchannels, but structural changes over time with variable localization of these microvessels are not well understood in terms of CTO recanalization [21].

In a post-mortem study of 96 CTO lesions, 49% exhibited residual <99% lumen stenosis by histologic criteria despite angiographically documented total occlusions [22]. In this cohort, adventitia and intimal plaque of total occlusions were the prevalent zones of inflammation and neovascularization. Furthermore, the results revealed in CTOs of all ages a close relation between cellular inflammation and vessel wall neovascularization in terms of location and intensity with an increase in numbers of neovascular channels rather than with an increase in their size.

Munce et al. found two histological types of microvessels in a rabbit model with induced femoral occlusion: a circumferentially oriented "extravascular" and a longitudinally oriented "intravascular" one. Interestingly, extravascular vessels around the occluded artery developed to a maximum at an early time point, followed by a slow regression over time, while intravascular vessel formation within the central body of the occlusion was delayed, and these vessels became thinner and more tortuous over time. Strongly angulated connections between the intra and extravascular microvessels were constantly present, which could explain deviation of the guidewire into extravascular channels during CTO recanalization [21].

Katsuragawa et al. found different histomorphological features in CTOs with tapering of the proximal occlusion point compared to those with a blunt proximal cap [19]. A total of 80% of the tapering-type lesions had shorter occluded segments and showed small recanalized areas with surrounding loose fibrous tissue along the occluded segment. In lesions with a blunt proximal cap, recanalization was rare, and a side branch was frequently found proximal to the occluded segment and easily entered by the guidewire, instead of the occlusion. These features influence penetration of the proximal cap and crossing of the guidewire through the occluded segment and explain why the tapering type of occlusion is favorable for angioplasty.

3.2. Remodeling in CTO

As atherosclerotic lesions develop in arteries, two types of remodeling can occur [23]. Positive remodeling is a compensatory process in which the arterial wall grows outward in an attempt to maintain a constant lumen diameter. Negative remodeling is angiographically defined as the ratio of the occluded vessel diameter to the diameter of the contiguous normal vessel <1 and was found to be the strongest predictor of failed antegrade CTO PCI [24, 25]. In negative remodeling, an early phase where fibrin-rich organizing thrombus becomes a proteoglycan-rich thrombus and a late phase where proteoglycan-rich thrombus within the CTO body is replaced by dense collagen, thus complicating antegrade wiring, were found [15].

4. Coronary collaterals

Collaterals are interarterial connections that exist during prenatal development of the coronary circulation and regress in most individuals [26]. They develop in a native occluded vessel through positive remodeling. With the low postocclusive pressure regions being interconnected by collateral vessels, pressure gradient along the occluded segment causes pulsatile shear stress and activates proliferation of vascular smooth muscle and endothelial cells. A complex interplay of actin-binding proteins, integrins and connexions, transcription factors, and mitogen-activated kinases finally leads to an increase in vascular diameter and tissue mass (positive remodeling), but still, the degree of functional restoration of blood flow capacity remains incomplete and ends at approximately 30% of maximal conductance in coronary vessels [27, 28].

The diameter of interarterial connections is usually below the spatial resolution of modern digital angiographic imaging systems (>200 μm) and ranges between 40 and 200 μm. Most of these connecting microvessels have been observed to be located intramyocardially, and only few reach the size of coronary side branches well above 1 mm in diameter [29].

It seems that occluded coronary arteries do not exclusively determine the level of functional collateral flow capacity and that some individuals without stenotic lesions do have immediately recruitable collateral flow to prevent myocardial ischemia during a brief coronary occlusion [30]. However, in patients without well-developed pre-existing interarterial connections, collaterals require between 2 and 12 weeks to fully reach functional capacity [31]. After successful CTO PCI, collateral function usually regresses in collaterals with small diameters but has the potential to recover in case of reocclusion [32].

4.1. Classification of collaterals in CTO

In 1985, Rentrop et al. developed an angiographic grading system to rate the effect of collaterals in filling the occluded arterial segment [33]. It distinguishes four degrees of collateral recipient artery filling by radiographic contrast medium, but in CTO with well-developed, spontaneously visible collaterals, it lacks further differentiation because most collaterals are Rentrop grade 3 (complete epicardial filling by collateral vessel of the target artery). The Werner classification adds an additional parameter to describe spontaneously visible collaterals and demonstrates a close association with clinical determinants of collateral adequacy [31]. Werner et al. graded collateral connections (CC) according to the angiographic visibility: CC0: no continuous connection between donor and recipient artery, CC1: continuous, thread-like connections (≥0.4 mm), and CC2: continuous, small side branch-like size of the collateral throughout its course (>1 mm). These CC grades are more practical to determine interventional collaterals suitable for retrograde CTO PCI (**Figure 2**).

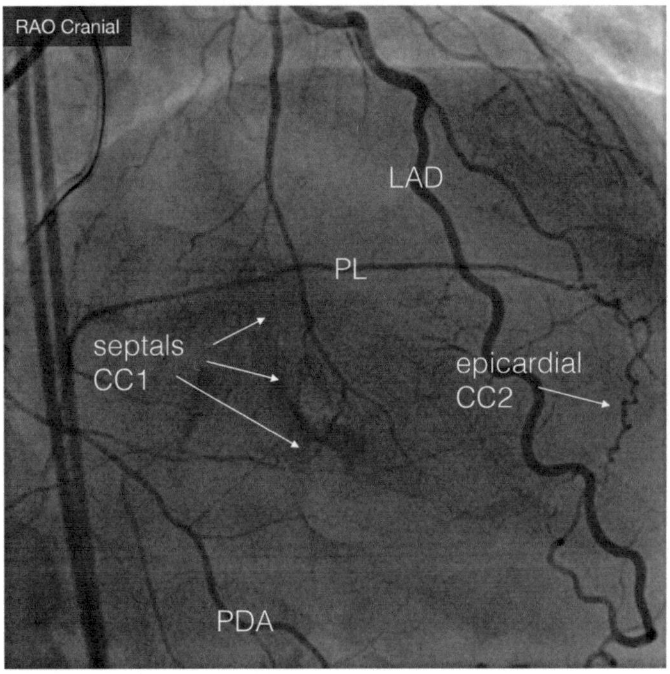

Collaterals (Werner classification)

CC0: invisible

CC1: threadlike <0.4mm
[collaterals in the lower septum from LAD to PDA]

CC2: small side branch like (>0.4mm)
[epicardial collateral from distal LAD to PLA]

Figure 2. Interventional collaterals according to the Werner classification.

4.2. Assessment of collateral function

Generally, collateral circulation in CTO is predominantly systolic and provides only approximately 50% of antegrade coronary flow, which itself is predominantly diastolic [34]. The assessment of collateral function in CTOs has a different quality than in nonoccluded lesions. Collateral blood pressure distal of a chronic occluded vessel is assessed by placing a piezo-resistive transducer beyond the occlusion, while the antegrade flow has not yet been re-established. This can be ensured by passing occlusive microcatheters over a recanalization guidewire and then exchanged for the pressure wire [29].

4.2.1. Collateral flow index (CFI)

Intracoronary (IC) flow velocity or pressure measurements to determine collateral flow is theoretically based on the fact that velocity or perfusion pressure signals with values above central venous pressure (CVP) obtained distal to an occluded vessel originates from collaterals [35]. Measurement of such signals provides the variables for the calculation of a CFI, which expresses the amount of flow via collaterals to the vascular region of interest as a fraction of the flow via the normally patent vessel. In contrast to qualitative assessment of collaterals, such as ST-segment changes and chest pain during PCI or the degree of collateral circulation on angiogram prior to PCI, intravascular flow velocity and pressure determination precisely reflect collateral blood flow. Approximately one-third of collateral flow to the occluded area relative to the patent vessel flow is needed to prevent myocardial ischemia at rest [28]. Noteworthy, the majority of patients with MI do not have enough of the collateral flow to avoid ischemia during coronary occlusion [36] and only 10% seem to have a recruitable CFI ≥ 0.4 [36]. Insufficient collateral flow indicated by a CFI ≤ 0.25 independently predicts long-term cardiac mortality [37], and only 10% seems to have a recruitable CFI ≥ 0.4 [36]. Above that, individuals with CTOs tend to have a higher CFI than those without, and the area at risk of myocardial infarction seems to be significantly associated with CFI.

4.2.2. Fractional flow reserve in the donor artery and coronary steal

Microvascular vasodilation might lead to reduced collateral blood flow during physical or pharmacological provocation in individuals with collateral-dependent blood supply. In order to generate coronary steal, Werner et al. describes, in reference to Gould et al., the following assumption: epicardial stenosis of the donor artery causes a pressure drop proximal to the collateral origin; the collateral resistance is significant, and the microvasculature distal to the occlusion lacks a vasodilatory reserve due to being already maximally dilated [38].

Therefore, Werner et al. measured fractional flow reserve in the donor artery (FFR_D) at the origin of the collaterals in patients with CTO and recorded coronary flow velocity and pressure during recanalization. Patients with steal had more severe regional dysfunction and those with steal but without an $FFR_D < 0.8$ tended to have an impaired microvascular function. The authors concluded that coronary steal mainly occurs as a result of hemodynamically significant donor artery lesions and might have an adverse effect on the preservation of myocardial function by collaterals.

In 50 patients who successfully underwent CTO recanalization compared to 50 matched non-CTO PCI subjects, patients with CTO and an intermediate donor artery stenosis showed a low FFR_D with a high frequency of ischemia in the donor artery territory, which was often normalized by successful CTO treatment, thus suggesting recanalization of CTO as a preferred therapeutic strategy. Reference: CCI 2014.

5. Myocardial viability and left ventricular function

It is in general difficult to predict which patient with stable ischemic heart disease will receive interventional or surgical revascularization in the long term, after initially being treated with optimal medical therapy (OMT). In the occluded artery trial (OAT), late opening of infarct-related arteries (IRA) post-MI in stable patients with persistent total occlusion and no severe inducible ischemia showed no difference in rates of reinfarction, death, or severe heart failure compared to OMT [39]. Nevertheless, the results of OAT in terms of CTO have to be interpreted with caution because total occlusions in this trial were subacute (3–28 days, median 8 days) and therefore did not meet the CTO definition of at least a 3-month duration. Furthermore, patients in OAT showed a relatively normal baseline LVEF of 48% and were rather asymptomatic, whereas CTOs considered for PCI should be symptomatic or have proof of ischemia and viability [40].

An ischemic burden above 12.5% favors PCI in patients with CTO undergoing pre- and post-interventional myocardial perfusion imaging, whereas subjects with mild pre-procedural ischemia (<6.25% of LV myocardium) tend to have increased ischemic burden after PCI [41]. Another magnetic resonance imaging (MRI) study significantly revealed reduction in inducible perfusion defects and improvement in segmental myocardial viability by successful CTO PCI compared to unsuccessful revascularization [42]. Furthermore, successful CTO PCI increases hyperemic and resting myocardial blood flow with enhanced regional contractility already 24 h after the procedure [43]. Patients with an infarction and a transmural involvement < 25% assessed by MRI show significant improvements in segmental wall thickening and a reduction of mean end-systolic and end-diastolic volumes after CTO PCI [44]. Finally, the diagnostic accuracy of pre-procedural contrast enhanced MRI in patients with CTO to detect myocardial infarction and to predict improvement of myocardial function after revascularization seems to be better by using a combined viability analysis rather than focusing on the widely used transmural extent of infarction [45].

6. Coronary computed tomography angiography

Coronary computed tomography angiography (CTA) is increasingly used to diagnose CAD and shows potential in predicting the probability of procedural success and clinical benefit in CTO PCI [46, 47]. In contrast to invasive coronary angiography, CTA offers better quantification of anatomical and morphological features in occluded vessels, especially in long lesions with pronounced tortuosity, and usually visualizes distal coronary segments more

http://dx.doi.org/10.5772/68067

precisely [48]. There are a number of CTA characteristics in CTO lesions to predict PCI failure. Some report calcifications >50% of the cross-sectional vessel area alone [49] or in combination with an occlusion length of >15 mm to be independent predictors of unsuccessful recanalization [50], while others revealed the ratio of calcification over the cross-sectional vessel area as being predictive for procedural failure [51]. Moreover, marked vessel tortuosity at the occlusion site seems to independently predict unsuccessful guidewire crossing [24] and multiple occlusions might have an adverse effect on revascularization's outcome, as reported from the CT-Registry of Chronic Total Occlusion Revascularization (CT-RECTOR), probably due to reduced feasibility in guiding the wire through the multiple entry and exit points [46].

Conclusively, CTA features in CTO, as described above, may be applicable to assess severity of the occlusion and to predict PCI outcome in order to guide treatment decision, especially in complex lesions.

7. Imaging in CTO

CTO interventions are technically challenging due to limitations in visualizing occluded arteries by angiography. As mentioned before, ambiguous proximal CTO cap, side branch at the occlusion site, extended tortuosity, or heavy calcification with limited visibility of distal path are important angiographic features which increase procedural difficulties during CTO recanalization [7]. Multislice computed tomography (MSCT) can provide useful pre-procedural information on the dimension of vessel calcification or tortuosity along the occluded segment but does not offer direct guidance during the procedure. Intravascular ultrasound (IVUS) and optical coherence tomography (OCT) can add visual guidance during CTO PCI to improve procedure time, safety, and efficacy.

7.1. Intravascular ultrasound

In contrast to OCT, IVUS can be operated in occluded vessels throughout the whole interventional procedure. It is used to identify the best wire entry point for penetration of proximal fibrous cap or to visualize the guidewire to check intraluminal position before balloon angioplasty or stent deployment.

The IVUS probe is usually advanced into a side branch originating proximal to the occlusion to determine the vessel course within the CTO segment [52]. Standard IVUS catheters cannot generate information of the vessel distal of the occlusion, and their use is limited by the diameter and angulation of side branches [53].

Besides its antegrade applications, IVUS is used in retrograde procedures to guide retrograde guidewire crossing and reverse controlled retrograde tracking techniques such as reverse CART to improve success rate and limit complications [52]. Generally, when using the retrograde approach in longer CTO lesions, IVUS guidance can reduce the incidence of subintimal wiring with consecutive side branch loss after stenting, angiographic extravasation, coronary hematoma, and perforation [54, 55].

Furthermore, the incidence of restenosis [56] or stent thrombosis after DES implantation [57] is related to minimum stent area detected by IVUS and malapposition due to aneurysm formation after subintimal DES implantation during CTO PCI, and it can be optimized with the help of IVUS [55].

Although IVUS facilitates CTO PCI and has the potential to reduce periprocedural complications, the clinical benefit of IVUS-guided CTO PCI has not yet been proven, and further studies are needed [52].

7.2. Optical coherence tomography

OCT is more sensitive than IVUS in detecting coronary dissection during PCI and improves stent deployment or detection of acute complications. Furthermore, resolution of OCT is high enough to visualize microvessels, the different layers of the vessel wall, and even collagen concentration in coronary arteries [58].

In contrast to IVUS, conventional OCT, at the cost of penetration depth, has a 10-fold higher imaging resolution as the main advantage but is unable to generate images in completely occluded vessels and does not allow real-time intracoronary imaging for guidance of wire crossing. However, optical coherence reflectometry used in a combined OCT and radiofrequency ablation device might be able to minimize the risk of perforation and increase the crossing potential of the guidewire in CTO PCI [59].

8. Percutaneous intervention of CTO

Complication rates of CTO PCI were traditionally too high to justify these procedures and success rates were based predominantly on individual operator skills and annual case volume [60, 61]. A review of the NHLBI Dynamic Registry revealed a decrease of CTO PCI attempts from 9.6% in 1997/1998 to 5.7% in 2004 [62]. With the introduction of coronary stents, procedural success rates increased substantially and became more consistent across CTO studies [63]. In-hospital MACE and 1-year target vessel, revascularization (TVR) rates have declined by approximately 50% over the years. Patients with successful recanalization of a single-vessel CTO experience a higher 10-year survival rate compared to matched patients with a single non-CTO lesion [64].

Among the patients randomized to PCI in the Synergy between PCI with Taxus and Cardiac Surgery (SYNTAX) trial, CTO lesions were present in 24% and exhibited a low success rate of only 53% [65]. Furthermore, the presence of CTO was the single most common reason for a patient to be referred to surgery, and the prevalence of CTO was almost doubled in the CABG registry.

A metaanalysis from 18,061 CTO patients treated in dedicated high-volume CTO PCI centers and expert operators reported 77% procedural success and a 3.1% risk for MACE [6], whereas an analysis from the National Cardiovascular Data Registry revealed CTO PCI in daily practice to be successful in only 59% [66].

http://dx.doi.org/10.5772/68067

We have recently seen dramatic improvements in outcomes from a series of single- and multiple-operator registries with procedural success of up to 98% and MACE rates as low as 1.7% [67–70]. These results were mainly achieved through constant refinement of interventional techniques and dedicated interventional tools, ongoing knowledge exchange, and the development of standardized treatment algorithms. Most of the current CTO crossing techniques were made possible by the introduction of microcatheters and specialized guidewires. Further advances in CTO PCI will be dependent on the interplay between the development of recanalization techniques and interventional armamentarium.

8.1. Indications for CTO PCI

Indications for CTO PCI are in principle identical to the standard PCI of non-CTO lesions and are based on detailed clinical assessments (**Figure 1**). High procedural success rates in conjunction with low complication rates improve risk/benefit ratio and are paramount for the acceptance and dissemination of CTO PCI. Successful CTO recanalization has the ability to relieve angina [71], reduce ischemia [41] and the need for CABG [72], improve exercise tolerance [73], electrical stability [74], left ventricular function [44], and tolerance of future ACS [13, 75], and possibly survival [76, 77] with a similar risk compared to regular PCI of non-CTO lesions [3]. **Table 1** summarizes the rationale for CTO PCI.

Asymptomatic patients with CTO demand additional ischemia and viability testing. As described above, cardiac MRI has the ability to quantify viable myocardium and detect transmural involvement and therefore may assist in patient selection and procedural planning [78].

Based on small retrospective studies and on expert consensus, American and European guidelines recommend CTO PCI in patients with evidence for substantial ischemia in a corresponding myocardial territory when performed by an experienced operator in case of adequate clinical indications and suitable anatomy with a class-IIa, evidence level B recommendation [79, 80].

Angina relief [71]
Reduction of ischemia [41]
Improvement of exercise tolerance [73]
Improvement of left ventricular function [44]
Improvement electric stability [74]
Improved tolerance of future ACS events [75]
Reduced need for CABG [72]
Increased long-term survival in successful versus failed cases [76, 77]

Table 1. Rationale for CTO PCI [226].

8.2. Radial access for CTO PCI

Radial access is feasible for contralateral injections in CTO PCI but may be challenging when microcatheters and techniques with additional equipment are used [81, 82]. However, based on the availability of sheathless-guiding catheters with a larger interventional lumen, the radial approach has become more frequently used for both the antegrade and retrograde approach.

8.3. Procedural success in patients with CTO undergoing PCI or CABG

In the early days of interventional cardiology, CTO PCI was associated with very low success and relatively high complication rates [83–87]. This leads to a high number of patients undergoing surgery, which was also seen in the SYNTAX and the BARI (Bypass Angioplasty Revascularization Investigation) trial, where the presence of a CTO was a strong predictor for referral to CABG [4, 88].

Procedural failures during CTO are mainly due to the incapacity to pass the lesion with a guidewire, followed by failed balloon crossing, the inability to dilate the lesion, or a vessel perforation [60, 66, 89–91]. Traditional predictors for CTO PCI failure are increasing age of the occlusion, small vessel diameter, presence of calcium or a blunt stump, proximal cap ambiguity, excessive tortuosity, long occlusion length, bridging collaterals, and absent visibility of the distal vessel [72, 89, 92–95]. Furthermore, these lesions show a higher mean Multicenter CTO Registry of Japan (J-CTO) score and have collaterals that are less likely suitable for the retrograde approach [96]. However, additional angiographic features such as multivessel disease, previous CABG, and side branch at the proximal occlusion point seem not to be predictive for procedural failure with novel guidewire techniques [97].

Over time, with the improvement of both equipment such as microcatheters and dedicated guidewires with greater torque response [98] and recanalization techniques such as retrograde procedures, safe and effective CTO PCI became possible [60] and most of the prior obstacles vanished [99].

Only limited randomized data are available on the outcomes of patients with CTO undergoing CABG [100–102]. CTOs represent a difficult lesion subset also for surgical revascularization, thus leading to incomplete revascularization with 31.9% of CTOs referred for CABG not being surgically revascularized and 7.5% with occluded bypass grafts after 1 year [103]. At least one CTO is found in more than 50% of patients with CABG [1, 104].

In SYNTAX, the presence of a CTO was the strongest independent predictor of incomplete revascularization with 51% in the PCI arm and one of the major anatomic predictors for referral to CABG [105]. Interestingly, CABG enhances the progression of atherosclerosis and increases the risk for new CTOs in native coronary arteries, which itself represents an independent predictor of death, MI, and repeat revascularization in these patients [102, 103]. Moreover, long-term patency of saphenous vein grafts (SVG) is limited and is significantly lower than for second-generation DES (70 vs 90% at 5 years, respectively) [106]. Therefore, CABG might only be considered when complete arterial revascularization can be achieved, and given the durability of LIMA-LAD grafts and superior patency of DES over SVGs to LCX or RCA, particularly in CTO cases, hybrid revascularization may represent future treatment options in selected patients [107, 108].

8.4. Predictive scores in CTO PCI

Scoring systems for CTO PCI are very helpful for case selection as well as to predict procedural efficiency and the probability for success and complications [109, 110]. The SYNTAX score, indeed, highly depends on the presence and specific features of CTO, with a single CTO contributing a substantial 10–15 points but is generally more suitable for diffused triple-vessel disease with and without involvement of the left main.

J-CTO [89] and CT-RECTOR [46] scores predict the likelihood of successful guidewire crossing within 30 minutes. The J-CTO score represents a standardized score of difficulty that predicts successful guidewire crossing within 30 minutes, is simple, easy to remember, and clinically applicable. However, the J-CTO score may be limited in some cases. The CL score considers both clinical and angiographic information, predicts success of a first antegrade attempt, and may be useful in centers where the retrograde or hybrid approach has not yet been implemented [111]. The progress CTO score includes four angiographic characteristics and should be applied when using the hybrid approach [112]. A comparison of these three scores for predicting success of CTO PCI showed a moderate performance in predicting technical outcome, with a favor for antegrade procedures [113]. A novel prediction model including age, ostial location, and collateral filling was also strongly associated with technical failure when using advanced recanalization technologies [70]. The ORA score, however, predicts technical failure by both antegrade and retrograde techniques and categorizes difficulty and success rate of CTO procedures into four groups.

Finally, the Mehran risk score is most widely used as a classic model for CIN after CTO PCI, but it is rather inconvenient in clinical practice because it was established only after contrast media exposure [114, 115].

8.5. Stents in CTO PCI

The use of bare-metal stents (BMS) after successful CTO PCI has been proven to be superior in terms of immediate angiographic success as well as long-term restenosis and reocclusion when compared with balloon angioplasty (POBA) alone [116–120]. DES in comparison to BMS shows again a significant reduction in TVR and adverse clinical events [121–126] although a trend toward a higher stent thrombosis rate was observed [127–129]. As a consequence, stent implantation following successful CTO PCI increased dramatically over time and reached nearly 100% at the turn of the millennium [130].

8.6. Bioresorbable vascular scaffolds in CTO

Bioresorbable vascular scaffolds (BVS) have potential long-term benefits compared with DES, thus being particularly reasonable in CTO [131]. A first feasibility analysis in 23 patients with selected and simple CTO lesions demonstrated excellent 6-month and 1-year follow-up after BVS implantation, but these initial results need to be confirmed in larger studies with further long-term follow-up [132].

8.7. Relevance of the target vessel of CTO PCI

Studies have shown the prognostic importance of the anterior wall of the left ventricle [133, 134]. In accordance with these findings, successful CTO PCI is associated with an improvement in long-term survival as compared to CTO PCI failure in the subpopulation of patients with LAD CTO [76] (cohort from 1980 to 2004, overall stent use < 20%, only three patients received DES).

Results from a contemporary multinational CTO registry suggest that successful PCI of a CTO in only the LAD and the LCX, but not the RCA, is associated with improved long-term survival [135]. Over 90% of patients included in this analysis received a stent, mostly DES, which likely resulted in higher long-term patency. Due to higher anatomical complexity, the LCX is the least commonly attempted target vessel in CTO PCI with a lower rate of procedural success and a trend toward higher MACE rates [89, 95, 97, 98, 136, 137].

8.8. CTO and STEMI

Patients presenting with acute STEMI show an incidence of CTO up to 13% and tend to suffer poor immediate and long-term prognosis [94, 130, 138–147]. Several trials revealed a concurrent CTO in a non-infarct-related artery (non-IRA) as an independent predictor of short- and long-term mortality in STEMI patients undergoing primary PCI [148–150]. A metaanalysis of seven observational studies including 14,117 patients with a concurrent CTO in a non-IRA artery presenting with STEMI found a three-fold increase in mortality in both single- and multi-vessel disease cases [75]. Furthermore, concurrent CTO in a non-IRA in MVD was significantly associated with residual left ventricular ejection fraction (LVEF) early after STEMI and further decrease of LVEF in the first year after the index STEMI [13], and this seems particularly true for a CTO of the LAD [151].

The acute closure of the donor artery during STEMI leads to extensive myocardial ischemia in a two-vessel area with consecutive hemodynamic instability [144, 148, 152–155]. This is even more pronounced if the culprit vessel has impaired collateral filling itself [156].

8.9. Complete revascularization in CTO PCI

The most common reason for incomplete revascularization in PCI is the presence of a CTO [157], and incomplete revascularization associated with CTO carries a worse outcome and a higher risk of death compared with complete revascularization [158, 159]. The potential benefit of successful CTO PCI has been derived from retrospective analyses and mainly includes improvement of LVF in preventing heart failure [160], reduction of arrhythmias, and, above all, reduction of mortality, MI, as well as the need for repeating revascularization procedures [161]. Therefore, complete revascularization strategies after the index PCI for STEMI should include CTO procedures.

The EXPLORE (Evaluating Xience and Left Ventricular Function in Percutaneous Coronary Intervention on Occlusions After ST-Elevation Myocardial Infarction) trial was the first randomized controlled trial evaluating whether patients with STEMI and concurrent CTO in a non-IRA benefit from additional CTO PCI shortly after primary PCI [151]. In agreement with earlier registry studies, EXPLORE reported a survival benefit only for successful CTO PCI of the LAD but not for the RCA or LCX [76, 135].

Migliorini et al. studied 330 high surgical risk patients undergoing PCI for unprotected left main disease (ULMD) with more than one-third having at least one CTO [162] and found the presence of a concurrent CTO of the RCA in patients undergoing PCI for ULMD to be a significant predictor for mortality. In contrast to other studies, CTO of both LAD and LCX were not found predictive of worse outcomes. The fact that RCA CTO were attempted less frequently (51%) than CTO of the other two main coronary arteries (79%) may explain the prognostic impact of the RCA in this study.

In the SYNTAX trial, incomplete revascularization was associated with a significant increase in 4-year mortality [105]. The presence of a CTO was less likely to result in complete revascularization in both the PCI and CABG arms and was the strongest independent predictor of incomplete revascularization in the PCI arm. The very low rate of complete revascularization in the PCI arm (34.3%) compared with the CABG arm (64.8%) was mostly related to CTO PCI failure in approximately 50%.

8.10. Restenosis after CTO PCI

Long subintimally placed stents may attribute to a higher restenosis rate. They are typically seen with the STAR technique [163] and are more frequent after retrograde wire crossing [164]. DES are consistently superior over BMS. Second-generation everolimus-eluting stents have lower rates of restenosis after CTO PCI compared with first-generation DES [165], and PCI of a CTO in stent restenosis shows generally a high success rate with good long-term results [166]. Many studies on restenosis after CTO PCI, however, did not have angiographic follow-up despite the fact that reocclusion can be completely silent after CTO PCI [121, 122, 129, 164, 165, 167–173].

9. Specialized CTO recanalization techniques

As described above, CTO remains one of the most difficult subsets in interventional treatment of CAD patients and is generally considered to be challenging during a revascularization approach because of high procedural complexity. With the introduction of innovative catheter-based devices and the development of standardized treatment algorithms, CTO PCI has been increasingly performed with high success and low complication rates. At this, a thorough assessment of specific lesion-related factors and the use of a systematic step-up interventional strategy contribute to lower periprocedural comorbidities with better post-procedural outcome [98, 174].

Currently, there are three major CTO crossing techniques: (1) antegrade wire escalation (AWE), (2) antegrade dissection re-entry (ADR), and (3) retrograde procedures including retrograde wire escalation (RWE) and retrograde dissection re-entry (RDR).

9.1. Antegrade techniques

9.1.1. Antegrade wire escalation

AWE is the most widely used CTO crossing technique and is appropriate for short occlusions or extended ones where a remaining microchannel is expected [174, 175]. However, AWE was found to be unlikely successful in complex lesions [176].

Classical antegrade techniques are single wire-based starting with a soft hydrophilic wire seeking for microchannels, followed by gradual escalation to harder and stiffer wires [98]. Higher penetrating force is needed in more fibrous and calcified lesions, and nonhydrophilic wires represent a good alternative for loose tissue or intimal plaque tracking [98]. However, strong angulated lesions with evidence of bridging collaterals usually exhibit a higher risk of perforation, and the use of stiffer wires with a higher tip load and penetration force in these cases should be cautious [174]. Furthermore, gradually increasing wire tip load with the goal of finding the safest wire has the potential to decrease risk of perforation [98].

When performing AWE, the guidewire is advanced to the occlusion point, advanced across the lesion, and followed by the microcatheter that adds support and increases penetration power, allows wire exchange or wire reshaping, and finally maintains position once the lesion is crossed to place an extra support wire for balloon dilatation and stenting [69]. In case of subintimal positioning, the wire is guided back into the true lumen by different techniques or withdrawn and redirected if it leaves the target vessel [174].

Parallel wire techniques facilitate re-entry of the true lumen by leaving the first wire in the subintimal space to seal the false track and act as a marker. Continued manipulation of this wire close to the distal cap should be avoided as it can cause subintimal hematoma that compresses the distal true lumen and complicate re-entry. A second penetrating wire is therefore introduced using a microcatheter, and an attempt is made at redirection into the true lumen. Double lumen microcatheters contain both a monorail and an OTW port and are ideally suited for parallel wiring techniques.

Seesaw wiring involves simultaneous use of two microcatheters and wires and has the advantage of avoiding the need for complex exchange of OTW microcatheters. Also, wires can be reshaped and their roles switched promptly.

9.1.2. Antegrade dissection re-entry

ADR techniques make intentional use of a dissection plane in the subintimal space for crossing CTOs. This concept was first introduced by Antonio Colombo who originally advanced a knuckled guidewire through the subintimal space until it spontaneously re-entered into the distal true lumen (subintimal tracking and re-entry technique) [177]. However, high restenosis and reocclusion rates are found in extensive subintimally stented lesions [165]. Therefore, ADR should not be enforced as a first-line technique. The mini-STAR was presented as bail-out technique and includes limited subintimal tracking distances [178] associated with improved outcomes [179]. Dedicated subintimal tracking and re-entry devices such as the CrossBoss catheter and Stingray balloon allow controlled re-entry into the distal true lumen from the subintimal space [180, 181].

9.2. Retrograde techniques

As complexity rises, advanced techniques are needed to improve procedural success. The retrograde approach has the ability to significantly increase success rates, particularly in challenging lesions (**Table 2**) and has become a widely used strategy for CTO PCI during recent years [182, 183]. Retrograde crossing of the CTO against the direction of blood flow is easier due to the softer, often tapered, and less ambiguous distal cap [15]. These properties in contrast to proximal cap morphology during an antegrade approach facilitate entering the CTO body with the retrograde guidewire. Additional advantages of the retrograde approach are found in the presence of ostial occlusions, unfavorable proximal cap (blunt stump, side branch), ambiguity of the occluded segment, poor distal target or distal bifurcation [184], and good interventional collaterals in post-CABG patients and in failed antegrade cases.

Retrograde CTO PCI can be performed via several collateral pathways including transseptal collaterals [185, 186], epicardial collaterals, and SVG [187]. Intraseptal collaterals are nonepicardial vessels, representing a safe route for CTO PCI with a lower risk of rupture, pericardial effusion, and tamponade [188]. The use of microcatheters seems to dramatically reduce injury to septal channels during a transseptal retrograde approach [189] and also increases the availability of additional routes through tortuous epicardial collaterals [190]. Previously, the CART technique with its retrograde approach was limited to the transseptal pathway in

Ostial occlusion
Unfavorable proximal cap: blunt stump, side branch
Anatomic ambiguity of CTO body
Poor distal target
Distal bifurcation [184]
Good interventional collaterals
Bifurcation at distal cap
Post-CABG patients (retrograde access over bypass)
After failed antegrade attempt

Table 2. Anatomical features favoring the retrograde approach.

nearly 80% and resulted in more balloon dilatations of the septal channels and a higher perforation rate [55, 191].

An in-hospital analysis of procedural and long-term outcomes from the European multicenter ERCTO registry demonstrated increased numbers of safe and successful retrograde procedures with good long-term outcomes [192]. However, the retrograde approach also seems to be independently associated with increased risk of periprocedural complications [193]. IVUS, as described above, can serve as a useful tool for the detection of procedure-related vessel damage and subintimal wire tracking to help guide retrograde CTO PCI [55].

9.3. The hybrid approach

The hybrid algorithm depicted in **Figure 3** represents a combined strategy comprising AWE/RWE and ADR/RDR techniques (**Table 3**) [194, 195]. The fundamental principles in hybrid procedures require a special mindset and great flexibility in the approach with the ability to perceive failure modes early to quickly change strategy and to come back to abandoned strategies, if necessary. Experienced CTO operators aim for efficiency and look for multiple strategies with several options and different techniques. This skillset can be taught and transferred with implementation of the hybrid algorithm, ideally in a broader setting with operators of different experience levels to improve technical success while maintaining low complication rates. The adoption of only a few strategies will limit the patients who can be treated on the basis of coronary anatomy [82, 176, 186, 196, 197].

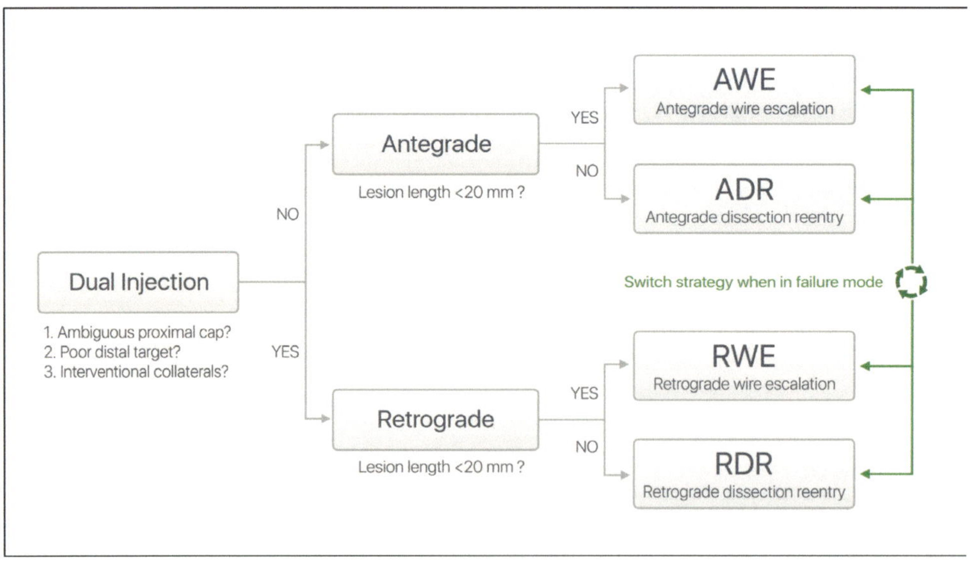

Figure 3. The Hybrid Algorithm. Adapted from Ref. [194].

Antegrade	
	Wire escalation facilitated by antegrade microcatheters [98]
	Subintimal tracking and re-entry (STAR) [177]
	miniSTAR [178]
	Balloon anchoring [227]
	Limited antegrade subintimal tracking (LAST) [228]
	Subintimal dissection/re-entry strategies (ADR) [196]
	Facilitated Antegrade Steering Technique (FAST) [180]
Retrograde	
	Collateral wire passage (marker wire)
	Septal surfing [229]
	Microcatheter-assisted retrograde wiring [69]
	Rendezvous
	Tip-in technique [230]
	Kissing wires (antegrade and retrograde wires)
	Knuckle wires
	controlled antegrade and retrograde tracking and dissection (CART) [231, 191]
	Confluent balloon technique [232]
	Guide extensions
	Externalization
	Snaring
Combined antegrade and retrograde techniques	
	Reverse CART [69]
	deflate, retract, and advance into the fenestration technique (DRAFT) [233]
	IVUS guiding

Table 3. Contemporary antegrade and retrograde techniques [195].

10. Complications

CTO PCI has long been associated with high complication rates with one-third of failed CTO PCI attributable to periprocedural complications [96, 183]. The prognostic value of periprocedural MI in non-CTO PCI depends on the extent of irreversible myocardial injury and correlates well with the release of cardiac biomarkers [198, 199]. MI after successful CTO PCI has been associated with increased long-term mortality and is considered as one of the most common yet unrecognized complications in CTO PCI [6]. However, its prognostic value remains controversial. Most of the myocardial injuries during CTO PCI are relatively limited to absent electrocardiographic or echocardiographic changes, and the prognosis in such "asymptomatic" patients is much more dependent on the procedural success. However, techniques unique to CTO PCI add to the risk of MI compared with PCI of non-CTO lesions [6, 200–203]. Hereby, periprocedural MI may occur from shearing off the collateral circulation, obstructing or dissecting the proximal epicardial artery or sidebranch[204], collateral vessel compromise, donor artery ischemia during balloon anchoring, compression of the lumen by subintimal hematoma, thrombus formation, air embolization, or perforation [193].

Altogether, the complexity of the procedure correlates with the risk of periprocedural MI. However, its pathophysiological mechanisms are considered to be multifactorial and not fundamentally different from non-CTO PCI [201, 205–210].

Classic safety equipment should be readily available in the catheter laboratory and includes transthoracic echo, coils, pericardial drains, and stent grafts. New techniques usually provoke new complications asking for specific treatment solutions [211, 212].

11. Interventional armamentarium

Technical difficulties during CTO PCI with high procedural failure rates have been lately overcome by introducing a growing number of innovative devices that address a very specific problem associated within a particular recanalization algorithm [213]. In order to perform CTO PCI successfully, it is paramount to know the availability, utilization properties, and technical limitations of each individual hardware.

11.1. Guidewires

Guidewires provide the primary and most critical piece of equipment to successfully perform CTO PCI. Innovation and repetitive iteration over the last 30 years lead to a wide range of primary, secondary, and tertiary design elements that directly influence endoluminal performance, especially in occluded lesions with specific anatomical properties [214]. At this, there is an individual demand for a specific wire spectrum during CTO recanalization with specific lesion characteristics, whereas in non-CTO PCI, usually one work horse wire serves for everything.

Tip load is measured in grams and defined by the amount of force the guidewire can create at the tip, whereas penetration power is the ability to penetrate the tissue and is defined by the ratio of tip load over tip area. CTO guidewires with tapered tips exhibit higher penetration power than their nontapered counterparts with equal tip load. Additional penetration force is generated with a microcatheter, in small vessels or tight lesions proximal to the tip, and by lateral support of the coating.

The coating, generally applied to the surface of the guidewire, can be a polymer jacket, a hydrophilic or hydrophobic film, or any combination of the above, and modifies pushability, trackability, and steerability.

http://dx.doi.org/10.5772/68067

The introduction of composite core dual coil guidewires with a second coil layer twisted in opposite turns around the first coil dramatically improved torque transmission and steering capabilities in tortuous arteries and opened new frontiers in CTO PCI, especially in hard calcified tortuous vessels.

Flexibility defines how well a guidewire advances around a sharp corner and is characterized by the core tapering length and the coil structure at the distal end of the wire. Gradually, long-tapered wires better follow tortuous, sharp-bended vessels but provide less support to other gear following. Shorter tapers, however, provide greater support near the tip but exhibit also greater tendency to prolaps.

Spring coils generally affect not only support, trackability, and visibility but also have an impact on the guidewire diameter and provide tactile feedback.

11.2. Microcatheters

After successful crossing of the CTO lesion with a dedicated CTO guidewire, the microcatheter is advanced past the occlusion to exchange the guidewire for a work horse wire or extra support guidewire in heavily calcified lesions of tortuous vessels, followed by balloon angioplasty and stenting. Special trapping techniques for hydrophilic wires and flushing techniques for non-hydrophilic wires are used to exchange individual microcatheters. Over the years, several microcatheters have been developed to dilate microchannels, to improve back-up support and torque transmission, and to facilitate guidewire exchange or reshaping. Furthermore, wire directability and penetration capacity can be maximized with the combined use of a microcatheter and a stiff-tapered penetration wire [215].

11.3. Angioplasty balloons

Very low profile angioplasty balloons with hydrophilic coating are available to cross tight and calcified lesions. However, with increasing use of retrograde and subintimal tracking techniques, these small balloons become less crucial to successfully cross the lesion.

11.4. Additional tools

In addition to the aforementioned devices, dedicated re-entry systems such as the Stingray balloon have been invented facilitating selected cases through controlled antegrade subintimal re-entry [216, 217]. Other novel applications and techniques are constantly being developed [218]. In complex cases, adjunctive use of several sophisticated devices may be cumbersome [219].

12. Clinical outcome data

Successful CTO PCI and improvement in survival strongly depend on the target vessel. So far, only CTO PCI of the LAD seems to be associated with improved long-term survival [76]. From a 20-year experience of CTO PCI, Suero et al. reported improved procedural and long-term outcome [64] which was in line with more recent data from Aziz et al. who revealed CTO failure as an independent predictor of death and a higher rate of subsequent CABG (3.2 vs. 21.7%, $P < 0.001$) [140]. The result from Aziz could be confirmed by Mehran et al. (long-term clinical outcomes in 1791 patients who underwent PCI of 1852 CTOs) and Jones et al. (6996 patients underwent elective PCI for stable angina with 11.9% for CTO) who both demonstrated an association of successful CTO revascularization with reduced long-term cardiac mortality (all-cause mortality: 17.2% for unsuccessful CTO PCI vs 4.5% for successful CTO PCI [220], and 8.6 vs. 6.0%, [221] respectively) and the need for CABG surgery at a 5-year follow-up (with similar rates as Suero et al.) [220, 221]. Other studies, however, did not show a mortality benefit for successful CTO PCI compared with failed PCI [222].

In the Swedish Coronary Angiography and Angioplasty Registry (SCAAR), CTO was associated with increased overall mortality and considered to be the highest risk in patients under 60 years of age. Furthermore, the risk attributable to CTO was highest in the STEMI subgroup, and the authors reported no interaction between CTO and either diabetes or sex [223].

A metaanalysis of CTO PCI on clinical outcomes including 13 observational studies and 7288 patients with a weighted average follow-up of 6 years [77] showed a significant lower mortality, residual or recurrent angina, and subsequently CABG rate after successful CTO PCI.

Another meta-analysis of procedural effects on clinical outcomes after CTO PCI in over 12,000 patients with a mean follow-up of 3.7 ± 2.1 years [224] showed a PCI success rate of 71.2% with a significant reduction of all-cause mortality and MACE in this group. Nevertheless, successful CTO PCI was associated with a higher risk of TVR but reduction of subsequent CABG. Recently, Christakopoulos et al. reported from the largest metaanalysis, including over 28,000 patients [225] as well an improvement of clinical outcomes (mortality, MI, CABG, stroke, and angina but not TVR) after successful PCI, regardless of the revascularization technique (balloon angioplasty, BMS, or DES).

13. Ongoing randomized CTO trials

Most of the clinical outcome data of CTO interventions derives from retrospective analyses and registry data. Prospective randomized controlled trials such as the DECISION-CTO trial (Drug-Eluting Stent Implantation Versus Optimal Medical Treatment in Patients with Chronic Total Occlusion) and the EURO-CTO trial (European Study on the Utilization of Revascularization versus Optimal Medical Therapy for the Treatment of Chronic Total Coronary Occlusions) are largely missing and eagerly awaited. Other trials such as the REVASC trial investigate left ventricular function before and after successful CTO PCI.

http://dx.doi.org/10.5772/68067

Abbreviations

ACS	Acute coronary syndrome
ADR	Antegrade dissection and re-entry
AMI	Acute myocardial infarction
AWE	Antegrade wire escalation
BARI	Bypass Angioplasty Revascularization Investigation
BMS	Bare-metal stent
BVS	Bioresorbable vascular scaffold
CABG	Coronary aortic bypass graft
CAD	Coronary artery disease
CART	Controlled antegrade and retrograde tracking and dissection
CART	Controlled antegrade and retrograde subintimal tracking
CC	Collateral connections
CFI	Collateral flow index
CT-RECTOR	CT-Registry of chronic total occlusion revascularization
CTA	Coronary computed tomography angiography
CTO	Chronic total occlusion
CVP	Central venous pressure
DECISION-CTO	Drug-eluting stent implantation versus optimal medical treatment in patients with chronic total occlusion
DES	Drug-eluting stent
EURO-CTO	European study on the utilization of revascularization versus optimal medical therapy for the treatment of chronic total coronary occlusions
FFR_D	Fractional flow reserve in the donor artery
HF	Heart failure
IRA	Infarct related artery
ISR	In-stent restenosis
IVUS	Intravascular ultrasound
J-CTO	Multicenter CTO Registry of Japan
LAD	Left anterior descending artery
LAST	Limited antegrade subintimal tracking
LAST	Limited antegrade subintimal tracking
LCX	Left circumflex artery

LVEF	Left ventricular ejection fraction
MACE	Major adverse cardiac event
MI	Myocardial infarction
MRI	Magnetic resonance imaging
MSCT	Multislice computed tomography
MVD	Multi-vessel disease
NHLBI	National Heart, Lung, and Blood Institute
OAT	Open artery trial
OCT	Optical coherence tomography
OMT	Optimal medical therapy
PCI	Percutaneous coronary intervention
POBA	Plain old balloon angioplasty
RCA	Right coronary artery
RCT	Randomized controlled trial
RDR	Retrograde dissection and re-entry
REVASC	Recovery of left ventricular function in chronic total occluded coronary arteries
RWE	Retrograde wire escalation
SCAAR	Swedish Coronary Angiography and Angioplasty Registry
STAR	Subintimal Tracking and Re-entry
STEMI	ST-segment elevation myocardial infarction
STRAW	Subintimal TRAnscatheter withdrawal technique
SVG	Saphenous vein grafts
SYNTAX	Synergy Between PCI with Taxus and Cardiac Surgery
TIMI	Thrombolysis In myocardial infarction
TVR	Target vessel revascularization
ULMD	Unprotected left main disease

Author details

Gregor Leibundgut[1*] and Mathias Kaspar[2]

*Address all correspondence to: kardiologie@mac.com

1 Department of Cardiology, University Hospital, Kantonsspital Baselland, Liestal, Switzerland

2 Department of Angiology, Kantonsspital Luzern, Luzern, Switzerland

References

[1] Fefer P, Knudtson ML, Cheema AN, et al. Current perspectives on coronary chronic total occlusions. J Am Coll Cardiol 2012;59:991-997.

[2] Råmunddal T, Hoebers LP, Hoebers L, et al. Chronic total occlusions in Sweden – a report from the Swedish Coronary Angiography and Angioplasty Registry (SCAAR). PLoS One 2014;9:e103850.

[3] Grantham JA, Grantham JA, Marso SP, et al. Chronic total occlusion angioplasty in the United States. J Am Coll Cardiol Intv 2009;2:479-486.

[4] Srinivas VS. Contemporary percutaneous coronary intervention versus balloon angioplasty for multivessel coronary artery disease: a comparison of the national heart, lung and blood institute dynamic registry and the Bypass Angioplasty Revascularization Investigation (BARI) study. Circulation 2002;106:1627-1633.

[5] Christofferson RD, Lehmann KG, Martin GV, Every N, Caldwell JH, Kapadia SR. Effect of chronic total coronary occlusion on treatment strategy. Am J Cardiol 2005;95:1088-1091.

[6] Patel VG, Brayton KM, Tamayo A, et al. Angiographic success and procedural complications in patients undergoing percutaneous coronary chronic total occlusion interventions: a weighted meta-analysis of 18,061 patients from 65 studies. J Am Coll Cardiol Intv 2013;6:128-136.

[7] Stone GW, Kandzari DE, Mehran R, et al. Percutaneous recanalization of chronically occluded coronary arteries: a consensus document: part I. Circulation 2005;112:2364-2372.

[8] Stone GW, Reifart NJ, Moussa I, et al. Percutaneous recanalization of chronically occluded coronary arteries: a consensus document: part II. Circulation 2005;112:2530-2537.

[9] Hoebers LP, Claessen BE, Dangas GD, Råmunddal T, Mehran R, Henriques JPS. Contemporary overview and clinical perspectives of chronic total occlusions. Nat Rev Cardiol 2014;11:458-469.

[10] Barlis P, Kaplan S, Dimopoulos K, Tanigawa J, Schultz C, Di Mario C. An indeterminate occlusion duration predicts procedural failure in the recanalization of coronary chronic total occlusions. Catheter Cardiovasc Interv 2008;71:621-628.

[11] Irving J. CTO pathophysiology: how does this affect management? Curr Cardiol Rev 2014;10:99-107.

[12] Szwoch M, Ambroch-Dorniak K, Sominka D, et al. Comparison the effects of recanalisation of chronic total occlusion of the right and left coronary arteries on the autonomic nervous system function. Kardiol Pol 2009;67:467-474.

[13] Claessen BEPM, van der Schaaf RJ, Verouden NJ, et al. Evaluation of the effect of a concurrent chronic total occlusion on long-term mortality and left ventricular function

in patients after primary percutaneous coronary intervention. J Am Coll Cardiol Intv 2009;2:1128-1134.

[14] Cohen HA, Williams DO, Holmes DR, et al. Impact of age on procedural and 1-year outcome in percutaneous transluminal coronary angioplasty: a report from the NHLBI Dynamic Registry. Am Heart J 2003;146:513-519.

[15] Sakakura K, Nakano M, Otsuka F, et al. Comparison of pathology of chronic total occlusion with and without coronary artery bypass graft. Eur Heart J 2014;35:1683-1693.

[16] Garcia S, Chadi Alraies M, Karatasakis A, et al. Coronary artery spatial distribution of chronic total occlusions: insights from a large US registry. Catheter Cardiovasc Interv 2016. [Epub ahead of print].

[17] Wang JC, Normand S-LT, Mauri L, Kuntz RE. Coronary artery spatial distribution of acute myocardial infarction occlusions. Circulation 2004;110:278-284.

[18] Tran P, Phan H, Shah SR, Latif F, Nguyen T. Applied pathology for interventions of coronary chronic total occlusion. Curr Cardiol Rev 2015;11:273-276.

[19] Katsuragawa M, Fujiwara H, Miyamae M, Sasayama S. Histologic studies in percutaneous transluminal coronary angioplasty for chronic total occlusion: comparison of tapering and abrupt types of occlusion and short and long occluded segments. J Am Coll Cardiol 1993;21:604-611.

[20] Schultz A, Lavie L, Hochberg I, et al. Interindividual heterogeneity in the hypoxic regulation of VEGF: significance for the development of the coronary artery collateral circulation. Circulation 1999;100:547-552.

[21] Munce NR, Strauss BH, Qi X, et al. Intravascular and extravascular microvessel formation in chronic total occlusions a micro-CT imaging study. JACC Cardiovasc Imag 2010;3:797-805.

[22] Srivatsa SS, Edwards WD, Boos CM, et al. Histologic correlates of angiographic chronic total coronary artery occlusions: influence of occlusion duration on neovascular channel patterns and intimal plaque composition. J Am Coll Cardiol 1997;29:955-963.

[23] Cilla M, Peña E, Martínez MA, Kelly DJ. Comparison of the vulnerability risk for positive versus negative atheroma plaque morphology. J Biomech 2013;46:1248-1254.

[24] Ehara M, Ehara M, Terashima M, et al. Impact of multislice computed tomography to estimate difficulty in wire crossing in percutaneous coronary intervention for chronic total occlusion. J Invas Cardiol 2009;21:575-582.

[25] Luo C, Huang M, Li J, et al. Predictors of interventional success of antegrade PCI for CTO. JACC Cardiovasc Imag 2015;8:804-813.

[26] Vo MN, Brilakis ES, Kass M, Ravandi A. Physiologic significance of coronary collaterals in chronic total occlusions. Can J Physiol Pharmacol 2015;93:867-871.

[27] Schaper W. Collateral circulation: past and present. Basic Res Cardiol 2009;104:5-21.

[28] Seiler C. Role (of assessment) of the human collateral circulation in (characterizing) ischemic adaptation to repeated coronary occlusion. JAC 1998;31:1698-1699.

[29] Werner GS. The role of coronary collaterals in chronic total occlusions. Curr Cardiol Rev 2014;10:57-64.

[30] Wustmann K, Zbinden S, Windecker S, Meier B, Seiler C. Is there functional collateral flow during vascular occlusion in angiographically normal coronary arteries? Circulation 2003;107:2213-2220.

[31] Werner GS. Angiographic assessment of collateral connections in comparison with invasively determined collateral function in chronic coronary occlusions. Circulation 2003;107:1972-1977.

[32] Werner GS, Werner GS, Emig U, et al. Regression of collateral function after recanalization of chronic total coronary occlusions: a serial assessment by intracoronary pressure and Doppler recordings. Circulation 2003;108:2877-2882.

[33] Rentrop KP, Rentrop KP, Cohen M, et al. Changes in collateral channel filling immediately after controlled coronary artery occlusion by an angioplasty balloon in human subjects. JAC 1985;5:587-592.

[34] Werner GS, Richartz BM, Gastmann O, Ferrari M, Figulla HR. Immediate changes of collateral function after successful recanalization of chronic total coronary occlusions. Circulation 2000;102:2959-2965.

[35] Seiler C, Fleisch M, Garachemani A, Meier B. Coronary collateral quantitation in patients with coronary artery disease using intravascular flow velocity or pressure measurements. JAC 1998;32:1272-1279.

[36] Pohl T, Pohl T, Seiler C, et al. Frequency distribution of collateral flow and factors influencing collateral channel development. Functional collateral channel measurement in 450 patients with coronary artery disease. JAC 2001;38:1872-1878.

[37] Meier P, Gloekler S, Zbinden R, et al. Beneficial effect of recruitable collaterals: a 10-year follow-up study in patients with stable coronary artery disease undergoing quantitative collateral measurements. Circulation 2007;116:975-983.

[38] Werner GS, Werner GS, Fritzenwanger M, et al. Determinants of coronary steal in chronic total coronary occlusions donor artery, collateral, and microvascular resistance. J Am Coll Cardiol 2006;48:51-58.

[39] Hochman JS, Lamas GA, Buller CE, et al. Coronary intervention for persistent occlusion after myocardial infarction. N Engl J Med 2006;355:2395-2407.

[40] Werner GS, Werner GS, Di Mario C, et al. Chronic total coronary occlusions and the occluded artery trial. A critical appraisal. EuroIntervention 2008;4:23-27.

[41] Safley DM, Safley DM, Koshy S, et al. Changes in myocardial ischemic burden following percutaneous coronary intervention of chronic total occlusions. Catheter Cardiovasc Interv 2011;78:337-343.

[42] Pujadas S, Pujadas S, Martin V, et al. Improvement of myocardial function and perfusion after successful percutaneous revascularization in patients with chronic total coronary occlusion. Int J Cardiol 2013;169:147-152.

[43] Cheng ASH, Selvanayagam JB, Jerosch-Herold M, et al. Percutaneous treatment of chronic total coronary occlusions improves regional hyperemic myocardial blood flow and contractility. J Am Coll Cardiol Intv 2008;1:44-53.

[44] Baks T, van Geuns R-J, Duncker DJ, et al. Prediction of left ventricular function after drug-eluting stent implantation for chronic total coronary occlusions. J Am Coll Cardiol 2006;47:721-725.

[45] Kirschbaum SW, Kirschbaum SW, Rossi A, et al. Combining magnetic resonance viability variables better predicts improvement of myocardial function prior to percutaneous coronary intervention. Int J Cardiol 2012;159:192-197.

[46] Opolski MP, Opolski MP, Achenbach S, et al. Coronary computed tomographic prediction rule for time-efficient guidewire crossing through chronic total occlusion: insights from the CT-RECTOR multicenter registry (Computed Tomography Registry of Chronic Total Occlusion Revascularization). J Am Coll Cardiol Intv 2015;8:257-267.

[47] Opolski MP, Achenbach S. CT Angiography for revascularization of CTO. JACC Cardiovasc Imag 2015;8:846-858.

[48] Magro M, Schultz C, Simsek C, et al. Computed tomography as a tool for percutaneous coronary intervention of chronic total occlusions. EuroIntervention 2010;6(Suppl G):G123-G131.

[49] Soon KH, Soon KH, Cox N, et al. CT coronary angiography predicts the outcome of percutaneous coronary intervention of chronic total occlusion. J Interv Cardiol 2007;20:359-366.

[50] Mollet NR, Hoye A, Lemos PA, et al. Value of preprocedure multislice computed tomographic coronary angiography to predict the outcome of percutaneous recanalization of chronic total occlusions. Am J Cardiol 2005;95:240-243.

[51] Cho JR, Kim YJ, Ahn C-M, et al. Quantification of regional calcium burden in chronic total occlusion by 64-slice multi-detector computed tomography and procedural outcomes of percutaneous coronary intervention. Int J Cardiol 2010;145:9-14.

[52] Galassi AR, Galassi AR, Sumitsuji S, et al. Utility of intravascular ultrasound in percutaneous revascularization of chronic total occlusions: an overview. JCIN 2016;9:1979-1991.

[53] Dato I, Hamilton-Craig C, Camaioni C, Porto I. Intracoronary imaging in chronic total occlusions. Interv Cardiol 2010;2:369-376.

[54] Biondi-Zoccai GGL, Bollati M, Moretti C, et al. Retrograde percutaneous recanalization of coronary chronic total occlusions: outcomes from 17 patients. Int J Cardiol 2008;130:118-120.

[55] Tsujita K, Tsujita K, Maehara A, et al. Intravascular ultrasound comparison of the retrograde versus antegrade approach to percutaneous intervention for chronic total coronary occlusions. J Am Coll Cardiol Intv 2009;2:846-854.

[56] Sonoda S, Morino Y, Ako J, et al. Impact of final stent dimensions on long-term results following sirolimus-eluting stent implantation: serial intravascular ultrasound analysis from the sirius trial. JAC 2004;43:1959-1963.

[57] Okabe T, Mintz GS, Buch AN, et al. Intravascular ultrasound parameters associated with stent thrombosis after drug-eluting stent deployment. Am J Cardiol 2007;100:615-620.

[58] Giattina SD, Courtney BK, Herz PR, et al. Assessment of coronary plaque collagen with Polarization Sensitive Optical Coherence Tomography (PS-OCT). Int J Cardiol 2006;107:400-409.

[59] Hoye A, Onderwater E, Cummins P, Sianos G, Serruys PW. Improved recanalization of chronic total coronary occlusions using an optical coherence reflectometry-guided guidewire. Catheter Cardiovasc Interv 2004;63:158-163.

[60] Kinoshita I, Katoh O, Nariyama J, et al. Coronary angioplasty of chronic total occlusions with bridging collateral vessels: immediate and follow-up outcome from a large single-center experience. JAC 1995;26:409-415.

[61] Shah PB. Management of coronary chronic total occlusion. Circulation 2011;123:1780-1784.

[62] Abbott JD, Abbott JD, Kip KE, et al. Recent trends in the percutaneous treatment of chronic total coronary occlusions. Am J Cardiol 2006;97:1691-1696.

[63] Prasad A, Galassi AR, Rihal CS, et al. Trends in outcomes after percutaneous coronary intervention for chronic total occlusions: a 25-year experience from the Mayo Clinic. J Am Coll Cardiol 2007;49:1611-1618.

[64] Suero JA, Marso SP, Jones PG, et al. Procedural outcomes and long-term survival among patients undergoing percutaneous coronary intervention of a chronic total occlusion in native coronary arteries: a 20-year experience. JAC 2001;38:409-414.

[65] Serruys PW. SYNTAX trial: chronic total occlusion subsets. Washington, DC: Cardiovascular Research Technologies; 2009.

[66] Brilakis ES, Banerjee S, Karmpaliotis D, et al. Procedural outcomes of chronic total occlusion percutaneous coronary intervention: a report from the NCDR (National Cardiovascular Data Registry). J Am Coll Cardiol Intv 2015;8:245-253.

[67] Christopoulos G, Karmpaliotis D, Alaswad K, et al. Application and outcomes of a hybrid approach to chronic total occlusion percutaneous coronary intervention in a contemporary multicenter US registry. Int J Cardiol 2015;198:222-228.

[68] Kandzari DE, Kini AS, Karmpaliotis D, et al. Safety and effectiveness of everolimus-eluting stents in chronic total coronary occlusion revascularization. J Am Coll Cardiol Intv 2015;8:761-769.

[69] Tsuchikane E, Katoh O, Kimura M, Nasu K, Kinoshita Y, Suzuki T. The first clinical experience with a novel catheter for collateral channel tracking in retrograde approach for chronic coronary total occlusions. J Am Coll Cardiol Intv 2010;3:165-171.

[70] Galassi AR, Boukhris M, Azzarelli S, Castaing M, Marzà F, Tomasello SD. Percutaneous coronary revascularization for chronic total occlusions: a novel predictive score of technical failure using advanced technologies. J Am Coll Cardiol Intv 2016;9:911-922.

[71] Grantham JA, Jones PG, Cannon L, Spertus JA. Quantifying the early health status benefits of successful chronic total occlusion recanalization: results from the FlowCardia's Approach to Chronic Total Occlusion Recanalization (FACTOR) trial. Circ Cardiovasc Qual Outcomes 2010;3:284-290.

[72] Noguchi T, Miyazaki S, Morii I, Daikoku S, Goto Y, Nonogi H. Percutaneous transluminal coronary angioplasty of chronic total occlusions. Determinants of primary success and long-term clinical outcome. Catheter Cardiovasc Interv 2000;49:258-264.

[73] Finci L, Finci L, Meier B, et al. Long-term results of successful and failed angioplasty for chronic total coronary arterial occlusion. Am J Cardiol 1990;66:660-662.

[74] Nombela-Franco L, Mitroi CD, Fernández Lozano I, et al. Ventricular arrhythmias among implantable cardioverter-defibrillator recipients for primary prevention: impact of chronic total coronary occlusion (VACTO Primary Study). Circ Arrhythm Electrophysiol 2012;5:147-154.

[75] O'Connor SA, O'Connor SA, Garot P, et al. Meta-analysis of the impact on mortality of noninfarct-related artery coronary chronic total occlusion in patients presenting with ST-segment elevation myocardial infarction. Am J Cardiol 2015;116:8-14.

[76] Safley DM, House JA, Marso SP, Grantham JA, Rutherford BD. Improvement in survival following successful percutaneous coronary intervention of coronary chronic total occlusions: variability by target vessel. J Am Coll Cardiol Intv 2008;1:295-302.

[77] Joyal D, Afilalo J, Rinfret S. Effectiveness of recanalization of chronic total occlusions: a systematic review and meta-analysis. Am Heart J 2010;160:179-187.

[78] Shan K, Constantine G, Sivananthan M, Flamm SD. Role of cardiac magnetic resonance imaging in the assessment of myocardial viability. Circulation 2004;109:1328-1334.

[79] Levine GN, Bates ER, Blankenship JC, et al. 2011 ACCF/AHA/SCAI guideline for percutaneous coronary intervention. A report of the American College of Cardiology Foundation/American Heart Association Task Force on practice guidelines and the society for cardiovascular angiography and interventions. J Am Coll Cardiol 2011;58:e44-122.

[80] Authors/Task Force Members, Windecker S, Kolh P, et al. 2014 ESC/EACTS guidelines on myocardial revascularization: the task force on myocardial revascularization of the European Society of Cardiology (ESC) and the European Association for Cardio-Thoracic Surgery (EACTS) * Developed with the special contribution of the European Association of Percutaneous Cardiovascular Interventions (EAPCI). Eur Heart J 2014;35:2541-2619.

[81] Rathore S, Hakeem A, Pauriah M, Roberts E, Beaumont A, Morris JL. A comparison of the transradial and the transfemoral approach in chronic total occlusion percutaneous coronary intervention. Catheter Cardiovasc Interv 2009;73:883-887.

[82] Rinfret S, Rinfret S, Joyal D, et al. Retrograde recanalization of chronic total occlusions from the transradial approach; early Canadian experience. Catheter Cardiovasc Interv 2011;78:366-374.

[83] Holmes DR, Vlietstra RE, Reeder GS, et al. Angioplasty in total coronary artery occlusion. JAC 1984;3:845-849.

[84] Kereiakes DJ, Selmon MR, McAuley BJ, McAuley DB, Sheehan DJ, Simpson JB. Angioplasty in total coronary artery occlusion: experience in 76 consecutive patients. JAC 1985;6:526-533.

[85] Melchior JP, Meier B, Urban P, et al. Percutaneous transluminal coronary angioplasty for chronic total coronary arterial occlusion. Am J Cardiol 1987;59:535-538.

[86] Stone GW, Rutherford BD, McConahay DR, et al. Procedural outcome of angioplasty for total coronary artery occlusion: an analysis of 971 lesions in 905 patients. JAC 1990;15:849-856.

[87] Maiello L, Colombo A, Gianrossi R, et al. Coronary angioplasty of chronic occlusions: factors predictive of procedural success. Am Heart J 1992;124:581-584.

[88] Serruys PW, Morice M-C, Kappetein AP, et al. Percutaneous coronary intervention versus coronary-artery bypass grafting for severe coronary artery disease. N Engl J Med 2009;360:961-972.

[89] Morino Y, Abe M, Morimoto T, et al. Predicting successful guidewire crossing through chronic total occlusion of native coronary lesions within 30 minutes: the J-CTO (Multicenter CTO Registry in Japan) score as a difficulty grading and time assessment tool. J Am Coll Cardiol Intv 2011;4:213-221.

[90] de Labriolle A, Bonello L, Roy P, et al. Comparison of safety, efficacy, and outcome of successful versus unsuccessful percutaneous coronary intervention in "true" chronic total occlusions. Am J Cardiol 2008;102:1175-1181.

[91] Baykan AO, Gür M, Acele A, et al. Predictors of successful percutaneous coronary intervention in chronic total coronary occlusions. Adv Interv Cardiol 2016;12:17-24.

[92] Tan KH, Sulke N, Taub NA, Watts E, Karani S, Sowton E. Determinants of success of coronary angioplasty in patients with a chronic total occlusion: a multiple logistic regression model to improve selection of patients. Br Heart J 1993;70:126-131.

[93] Suzuki T, Hosokawa H, Yokoya K, et al. Time-dependent morphologic characteristics in angiographic chronic total coronary occlusions. Am J Cardiol 2001;88:167-9, A5-6.

[94] Olivari Z, Rubartelli P, Piscione F, et al. Immediate results and one-year clinical outcome after percutaneous coronary interventions in chronic total occlusions: data from a multicenter, prospective, observational study (TOAST-GISE). JAC 2003;41:1672-1678.

[95] Dong S, Smorgick Y, Nahir M, et al. Predictors for successful angioplasty of chronic totally occluded coronary arteries. J Interv Cardiol 2005;18:1-7.

[96] Sapontis J, Christopoulos G, Grantham JA, et al. Procedural failure of chronic total occlusion percutaneous coronary intervention: insights from a multicenter US registry. Catheter Cardiovasc Interv 2015;85:1115-1122.

[97] Rathore S, Matsuo H, Terashima M, et al. Procedural and in-hospital outcomes after percutaneous coronary intervention for chronic total occlusions of coronary arteries 2002 to 2008: impact of novel guidewire techniques. J Am Coll Cardiol Intv 2009;2:489-497.

[98] Sumitsuji S, Inoue K, Ochiai M, Tsuchikane E, Ikeno F. Fundamental wire technique and current standard strategy of percutaneous intervention for chronic total occlusion with histopathological insights. J Am Coll Cardiol Intv 2011;4:941-951.

[99] Danek BA, Karatasakis A, Karmpaliotis D, et al. Effect of lesion age on outcomes of chronic total occlusion percutaneous coronary intervention: insights from a contemporary US multicenter registry. Can J Cardiol 2016;32:1433-1439.

[100] Fefer P, Fefer P, Gannot S, et al. Impact of coronary chronic total occlusions on long-term mortality in patients undergoing coronary artery bypass grafting. Interact Cardiovasc Thorac Surg 2014;18:713-716.

[101] Banerjee S, Master RG, Peltz M, et al. Influence of chronic total occlusions on coronary artery bypass graft surgical outcomes. J Cardiac Surg 2012;27:662-667.

[102] Pereg D, Fefer P, Samuel M, et al. Long-term follow-up of coronary artery bypass patients with preoperative and new postoperative native coronary artery chronic total occlusion. Can J Cardiol 2016;32:1326-1331.

[103] Pereg D, Fefer P, Samuel M, et al. Native coronary artery patency after coronary artery bypass surgery. J Am Coll Cardiol Intv 2014;7:761-767.

[104] Mashayekhi K, Büttner HJ. Chronic coronary occlusions: when and how should revascularization be performed?. Herz 2016;41:585-590.

[105] Farooq V, Serruys PW, Garcia-Garcia HM, et al. The negative impact of incomplete angiographic revascularization on clinical outcomes and its association with total occlusions: the SYNTAX (Synergy Between Percutaneous Coronary Intervention with Taxus and Cardiac Surgery) trial. J Am Coll Cardiol 2013;61:282-294.

[106] Tatoulis J, Buxton BF, Fuller JA. Patencies of 2,127 arterial to coronary conduits over 15 years. Ann Thorac Surg 2004;77:93-101.

[107] Shen L, Hu S, Wang H, et al. One-stop hybrid coronary revascularization versus coronary artery bypass grafting and percutaneous coronary intervention for the treatment of multivessel coronary artery disease: 3-year follow-up results from a single institution. J Am Coll Cardiol 2013;61:2525-2533.

[108] Panoulas VF, Colombo A, Margonato A, Maisano F. Hybrid coronary revascularization. J Am Coll Cardiol 2015;65:85-97.

http://dx.doi.org/10.5772/68067

[109] Karatasakis A, Karatasakis A, Danek BA, Danek BA, Brilakis ES, Brilakis ES. Scoring systems for chronic total occlusion percutaneous coronary intervention: if you fail to prepare you are preparing to fail. J Thorac Dis 2016;8:E1096-E1099.

[110] Boukhris M, Mashayekhi K, Elhadj ZI, Galassi AR. Predictive scores in chronic total occlusions percutaneous recanalization: only fashionable or really useful? J Thorac Dis 2016;8:1037-1041.

[111] Alessandrino G, Chevalier B, Lefevre T, et al. A clinical and angiographic scoring system to predict the probability of successful first-attempt percutaneous coronary intervention in patients with total chronic coronary occlusion. J Am Coll Cardiol Intv 2015;8:1540-1548.

[112] Christopoulos G, Kandzari DE, Yeh RW, et al. Development and validation of a novel scoring system for predicting technical success of chronic total occlusion percutaneous coronary interventions: the PROGRESS CTO (Prospective Global Registry for the Study of Chronic Total Occlusion Intervention) score. J Am Coll Cardiol Intv 2016;9:1-9.

[113] Karatasakis A, Danek BA, Karmpaliotis D, et al. Comparison of various scores for predicting success of chronic total occlusion percutaneous coronary intervention. Int J Cardiol 2016;224:50-56.

[114] Mehran R, Aymong ED, Nikolsky E, et al. A simple risk score for prediction of contrast-induced nephropathy after percutaneous coronary intervention: development and initial validation. JAC 2004;44:1393-1399.

[115] Liu Y, Liu Y-H, Chen J-Y, et al. A simple pre-procedural risk score for contrast-induced nephropathy among patients with chronic total occlusion undergoing percutaneous coronary intervention. Int J Cardiol 2015;180:69-71.

[116] Rubartelli P, Rubartelli P, Niccoli L, et al. Stent implantation versus balloon angioplasty in chronic coronary occlusions: results from the GISSOC trial. Gruppo Italiano di Studio sullo Stent nelle Occlusioni Coronariche. JAC 1998;32:90-96.

[117] Rubartelli P, Verna E, Niccoli L, et al. Coronary stent implantation is superior to balloon angioplasty for chronic coronary occlusions: six-year clinical follow-up of the GISSOC trial. JAC 2003;41:1488-1492.

[118] Tamai H, Tamai H, Berger PB, et al. Frequency and time course of reocclusion and restenosis in coronary artery occlusions after balloon angioplasty versus Wiktor stent implantation: results from the Mayo-Japan Investigation for Chronic Total Occlusion (MAJIC) trial. Am Heart J 2004;147:E9.

[119] Claessen BE, Lotan C, Dangas GD, et al. Stents in total occlusion for restenosis prevention. The multicentre randomized STOP study. Eur Heart J 2000;21:1960-1966.

[120] Rahel BM, Suttorp MJ, Laarman GJ, et al. Primary stenting of occluded native coronary arteries: final results of the Primary Stenting of Occluded Native Coronary Arteries (PRISON) study. Am Heart J 2004;147:e22.

[121] Lotan C, Almagor Y, Kuiper K, Suttorp MJ, Wijns W. Sirolimus-eluting stent in chronic total occlusion: the SICTO study. J Interv Cardiol 2006;19:307-312.

[122] Suttorp MJ, Laarman GJ, Rahel BM, et al. Primary Stenting of Totally Occluded Native Coronary Arteries II (PRISON II): a randomized comparison of bare metal stent implantation with sirolimus-eluting stent implantation for the treatment of total coronary occlusions. Circulation 2006;114:921-928.

[123] Rahel BM, Rahel BM, Laarman GJ, et al. Three-year clinical outcome after primary stenting of totally occluded native coronary arteries: a randomized comparison of bare-metal stent implantation with sirolimus-eluting stent implantation for the treatment of total coronary occlusions (Primary Stenting of Totally Occluded Native Coronary Arteries [PRISON] II study). Am Heart J 2009;157:149-155.

[124] de Felice F, de Felice F, Fiorilli R, et al. 3-year clinical outcome of patients with chronic total occlusion treated with drug-eluting stents. J Am Coll Cardiol Intv 2009;2:1260-1265.

[125] Shen ZJ, Garcia-Garcia HM, Garg S, et al. Five-year clinical outcomes after coronary stenting of chronic total occlusion using sirolimus-eluting stents: insights from the rapamycin-eluting stent evaluated at Rotterdam Cardiology Hospital-(Research) registry. Catheter Cardiovasc Interv 2009;74:979-986.

[126] Han Y-L, Zhang J, Li Y, et al. Long-term outcomes of drug-eluting versus bare-metal stent implantation in patients with chronic total coronary artery occlusions. Chin Med J 2009;122:643-647.

[127] Colmenarez HJ, Escaned J, Fernández C, et al. Efficacy and safety of drug-eluting stents in chronic total coronary occlusion recanalization: a systematic review and meta-analysis. J Am Coll Cardiol 2010;55:1854-1866.

[128] Yang S-S, Tang L, Ge G-G, et al. Efficacy of drug-eluting stent for chronic total coronary occlusions at different follow-up duration: a systematic review and meta-analysis. Eur Rev Med Pharmacol Sci 2015;19:1101-1116.

[129] Garcia-Garcia HM, Daemen J, Kukreja N, et al. Three-year clinical outcomes after coronary stenting of chronic total occlusion using sirolimus-eluting stents: insights from the rapamycin-eluting stent evaluated at rotterdam cardiology hospital—(RESEARCH) registry. Catheter Cardiovasc Interv 70:635-639.

[130] Hoye A, van Domburg RT, Sonnenschein K, Serruys PW. Percutaneous coronary intervention for chronic total occlusions: the Thoraxcenter experience 1992-2002. Eur Heart J 2005;26:2630-2636.

[131] Onuma Y, Serruys PW. Bioresorbable scaffold: the advent of a new era in percutaneous coronary and peripheral revascularization? Circulation 2011;123:779-797.

[132] Vaquerizo B, Vaquerizo B, Barros A, et al. Bioresorbable everolimus-eluting vascular scaffold for the treatment of chronic total occlusions: CTO-ABSORB pilot study. EuroIntervention 2015;11:555-563.

http://dx.doi.org/10.5772/68067

[133] Elhendy A, Mahoney DW, Khandheria BK, Paterick TE, Burger KN, Pellikka PA. Prognostic significance of the location of wall motion abnormalities during exercise echocardiography. J Am Coll Cardiol 2002;40:1623-1629.

[134] Henriques JPS. Primary percutaneous coronary intervention versus thrombolytic treatment: long term follow up according to infarct location. Heart 2006;92:75-79.

[135] Claessen BE, Dangas GD, Godino C, et al. Impact of target vessel on long-term survival after percutaneous coronary intervention for chronic total occlusions. Catheter Cardiovasc Interv 2013;82:76-82.

[136] Christopoulos G, Karmpaliotis D, Wyman MR, et al. Percutaneous intervention of circumflex chronic total occlusions is associated with worse procedural outcomes: insights from a Multicentre US Registry. Can J Cardiol 2014;30:1588-1594.

[137] Hasegawa T, Godino C, Basavarajaiah S, et al. Differences in the clinical and angiographic characteristics of chronic total occlusion lesions in the three major coronary arteries. J Interv Cardiol 2014;27:44-49.

[138] van der Schaaf RJ, Vis MM, Sjauw KD, et al. Impact of multivessel coronary disease on long-term mortality in patients with ST-elevation myocardial infarction is due to the presence of a chronic total occlusion. Am J Cardiol 2006;98:1165-1169.

[139] Moreno R, Moreno R, Conde C, et al. Prognostic impact of a chronic occlusion in a noninfarct vessel in patients with acute myocardial infarction and multivessel disease undergoing primary percutaneous coronary intervention. J Invas Cardiol 2006;18: 16-19.

[140] Aziz S, Stables RH, Grayson AD, Perry RA, Ramsdale DR. Percutaneous coronary intervention for chronic total occlusions: improved survival for patients with successful revascularization compared to a failed procedure. Catheter Cardiovasc Interv 2007;70:15-20.

[141] Valenti R, Migliorini A, Signorini U, et al. Impact of complete revascularization with percutaneous coronary intervention on survival in patients with at least one chronic total occlusion. Eur Heart J 2008;29:2336-2342.

[142] Lexis CPH, Rentrop KP, van der Horst ICC, et al. Impact of chronic total occlusions on markers of reperfusion, infarct size, and long-term mortality: a substudy from the TAPAS-trial. Catheter Cardiovasc Interv 2011;77:484-491.

[143] Tajstra M, Gasior M, Gierlotka M, et al. Comparison of five-year outcomes of patients with and without chronic total occlusion of noninfarct coronary artery after primary coronary intervention for ST-segment elevation acute myocardial infarction. Am J Cardiol 2012;109:208-213.

[144] Gierlotka M, Tajstra M, Gasior M, et al. Impact of chronic total occlusion artery on 12-month mortality in patients with non-ST-segment elevation myocardial infarction treated by percutaneous coronary intervention (from the PL-ACS Registry). Int J Cardiol 2013;168:250-254.

[145] Mozid AM, Mozid AM, Mohdnazri S, et al. Impact of a chronic total occlusion in a non-infarct related artery on clinical outcomes following primary percutaneous intervention in acute ST-elevation myocardial infarction. J Invas Cardiol 2014;26:13-16.

[146] Shi G, Shi G, He P, et al. Evaluation of the effect of concurrent chronic total occlusion and successful staged revascularization on long-term mortality in patients with ST-elevation myocardial infarction. Sci World J 2014;2014:756080-756089.

[147] Lesiak M, Cugowska M, Araszkiewicz A, et al. Impact of the presence of chronically occluded coronary artery on long-term prognosis of patients with acute ST-segment elevation myocardial infarction. Cardiol J 2016. [Epub ahead of print].

[148] Claessen BE, Dangas GD, Weisz G, et al. Prognostic impact of a chronic total occlusion in a non-infarct-related artery in patients with ST-segment elevation myocardial infarction: 3-year results from the HORIZONS-AMI trial. Eur Heart J 2012;33:768-775.

[149] Hoebers LPC, Hoebers LPC, Elias J, et al. The impact of the location of a chronic total occlusion in a non-infarct-related artery on long-term mortality in ST-elevation myocardial infarction patients. EuroIntervention 2016;12:423-430.

[150] Watanabe H, Morimoto T, Shiomi H, et al. Chronic total occlusion in non-infarct-related artery is closely associated with increased five-year mortality in patients with ST-segment elevation acute myocardial infarction undergoing primary percutaneous coronary intervention (From the CREDO-Kyoto AMI registry). EuroIntervention 2017;12:e1874-e1882.

[151] Henriques JPS, Hoebers LP, Råmunddal T, et al. Percutaneous intervention for concurrent chronic total occlusions in patients with STEMI. J Am Coll Cardiol 2016;68: 1622-1632.

[152] Bataille Y, Bataille Y, Déry J-P, et al. Deadly association of cardiogenic shock and chronic total occlusion in acute ST-elevation myocardial infarction. Am Heart J 2012;164: 509-515.

[153] Hoebers LP, Hoebers LP, Vis MM, et al. The impact of multivessel disease with and without a co-existing chronic total occlusion on short- and long-term mortality in ST-elevation myocardial infarction patients with and without cardiogenic shock. Eur J Heart Fail 2013;15:425-432.

[154] Claessen BEPM, Claessen BEPM, Hoebers LP, et al. Prevalence and impact of a chronic total occlusion in a non-infarct-related artery on long-term mortality in diabetic patients with ST elevation myocardial infarction. Heart 2010;96:1968-1972.

[155] Fujii T, Sakai K, Nakano M, et al. Impact of the origin of the collateral feeding donor artery on short-term mortality in ST-elevation myocardial infarction with comorbid chronic total occlusion. Int J Cardiol 2016;218:158-163.

[156] Fujii T, Boukhris M, Nakano M, et al. Collateral filling efficiency of comorbid chronic total occlusion segment on short-term mortality in ST-elevation myocardial infarction. Int J Cardiol 2017;230:346-352.

[157] Head SJ, Mack MJ, Holmes DR, et al. Incidence, predictors and outcomes of incomplete revascularization after percutaneous coronary intervention and coronary artery bypass grafting: a subgroup analysis of 3-year SYNTAX data. Eur J Cardio-thorac Surg 2012;41:535-541.

[158] Hannan EL, Racz M, Holmes DR, et al. Impact of completeness of percutaneous coronary intervention revascularization on long-term outcomes in the stent era. Circulation 2006;113:2406-2412.

[159] Hannan EL, Wu C, Walford G, et al. Incomplete revascularization in the era of drug-eluting stents: impact on adverse outcomes. J Am Coll Cardiol Intv 2009;2:17-25.

[160] Shaw LJ, Berman DS, Maron DJ, et al. Optimal medical therapy with or without percutaneous coronary intervention to reduce ischemic burden: results from the Clinical Outcomes Utilizing Revascularization and Aggressive Drug Evaluation (COURAGE) trial nuclear substudy. Circulation 2008;117:1283-1291.

[161] Garcia S, Sandoval Y, Roukoz H, et al. Outcomes after complete versus incomplete revascularization of patients with multivessel coronary artery disease: a meta-analysis of 89,883 patients enrolled in randomized clinical trials and observational studies. J Am Coll Cardiol 2013;62:1421-1431.

[162] Migliorini A, Migliorini A, Valenti R, et al. The impact of right coronary artery chronic total occlusion on clinical outcome of patients undergoing percutaneous coronary intervention for unprotected left main disease. J Am Coll Cardiol 2011;58:125-130.

[163] Godino C, Latib A, Economou FI, et al. Coronary chronic total occlusions: mid-term comparison of clinical outcome following the use of the guided-STAR technique and conventional anterograde approaches. Catheter Cardiovasc Interv 2012;79:20-27.

[164] Isaaz K, Gerbay A, Terreaux J, et al. Restenosis after percutaneous coronary intervention for coronary chronic total occlusion. The central role of an optimized immediate post-procedural angiographic result. Int J Cardiol 2016;224:343-347.

[165] Valenti R, Vergara R, Migliorini A, et al. Predictors of reocclusion after successful drug-eluting stent-supported percutaneous coronary intervention of chronic total occlusion. J Am Coll Cardiol 2013;61:545-550.

[166] la Torre Hernandez de JM, Rumoroso JR, Subinas A, et al. Percutaneous intervention in chronic total coronary occlusions caused by in-stent restenosis. Procedural results and long term clinical outcomes in the TORO (spanish registry of chronic TOtal occlusion secondary to an occlusive in stent RestenOsis) multicenter registry. EuroIntervention 2016. [Epub ahead of print].

[167] Ge L, Iakovou I, Cosgrave J, et al. Immediate and mid-term outcomes of sirolimus-eluting stent implantation for chronic total occlusions. Eur Heart J 2005;26:1056-1062.

[168] Migliorini A, Moschi G, Vergara R, Parodi G, Carrabba N, Antoniucci D. Drug-eluting stent-supported percutaneous coronary intervention for chronic total coronary occlusion. Catheter Cardiovasc Interv 67:344-348.

[169] Galassi AR, Tomasello SD, Costanzo L, Campisano MB, Barrano G, Tamburino C. Long-term clinical and angiographic results of sirolimus-eluting stent in complex coronary chronic total occlusion revascularization: the SECTOR registry. J Interv Cardiol 24:426-436.

[170] Isaaz K, Mayaud N, Gerbay A, et al. Long-term clinical outcome and routine angiographic follow-up after successful recanalization of complex coronary true chronic total occlusion with a long stent length: a single-center experience. J Invas Cardiol 2013;25:323-329.

[171] Park H-J, Kim HY, Lee J-M, et al. Randomized comparison of the efficacy and safety of otarolimus-eluting stents vs. sirolimus-eluting stents for percutaneous coronary intervention in chronic total occlusion. Circ J 2012;76:868-875.

[172] Rubartelli P, Petronio AS, Guiducci V, et al. Comparison of sirolimus-eluting and bare metal stent for treatment of patients with total coronary occlusions: results of the GISSOC II-GISE multicentre randomized trial. Eur Heart J 2010;31:2014-2020.

[173] Kelbæk H, Helqvist S, Thuesen L, et al. Sirolimus versus bare metal stent implantation in patients with total coronary occlusions: subgroup analysis of the Stenting Coronary Arteries in Non-Stress/Benestent Disease (SCANDSTENT) trial. Am Heart J 2006;152:882-886.

[174] Lim MCL. Antegrade techniques for chronic total occlusions. Curr Cardiol Rev 2015;11:285.

[175] Touma G, Ramsay D, Weaver J. Chronic total occlusions – current techniques and future directions. IJC Heart Vasc 2015;7:28-39.

[176] Maeremans J, Maeremans J, Walsh S, et al. The hybrid algorithm for treating chronic total occlusions in Europe. JAC 2016;68:1958-1970.

[177] Colombo A, Mikhail GW, Michev I, et al. Treating chronic total occlusions using subintimal tracking and reentry: the STAR technique. Catheter Cardiovasc Interv 2005;64:407-411; discussion 412.

[178] Galassi AR, Galassi AR, Tomasello SD, et al. Mini-STAR as bail-out strategy for percutaneous coronary intervention of chronic total occlusion. Catheter Cardiovasc Interv 2012;79:30-40.

[179] Brilakis ES, Banerjee S. Dancing with the "STAR": the role of subintimal dissection/reentry strategies in coronary chronic total occlusion interventions. Catheter Cardiovasc Interv 2012;79:28-29.

[180] Whitlow PL, Burke MN, Lombardi WL, et al. Use of a novel crossing and re-entry system in coronary chronic total occlusions that have failed standard crossing techniques: results of the FAST-CTOs (Facilitated Antegrade Steering Technique in Chronic Total Occlusions) trial. J Am Coll Cardiol Intv 2012;5:393-401.

[181] Mogabgab O, Patel VG, Michael TT, et al. Long-term outcomes with use of the CrossBoss and stingray coronary CTO crossing and re-entry devices. J Invas Cardiol 2013;25:579-585.

[182] Joyal D, Thompson CA, Grantham JA, Buller CEH, Rinfret S. The retrograde technique for recanalization of chronic total occlusions: a step-by-step approach. J Am Coll Cardiol Intv 2012;5:1-11.

[183] Sabbagh El A, Patel VG, Jeroudi OM, et al. Angiographic success and procedural complications in patients undergoing retrograde percutaneous coronary chronic total occlusion interventions: a weighted meta-analysis of 3,482 patients from 26 studies. Int J Cardiol 2014;174:243-248.

[184] Kotsia A, Christopoulos G, Brilakis ES. Use of the retrograde approach for preserving the distal bifurcation after antegrade crossing of a right coronary artery chronic total occlusion. J Invas Cardiol 2014;26:E48-E49.

[185] Rathore S, Katoh O, Matsuo H, et al. Retrograde percutaneous recanalization of chronic total occlusion of the coronary arteries: procedural outcomes and predictors of success in contemporary practice. Circ Cardiovasc Interv 2009;2:124-132.

[186] Karmpaliotis D, Michael TT, Brilakis ES, et al. Retrograde coronary chronic total occlusion revascularization: procedural and in-hospital outcomes from a multicenter registry in the United States. J Am Coll Cardiol Intv 2012;5:1273-1279.

[187] Brilakis ES, Brilakis ES, Banerjee S, Banerjee S, Lombardi WL, Lombardi WL. Retrograde recanalization of native coronary artery chronic occlusions via acutely occluded vein grafts. Catheter Cardiovasc Interv 2010;75:109-113.

[188] Otsuji S, Otsuji S, Terasoma K, Terasoma K, Takiuchi S, Takiuchi S. Retrograde recanalization of a left anterior descending chronic total occlusion via an ipsilateral intraseptal collateral. J Invas Cardiol 2008;20:312-316.

[189] Tsuchikane E, Yamane M, Mutoh M, et al. Japanese multicenter registry evaluating the retrograde approach for chronic coronary total occlusion. Catheter Cardiovasc Interv 2013;82:E654-E661.

[190] Mashayekhi K, Behnes M, Valuckiene Z, et al. Comparison of the ipsi-lateral versus contra-lateral retrograde approach of percutaneous coronary interventions in chronic total occlusions. Catheter Cardiovasc Interv 2017;89:649-655.

[191] Kimura M, Kimura M, Katoh O, et al. The efficacy of a bilateral approach for treating lesions with chronic total occlusions the CART (controlled antegrade and retrograde subintimal tracking) registry. J Am Coll Cardiol Intv 2009;2:1135-1141.

[192] Galassi AR, Sianos G, Werner GS, et al. Retrograde recanalization of chronic total occlusions in Europe: procedural, in-hospital, and long-term outcomes from the multicenter ERCTO registry. J Am Coll Cardiol 2015;65:2388-2400.

[193] Patel VG, Michael TT, Mogabgab O, et al. Clinical, angiographic, and procedural predictors of periprocedural complications during chronic total occlusion percutaneous coronary intervention. J Invas Cardiol 2014;26:100-105.

[194] Brilakis ES, Grantham JA, Rinfret S, et al. A percutaneous treatment algorithm for crossing coronary chronic total occlusions. JCIN 2012;5:367-379.

[195] Michael TT, Mogabgab O, Fuh E, et al. Application of the "hybrid approach" to chronic total occlusion interventions: a detailed procedural analysis. J Interv Cardiol 2014;27:36-43.

[196] Michael TT, Michael TT, Papayannis A, et al. Subintimal dissection/re-entry strategies in coronary chronic total occlusion interventions. Circ Cardiovasc Interv 2012;5:729-738.

[197] Rinfret S, Ribeiro HB, Nguyen CM, Nombela-Franco L, Ureña M, Rodés-Cabau J. Dissection and re-entry techniques and longer-term outcomes following successful percutaneous coronary intervention of chronic total occlusion. Am J Cardiol 2014;114:1354-1360.

[198] Ricciardi MJ, Wu E, Davidson CJ, et al. Visualization of discrete microinfarction after percutaneous coronary intervention associated with mild creatine kinase-MB elevation. Circulation 2001;103:2780-2783.

[199] Selvanayagam JB. Troponin elevation after percutaneous coronary intervention directly represents the extent of irreversible myocardial injury: insights from cardiovascular magnetic resonance imaging. Circulation 2005;111:1027-1032.

[200] Galassi AR, Tomasello SD, Reifart N, et al. In-hospital outcomes of percutaneous coronary intervention in patients with chronic total occlusion: insights from the ERCTO (European Registry of Chronic Total Occlusion) registry. EuroIntervention 2011;7:472-479.

[201] Lo N, Michael TT, Moin D, et al. Periprocedural myocardial injury in chronic total occlusion percutaneous interventions: a systematic cardiac biomarker evaluation study. J Am Coll Cardiol Intv 2014;7:47-54.

[202] Kim SM, Gwon H-C, Lee HJ, et al. Periprocedural myocardial infarction after retrograde approach for chronic total occlusion of coronary artery: demonstrated by cardiac magnetic resonance imaging. Korean Circ J 2011;41:747-749.

[203] Werner GS, Coenen A, Tischer K-H. Periprocedural ischaemia during recanalisation of chronic total coronary occlusions: the influence of the transcollateral retrograde approach. EuroIntervention 2014;10:799-805.

[204] Paizis I, Manginas A, Voudris V, Pavlides G, Spargias K, Cokkinos DV. Percutaneous coronary intervention for chronic total occlusions: the role of side-branch obstruction. EuroIntervention 2009;4:600-606.

[205] Lee S-W, Lee PH, Kang SH, et al. Determinants and prognostic significance of periprocedural myocardial injury in patients with successful percutaneous chronic total occlusion interventions. J Am Coll Cardiol Intv 2016;9:2220-2228.

[206] Chen S-L, Zhang J-J, Ye F, et al. Periprocedural myocardial infarction is associated with increased mortality in patients with coronary artery bifurcation lesions after implantation of a drug-eluting stent. Catheter Cardiovasc Interv 2015;85(Suppl 1):696-705.

[207] Park D-W, Kim Y-H, Yun S-C, et al. Frequency, causes, predictors, and clinical significance of peri-procedural myocardial infarction following percutaneous coronary intervention. Eur Heart J 2013;34:1662-1669.

[208] Topol EJ, Yadav JS. Recognition of the Importance of embolization in atherosclerotic vascular disease. Circulation 2000;101:570-580.

[209] Bhatt DL. Does creatinine kinase-MB elevation after percutaneous coronary intervention predict outcomes in 2005? Circulation 2005;112:906-915.

[210] Choi J-H, Chang S-A, Choi J-O, et al. Frequency of myocardial infarction and its relationship to angiographic collateral flow in territories supplied by chronically occluded coronary arteries clinical perspective. Circulation 2013;127:703-709.

[211] Brilakis ES, Karmpaliotis D, Patel V, Banerjee S. Complications of chronic total occlusion angioplasty. Interv Cardiol Clin 2012;1:373-389.

[212] Dash D. Complications encountered in coronary chronic total occlusion intervention: prevention and bailout. Indian Heart J 2016;68:737-746.

[213] Godino C, Sharp ASP, Carlino M, Colombo A. Crossing CTOs-the tips, tricks, and specialist kit that can mean the difference between success and failure. Catheter Cardiovasc Interv 2009;74:1019-1046.

[214] Buller CE. Coronary guidewires for chronic total occlusion procedures: function and design. Interv Cardiol 2013;5:533-540.

[215] Brilakis ES, Pereg D, Lombardi WB, et al. Use of the stingray guidewire and the venture catheter for crossing flush coronary chronic total occlusions due to in-stent restenosis. Catheter Cardiovasc Interv 2010;76:391-394.

[216] Werner GS, Werner GS. The BridgePoint devices to facilitate recanalization of chronic total coronary occlusions through controlled subintimal reentry. Expert Rev Med Devices 2011;8:23-29.

[217] Brilakis ES, Badhey N, Banerjee S. "Bilateral knuckle" technique and Stingray re-entry system for retrograde chronic total occlusion intervention. J Invas Cardiol 2011;23:E37-E39.

[218] Nicholson W, Harvey J, Dhawan R. E-CART (ElectroCautery-Assisted Re-enTry) of an aorto-ostial right coronary artery chronic total occlusion: first-in-man. J Am Coll Cardiol Intv 2016;9:2356-2358.

[219] Garcia-Garcia HM, Kukreja N, Daemen J, et al. Contemporary treatment of patients with chronic total occlusion: critical appraisal of different state-of-the-art techniques and devices. EuroIntervention 2007;3:188-196.

[220] Mehran R, Claessen BE, Godino C, et al. Long-term outcome of percutaneous coronary intervention for chronic total occlusions. J Am Coll Cardiol Intv 2011;4:952-961.

[221] Jones DA, Weerackody R, Rathod K, et al. Successful recanalization of chronic total occlusions is associated with improved long-term survival. J Am Coll Cardiol Intv 2012;5:380-388.

[222] Lee PH, Lee S-W, Park H-S, et al. Successful recanalization of native coronary chronic total occlusion is not associated with improved long-term survival. J Am Coll Cardiol Intv 2016;9:530-538.

[223] Råmunddal T, Hoebers LP, Henriques JPS, et al. Prognostic impact of chronic total occlusions: a report from SCAAR (Swedish Coronary Angiography and Angioplasty Registry). J Am Coll Cardiol Intv 2016;9:1535-1544.

[224] Khan MF, Wendel CS, Thai HM, Movahed MR. Effects of percutaneous revascularization of chronic total occlusions on clinical outcomes: a meta-analysis comparing successful versus failed percutaneous intervention for chronic total occlusion. Catheter Cardiovasc Interv 2013;82:95-107.

[225] Christakopoulos GE, Christopoulos G, Carlino M, et al. Meta-analysis of clinical outcomes of patients who underwent percutaneous coronary interventions for chronic total occlusions. Am J Cardiol 2015;115:1367-1375.

[226] White HD, Braunwald E. Applying the open artery theory: use of predictive survival markers. Eur Heart J 1998;19:1132-1139.

[227] Fujita S, Tamai H, Kyo E, et al. New technique for superior guiding catheter support during advancement of a balloon in coronary angioplasty: the anchor technique. Catheter Cardiovasc Interv 2003;59:482-488.

[228] Lombardi WL. Retrograde PCI: what will they think of next? J Invas Cardiol 2009;21:543.

[229] Dautov R, Ureña M, Nguyen CM, Gibrat C, Rinfret S. Safety and effectiveness of the surfing technique to cross septal collateral channels during retrograde chronic total occlusion percutaneous coronary intervention. EuroIntervention 2017;12:e1859-e1867.

[230] Vo MN, Ravandi A, Brilakis ES. "Tip-in" technique for retrograde chronic total occlusion revascularization. J Invas Cardiol 2015;27:E62-E64.

[231] Surmely J-F, Tsuchikane E, Katoh O, et al. New concept for CTO recanalization using controlled antegrade and retrograde subintimal tracking: the CART technique. J Invas Cardiol 2006;18:334-338.

[232] Zhang B, Zhang B, Wong A, Wong A. The confluent balloon technique for retrograde therapy of chronic total occlusion. Catheter Cardiovasc Interv 2011;78:60-64.

[233] Carlino M, Azzalini L, Colombo A. A novel maneuver to facilitate retrograde wire externalization during retrograde chronic total occlusion percutaneous coronary intervention. Catheter Cardiovasc Interv 2017;89:E7-E12.

Chapter 4

Chronic Total Occlusion (CTO): Scientific Benefit and Principal Interventional Approach

Michael Behnes and Kambis Mashayekhi

Additional information is available at the end of the chapter

http://dx.doi.org/10.5772/intechopen.68303

Abstract

Chronic total occlusion (CTO) of coronary arteries are found in about 20% of patients undergoing percutaneous coronary intervention (PCI) and in about 50% of post-CABG patients. Specialized centers can now achieve success rates of over 85%, which is a result of technical advancements in retrograde techniques irrespective of the CTO anatomy. Due to the complexity of retrograde CTO-techniques, a consensus paper issued by the EuroCTO-Club requires interventional cardiologists to have sufficient experience in antegrade approaches (>300 antegrade CTO-cases, 50/year) with additional retrograde training (25 retrograde cases each as first and second operator) before becoming an independent retrograde operator. The increased investment in time and technical resources may only be justified if the patient has a clear clinical benefit. However, technical advancements and the clearer evidence that complete revascularization can be achieved in patients with coronary multivessel disease have attracted growing interest in recent years from interventional cardiologists in treating CTO. The chapter will review current knowledge in the interventional treatment of CTO and focuses on indications and the potential benefits for the individual patient being based on the current state of scientific evidence.

Keywords: chronic total occlusion, CTO, percutaneous coronary intervention, PCI

1. Introduction

Chronic total occlusions (CTO) of coronary arteries are defined as a complete coronary arterial occlusion (thrombolysis in myocardial infarction, TIMI grade 0) being present for more than 3 months. About 20% of patients undergoing percutaneous coronary interventions (PCI) reveal a CTO, whereas in patients with prior coronary artery bypass grafting (CABG), CTOs are even more common in more than 50% [1]. Although registry data demonstrate an improvement of the patients' symptoms such as angina pectoris or dyspnea [2] and a reduction of adverse cardiac events [3, 4] after successful revascularization of a CTO, the overall clinical benefit is still under controversial debate, since prospective randomized controlled studies are still lacking [5, 6]. This is due partly to the greater complexity of catheter-based interventional techniques and the higher demand for materials compared to PCIs of nonchronically occlusive coronary lesions. In contrast, over the last decade, modern and novel developments of special techniques and materials increased the success rates of CTO revascularization in specialized centers toward more than 85% alongside acceptable low complication rates. This technical advance and the growing scientific evidence envisaging potential complete coronary revascularization in patients suffering from coronary multivessel disease [7, 8] have pushed CTO-PCIs into the spotlight of modern interventional cardiology.

2. Indication to revascularize a CTO

In more than 50% left ventricular (LV) function is still preserved in the territory of supply of the CTO artery [9], whereas the maintaining supply by collateral connections (CCs) is sufficient for only 20% of CTO patients while preventing exercise-induced myocardial ischemia [10, 11]. The fractional flow reserve (FFR) distally of the CTO lesion is usually less than 0.5 reflecting an insufficient collateral circulation [12]. Accordingly, exercise-testing oftentimes reveals an exercise-induced myocardial ischemia in the territory of supply of the chronically occluded coronary artery.

No prospective randomized controlled studies have been published yet evaluating clinical endpoints in patients with CTO-PCI compared to patients being treated conservatively by optimal medical therapy. However, there are numerous observational studies comparing a successful with unsuccessful CTO-PCI. A meta-analysis of these retrospective registry data show an improvement of angina pectoris and a decrease of consecutive need for CABG surgery after successful CTO-PCI [2].

Although symptoms' relief instead of prognostic benefit represents the primary indication for an elective CTO-PCI, the prognostic aspect is debated increasingly as a potential indication. Accordingly, there are still only retrospective cohort studies available suggesting a potential prognostic benefit after successful CTO-PCI [13]. The largest CTO registry from the UK database demonstrated a 30% improvement of long-term survival both for patients with successful PCI of at least one CTO as well as for those with complete coronary revascularization in 13,433 CTO patients [14].

Sub-analyses of the New York State Registry including more than 21,000 patients with elective coronary stent implantation showed that a complete revascularization was associated with an improved adjusted long-term survival compared to incomplete revascularization including CTOs [8]. These data support the concept targeting the complete revascularization including the revascularization of coronary CTOs.

Figure 1 shows own data from a recent monocentric analysis including 1,642 CTO-patients. The prognostic benefit of a CTO-PCI depends on the extend of coronary artery disease and is most prominent in patients with a coronary three-vessel disease [15].

http://dx.doi.org/10.5772/intechopen.68303

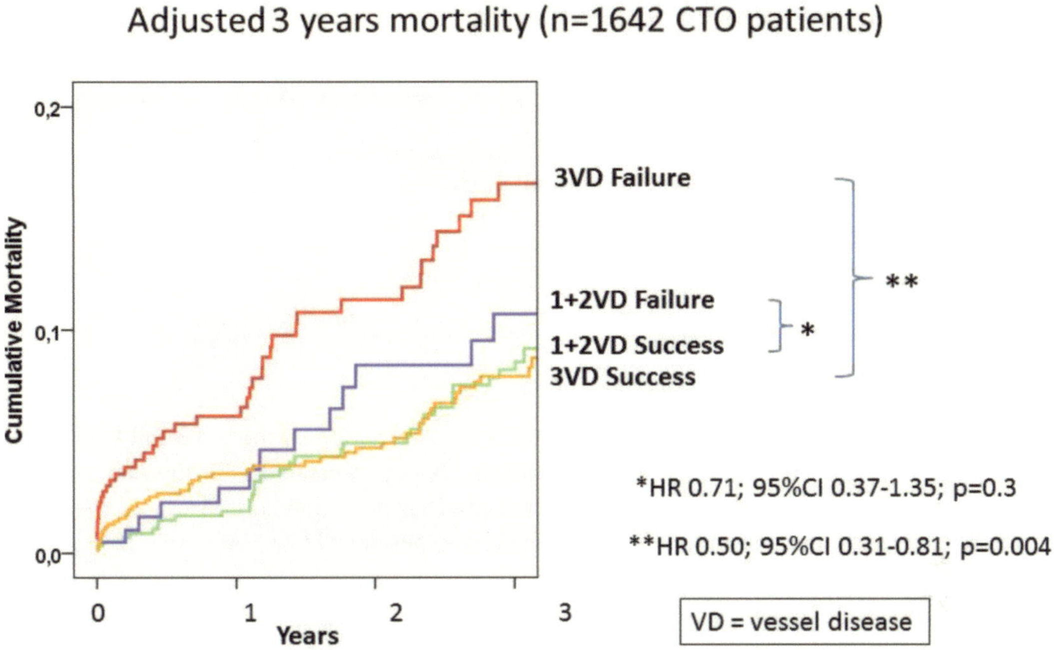

Figure 1. Adjusted 3-year mortality of 1,642 CTO patients presenting at the University Heart Centre Bad Krozingen, Germany. A clear prognostic benefit is shown for complete coronary revascularization, especially in patients with a coronary three-vessel disease including a CTO (HR, hazard ratio; CI, confidence interval) a CTO (HR, hazard ratio; CI, confidence interval) [15].

A main mechanism for a beneficial prognostic influence of a successful CTO-PCI may consist in an improved tolerance for future acute coronary syndromes. A sub-analysis from the HORIZONS-AMI-study showed that patients with an ST segment elevation myocardial infarction (STEMI) and a concomitant CTO revealed a significantly increased mortality both in the acute phase and within long-term follow-up, especially in the presence of a coronary three-vessel disease [16]. Another registry database demonstrated that the presence of a CTO was associated with the future development of malignant ventricular arrhythmias in patients with an ischemia-related LV dysfunction [17].

The so-called EURO-CTO-study has just finished the recruiting phase. It represents the first prospective and randomized CTO-study comparing CTO-PCIs with optimal medical treatment focusing on the improvement of predefined clinical endpoints (i.e., quality of live at 1 year, death or myocardial infarction at 3 years). Furthermore, the prospective DECISION-PCI-study from Korea randomizes CTO patients either to PCI or optimal medical treatment in order to evaluate the influence of CTO-PCI on cardiovascular mortality and future myocardial infarction at 5 years.

Whether LV function being assessed by cardiovascular magnetic resonance imaging (cMRI) might be improved is currently being evaluated within the REVASC-study, in which 200 patients with CTOs are randomized to PCI or optimal medical treatment. Within a prior smaller cMRI study, regional LV function depended on the extend of transmural scarring after myocardial infarction [18], whereas a further meta-analysis of registry data demonstrated an improvement of global LV ejection fraction (LVEF) of 4.7% [19].

3. Principal approaches during CTO-PCI

As shown in **Figure 2**, the principal factors on which the indication for revascularization of a CTO depends on comprise the following:

- Extend of patient's symptoms under optimal medical therapy.
- Exercise testing.
- Global and regional ventricular function and viability.
- Severity of coronary artery disease.
- Localization and morphology of the CTO.

Considering these factors before CTO-PCI allows the estimation of the potential benefit for the patient, as well as the technical severity and risk being associated with the intervention. Using the so-called J-CTO-score reveals optimal graduation of the complexity of the CTO-lesion itself and is more commonly being applied by experienced CTO operators [20].

The latest European guidelines for myocardial revascularization from the year 2014 [21] recommended a class IIa, with a level of evidence B (*"Percutaneous recanalization of CTOs may be considered in patients with suspected ischemia reduction in a corresponding myocardial territory and/or angina relief."*), and retrograde recanalization techniques are recommended only by a class IIB, level of evidence C (*"Retrograde recanalization of CTOs may be considered after a failed antegrade approach or as the primary approach for selected patients."*).

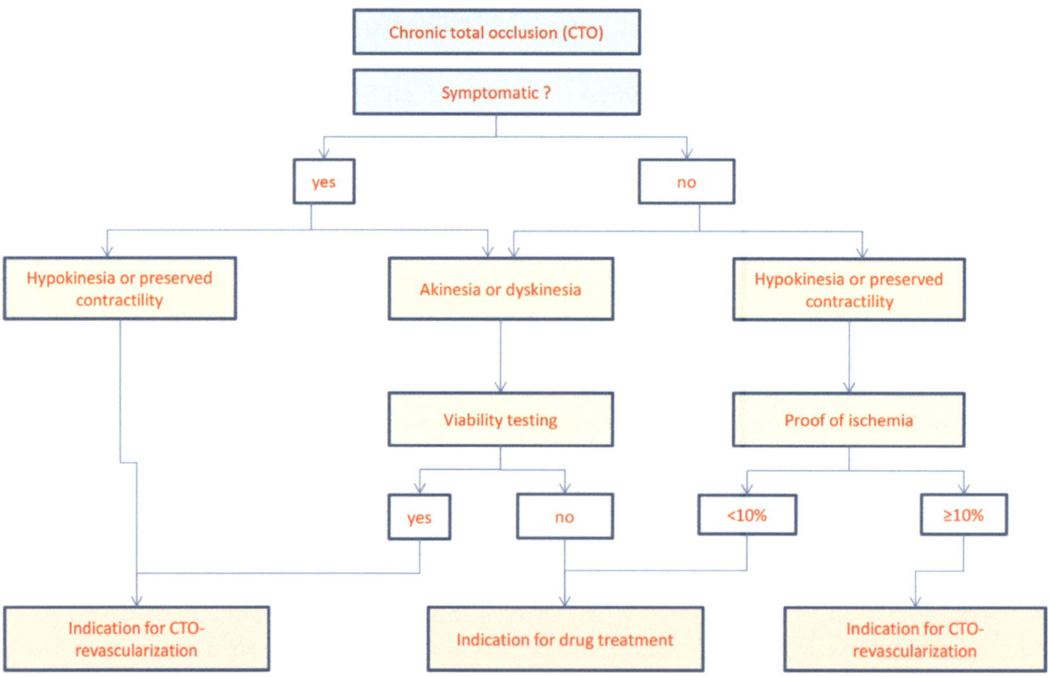

Figure 2. Indications for CTO-revascularization.

This lower recommendation class compared to the PCI of nonchronically occluded coronary lesions is in conflict to the nowadays very high success rates and low complication rates of CTO-PCIs being performed by experienced interventionalists. For instance, patients with prior CABG and a complex morphology of occluded native coronary arteries as well as consecutively occluded bypasses years after CABG surgery may benefit most from a technically demanding and long-lasting antegrade-retrograde but finally successful recanalization of native coronary arteries, as these patients may become free from limiting symptoms in daily life [22].

4. Antegrade recanalization techniques

The close cooperation of members of national and international CTO-expert groups such as the EuroCTO-club in collaboration with Japanese CTO-specialists refined and improved specific CTO techniques for more than 10 years. As a result, their experiences consolidated and were summarized including numerous publications about technical approaches and interventional steps in the so-called expert consensus statements [9, 23, 24].

The primary aim is to advance a coronary guide wire through the CTO lesion into the distal true lumen of the coronary artery. Most interventionalists at first apply a soft, polymer-jacked recanalization wire with a reduced tip diameter, which passes the CTO lesion in about 40% into the right direction usually through microchannels or soft tissue at the site of the occlusion. In the case of hard and severely calcified parts of the occlusion, a so-called "wire escalation strategy" is required using recanalization wires with increasing tip loads. Within a next step, a medium-heavy, very well guidable recanalization wire is used, when the course of the CTO lesion is unclear. In contrast, when the course of the CTO-lesion is recognizable again, a harder recanalization wire with a reduce tip diameter is used, which in turn reveals an increasing force to penetrate the CTO-tissue and is targeted actively into the true distal coronary arterial lumen. The correct distal position of the wire has to be confirmed in two different angulations by contralateral contrast injections through the contralateral coronary artery (i.e., from LCA in the case of RCA-CTO and from RCA in the case of LCA-CTO). This makes a double arterial access necessary for most CTO-PCIs. When the recanalization wire does not pass the distal end of the CTO into the true vessel lumen, the so-called "parallel-wire technique" may be applied. Here, the first wire marks the false pathway, whereas a second mostly harder wire is used additionally and usually enters then the distal lumen. A crucial technical device are microcatheters—catheters of very narrow diameters—which will be advanced over and to the tip of the recanalization wires. They secure the achieved recanalization pathway and thereby exchanging to other recanalization wires becomes possible.

After successful wire passage through the CTO-lesion, predilation with increasing balloon sizes will be performed with final implantation of drug-eluting coronary stents, which ensure valuable long-term results [25].

The success rates of the above-described antegrade recanalization techniques reach 55–80% depending of characteristics of patients and CTO lesions [26–29].

5. Retrograde recanalization techniques

In about 50% of CTOs, very complex occlusions are present being characterized by a straight nontapered proximal cap, long length or torturous course of the lesion, diffuse alterations of the distal vessel, or prior failures of recanalization attempts [20]. Retrograde recanalization techniques were introduced by Japanese CTO experts and have increased significantly the success rates of these complex CTOs without increasing peri-interventional complication rates [30–32]. The main goal of all retrograde techniques is to advance successfully a coronary wire to the distal end of the CTO lesion using collateral connections originating from the contra-lateral coronary artery. Additionally, ipsilateral retrograde techniques without using contra-lateral collaterals can be applied [33, 34]. **Figure 3** shows schematically an occlusion of the right coronary artery (RCA) and wire positioning using epi-myocardial collateral connections to the distal end of the CTO (**Figure 3A, B**). This retrograde wire marks exactly the distal end of the occlusion and can afterwards be targeted precisely by an antegrade wire, which will be able to be advanced antegradely and parallel to the retrograde "marker" wire into the distal vessel lumen (so-called "marker wire" technique, **Figure 3C, D**).

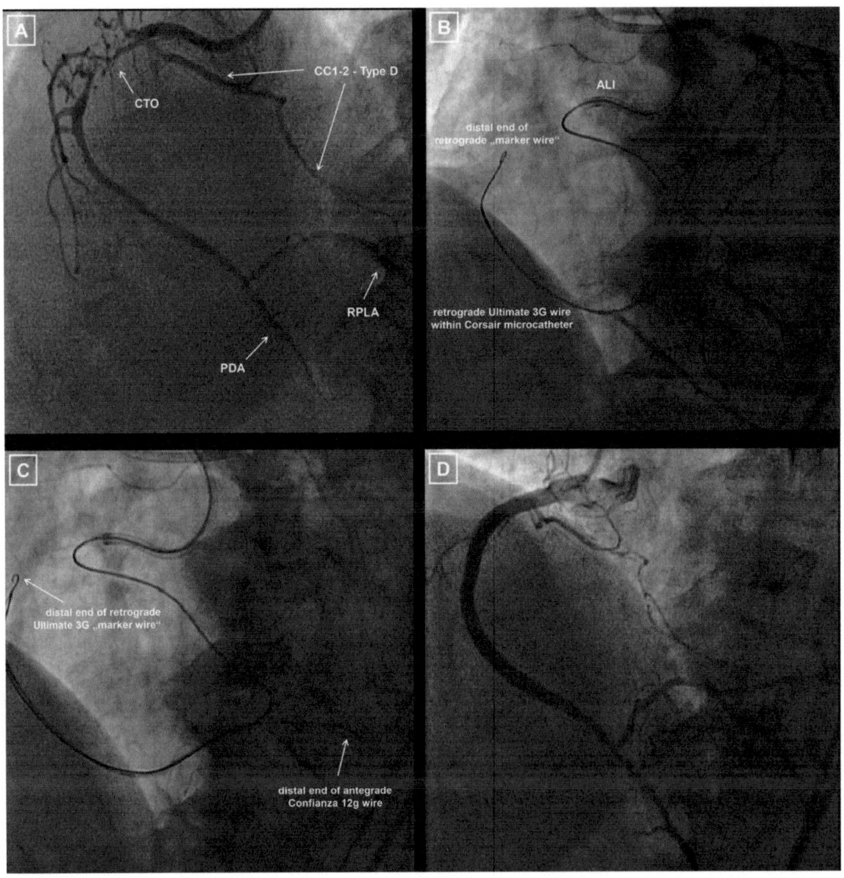

Figure 3. "Marker-wire" technique (CTO, chronic total occlusion) [34].

Occasionally, more complex retrograde techniques may be performed, such as the "reverse-CART" ("controlled antegrade and retrograde tracking")-technique [35, 36]. Here, balloon inflation over the antegrade wire creates space within the CTO lesion, which alleviates the entry of the retrograde wire, which may then advance parallel to the antegrade wire into the antegrade guiding catheter (**Figure 4A, B**). A consecutively introduced microcatheter protects

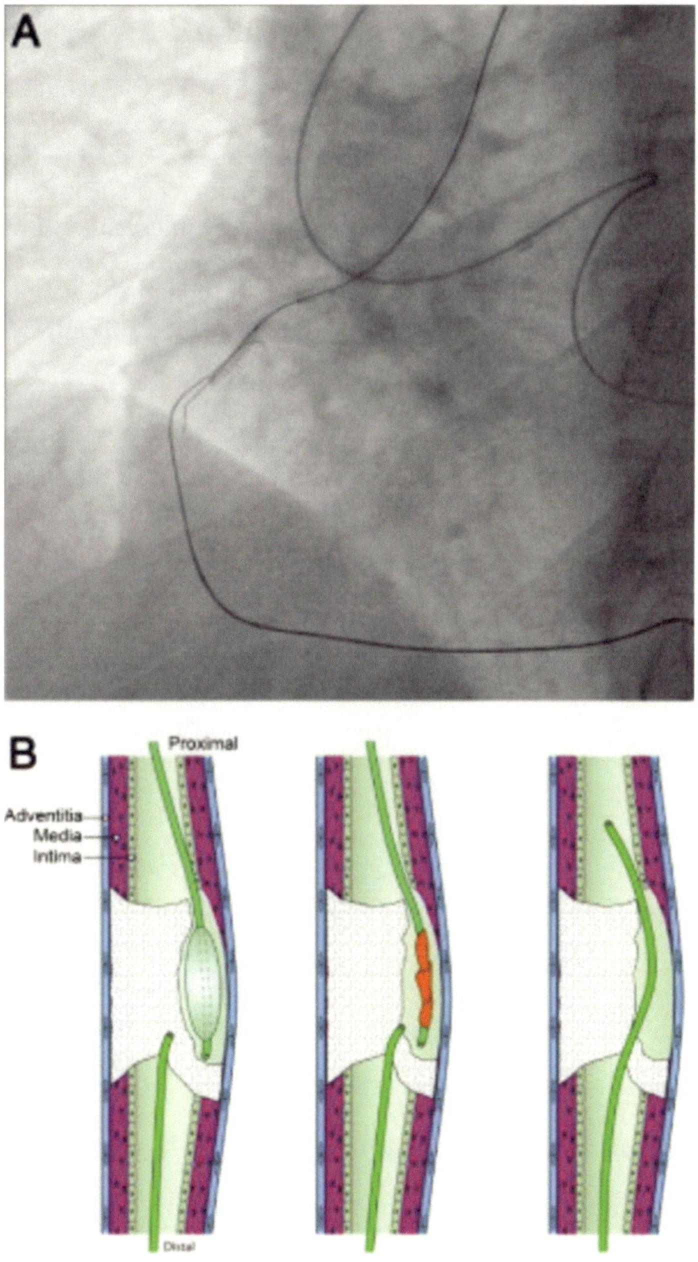

Figure 4. "Reverse-CART" ("controlled antegrade and retrograde tracking") technique [36].

coronary circulation, and within the microcatheter, a 330-cm long special externalization wire can be advanced from retrogradely and outside of the body (so-called "externalization"). After wire externalization, balloon dilation and stent implantation will then be performed antegradely using the externalization wire.

6. Recanalization strategies

Most CTO lesions can be recanalized by antegrade techniques. In about 30%, a retrograde technique is necessary due to the complex morphology of the CTO (**Figure 5**). An escalation of the recanalization strategy is valuable, because an antegrade attempt may be successful in the case of a complex morphology of the CTO. Retrograde methods reveal a high technical expertise and should only be performed independently by interventional cardiologists with sufficient training in antegrade techniques (i.e., >300 antegrade CTO-interventions, >50/year) and additional training in retrograde techniques (25 retrograde cases as second and primary operator each), as stated in a consensus document of the EuroCTO-club [9]. In the presence of high expertise in all recanalization techniques, availability of necessary specific materials and a possible widened indication up to 90% of CTOs can be recanalized. However, the high

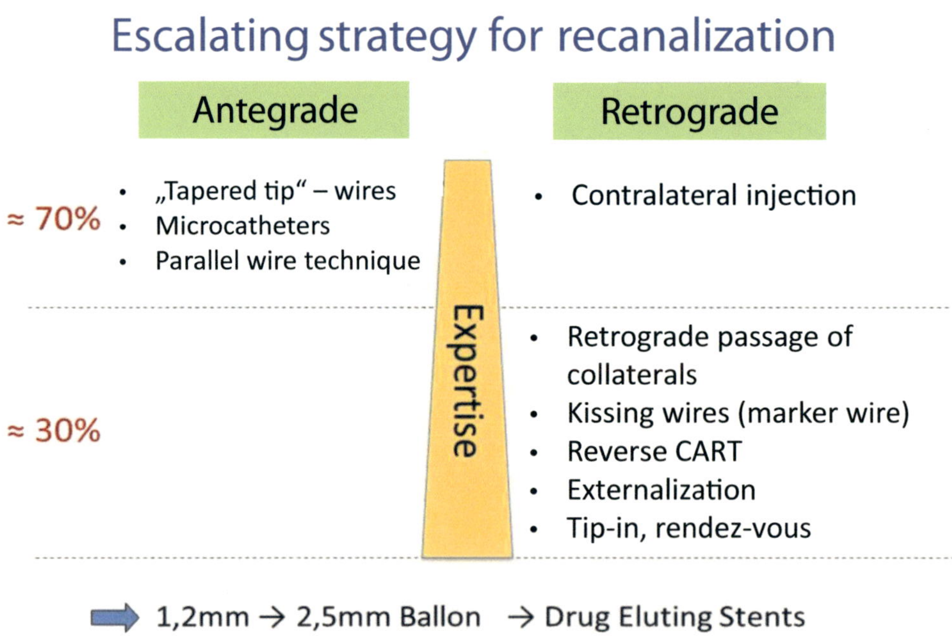

Figure 5. Escalating strategies for recanalization (CART, controlled antegrade and retrograde tracking).

technical demand and effort in time with longer radiation exposure are justified only in recognition of a presumed clinical benefit for the individual patient.

Author details

Michael Behnes[1]* and Kambis Mashayekhi[2]

*Address all correspondence to: michael.behnes@umm.de

1 First Department of Medicine, University Medical Centre Mannheim (UMM), Faculty of Medicine Mannheim, University of Heidelberg, Mannheim, Germany

2 Division of Cardiology and Angiology II, University Heart Center Freiburg Bad Krozingen, Bad Krozingen, Germany

References

[1] Fefer P, et al. Current perspectives on coronary chronic total occlusions: The Canadian Multicenter Chronic Total Occlusions Registry. Journal of the American College of Cardiology. 2012;**59**(11):991-997.

[2] Joyal D, Afilalo J, Rinfret S. Effectiveness of recanalization of chronic total occlusions: A systematic review and meta-analysis. American Heart Journal. 2010;**160**(1):179-187.

[3] Mehran R, et al. Long-term outcome of percutaneous coronary intervention for chronic total occlusions. JACC Cardiovascular Interventions. 2011;**4**(9):952-961.

[4] Pancholy SB, et al. Meta-analysis of effect on mortality of percutaneous recanalization of coronary chronic total occlusions using a stent-based strategy. American Journal of Cardiology. 2013;**111**(4):521-525.

[5] Galassi AR, et al. Appropriateness of percutaneous revascularization of coronary chronic total occlusions: An overview. European Heart Journal. 2016;**37**(35):2692-2700.

[6] Strauss BH, Shuvy M, Wijeysundera HC. Revascularization of chronic total occlusions: Time to reconsider? Journal of the American College of Cardiology. 2014;**64**(12):281-289.

[7] Garcia S, et al. Outcomes after complete versus incomplete revascularization of patients with multivessel coronary artery disease: A meta-analysis of 89,883 patients enrolled in randomized clinical trials and observational studies. Journal of the American College of Cardiology. 2013;**62**(16):1421-1431.

[8] Hannan EL, et al. Impact of completeness of percutaneous coronary intervention revascularization on long-term outcomes in the stent era. Circulation. 2006;**113**(20):2406-2412.

[9] Sianos G, et al. Recanalisation of chronic total coronary occlusions: 2012 consensus document from the EuroCTO club. EuroIntervention. 2012;**8**(1):139-145.

[10] Meier P, et al. Beneficial effect of recruitable collaterals: A 10-year follow-up study in patients with stable coronary artery disease undergoing quantitative collateral measurements. Circulation. 2007;**116**(9):975-983.

[11] Werner GS, et al. Angiographic assessment of collateral connections in comparison with invasively determined collateral function in chronic coronary occlusions. Circulation. 2003;**107**(15):1972-1977.

[12] Zimarino M, et al. Rapid decline of collateral circulation increases susceptibility to myocardial ischemia: The trade-off of successful percutaneous recanalization of chronic total occlusions. Journal of the American College of Cardiology. 2006;**48**(1):59-65.

[13] Khan MF, et al. Effects of percutaneous revascularization of chronic total occlusions on clinical outcomes: A meta-analysis comparing successful versus failed percutaneous intervention for chronic total occlusion. Catheter Cardiovascular Interventions. 2013;**82**(1):95-107.

[14] George S, et al. Long-term follow-up of elective chronic total coronary occlusion angioplasty: Analysis from the U.K. Central Cardiac Audit Database. Journal of the American College of Cardiology. 2014;**64**(3):235-243.

[15] Toma A, et al. Impact of multi-vessel versus single-vessel disease on outcomes after percutaneous coronary interventions for chronic total occlusions. Clinical Research in Cardiology. 2017 Feb 24. [Epub ahead of print]

[16] Claessen BE, et al. Gender differences in long-term clinical outcomes after percutaneous coronary intervention of chronic total occlusions. Journal of Invasive Cardiology. 2012;**24**(10):484-488.

[17] Nombela-Franco L, et al. Ventricular arrhythmias among implantable cardioverter-defibrillator recipients for primary prevention: Impact of chronic total coronary occlusion (VACTO Primary Study). Circulation: Arrhythmia and Electrophysiology. 2012;**5**(1): 147-154.

[18] Kirschbaum SW, et al. Contractile reserve in segments with nontransmural infarction in chronic dysfunctional myocardium using low-dose dobutamine CMR. JACC Cardiovascular Imaging. 2010;**3**(6):614-622.

[19] Hoebers LP, et al. Meta-analysis on the impact of percutaneous coronary intervention of chronic total occlusions on left ventricular function and clinical outcome. International Journal of Cardiology. 2015;**187**:90-96.

[20] Morino Y, et al. Predicting successful guidewire crossing through chronic total occlusion of native coronary lesions within 30 minutes: The J-CTO (Multicenter CTO Registry in Japan) score as a difficulty grading and time assessment tool. JACC Cardiovascular Interventions. 2011;**4**(2):213-221.

[21] Authors/Task Force M, et al. 2014 ESC/EACTS Guidelines on myocardial revascularization: The Task Force on Myocardial Revascularization of the European Society of Cardiology (ESC) and the European Association for Cardio-Thoracic Surgery (EACTS)

Developed with the special contribution of the European Association of Percutaneous Cardiovascular Interventions (EAPCI). European Heart Journal. 2014;**35**(37):2541-2619.

[22] Michael TT, et al. Impact of prior coronary artery bypass graft surgery on chronic total occlusion revascularisation: Insights from a multicentre US registry. Heart. 2013; **99**(20):1515-1518.

[23] Brilakis ES, et al. A percutaneous treatment algorithm for crossing coronary chronic total occlusions. JACC Cardiovascular Interventions. 2012;**5**(4):367-379.

[24] Galassi AR, et al. Retrograde recanalization of chronic total occlusions in Europe: Procedural, in-hospital, and long-term outcomes from the multicenter ERCTO registry. Journal of the American College of Cardiology. 2015;**65**(22):2388-2400.

[25] Saeed B, et al. Use of drug-eluting stents for chronic total occlusions: A systematic review and meta-analysis. Catheter Cardiovascular Interventions. 2011;**77**(3):315-332.

[26] Michael TT, et al. Procedural outcomes of revascularization of chronic total occlusion of native coronary arteries (from a multicenter United States registry). American Journal of Cardiology. 2013;**112**(4):488-492.

[27] Syrseloudis D, et al. Increase in J-CTO lesion complexity score explains the disparity between recanalisation success and evolution of chronic total occlusion strategies: Insights from a single-centre 10-year experience. Heart. 2013;**99**(7):474-479.

[28] Farooq V, et al. The negative impact of incomplete angiographic revascularization on clinical outcomes and its association with total occlusions: The SYNTAX (Synergy between Percutaneous Coronary Intervention with Taxus and Cardiac Surgery) trial. Journal of the American College of Cardiology. 2013;**61**(3):282-294.

[29] Galassi AR, et al. In-hospital outcomes of percutaneous coronary intervention in patients with chronic total occlusion: Insights from the ERCTO (European Registry of Chronic Total Occlusion) registry. EuroIntervention. 2011;**7**(4):472-479.

[30] Patel VG, et al. Angiographic success and procedural complications in patients undergoing percutaneous coronary chronic total occlusion interventions: A weighted meta-analysis of 18,061 patients from 65 studies. JACC Cardiovascular Interventions. 2013;**6**(2):128-136.

[31] Yamane M, et al. Contemporary retrograde approach for the recanalisation of coronary chronic total occlusion: On behalf of the Japanese Retrograde Summit Group. EuroIntervention. 2013;**9**(1):102-109.

[32] Muramatsu T, et al. Changing strategies of the retrograde approach for chronic total occlusion during the past 7 years. Catheter Cardiovascular Interventions. 2013;**81**(4): E178-E185.

[33] Mashayekhi K, et al. Comparison of the ipsi-lateral versus contra-lateral retrograde approach of percutaneous coronary interventions in chronic total occlusions. Catheter Cardiovascular Interventions. 2017;89(4):649-655.

[34] Mashayekhi K, et al. Novel retrograde approach for percutaneous treatment of chronic total occlusions of the right coronary artery using ipsilateral collateral connections: A European centre experience. EuroIntervention. 2016;**11**(11):e1231-e1236.

[35] Brilakis ES, et al. The retrograde approach to coronary artery chronic total occlusions: A practical approach. Catheter Cardiovascular Interventions. 2012;**79**(1):3-19.

[36] Joyal D, et al. The retrograde technique for recanalization of chronic total occlusions: A step-by-step approach. JACC Cardiovascular Interventions. 2012;**5**(1):1-11.

Section 3

Interventional Valve Treatment

Chapter 5

Percutaneous Balloon Mitral Valvuloplasty

Hamidreza Sanati and Ata Firoozi

Additional information is available at the end of the chapter

http://dx.doi.org/10.5772/67757

Abstract

Mitral stenosis (MS) is the most important long-term sequel of rheumatic fever (RF). MS is associated with deterioration of the functional status of the patients and worsens their long-term prognosis. Percutaneous balloon mitral valvuloplasty (BMV) is an effective and safe method in treating rheumatic MS when performed by an experienced operator in a carefully selected patient. A successful BMV procedure results in reducing the symptoms and improving the long-term outcome of the patients. Of the different proposed techniques, the Inoue balloon technique is the most frequently used. Appropriate patient selection using clinical and echocardiographic characteristics is of paramount importance for achieving acceptable final results. Complications are infrequent but can cause significant morbidity and even mortality. Special subgroups of patients might also benefit from BMV, including pregnant women, older patients with rigid valves, and those with mitral valve restenosis.

Keywords: balloon valvuloplasty, Inoue technique, mitral stenosis, rheumatic heart disease, transseptal catheterization

1. Introduction

Rheumatic fever (RF) develops as the consequence of autoimmune reaction to group A beta-hemolytic streptococcal pharyngeal infection [1]. Cardiac involvement is the most important manifestation of RF and mainly presents an acute endocarditis and valvulitis. The following inflammatory and hemodynamic changes involving the cardiac valves insulted by the acute RF could result in long-standing rheumatic heart disease (RHD). The natural course of RHD depends on the severity of the initial attack and the frequency of recurrences. Unlike in developed countries, RHD is not infrequently seen in many areas of the world. Indeed, some countries have reported persistently high or even increasing incidence of RF and subsequent RHD during the recent decades [2]. All cardiac valves could be involved in patients with RHD.

The mitral valve is almost always affected in clinically manifested patients, followed by the aortic and tricuspid valves. Mitral stenosis (MS) is the cardinal valvular lesion in RHD and is particularly amenable to transcatheter therapy when it is isolated or dominant and the anatomy is favorable. When left untreated, severe MS deteriorates the functional status of the patients and worsens their long-term outcomes [3]. Rarely, other etiologies might cause MS (i.e., connective tissue disorders, drugs, and congenital abnormalities). Today, degenerative calcified MS, failure of the bioprosthetic mitral valve, and overcorrection of mitral regurgitation (MR) are increasingly seen. Unlike rheumatic MS, these non-rheumatic mitral valve obstructions are not associated with commissural fusion and are not generally relieved by percutaneous balloon mitral valvuloplasty (BMV). When applied in correctly selected subjects and performed by experienced operators, a successful BMV procedure can improve symptoms and long-term survival of the patients and is, therefore, the method of choice in the treatment of patients with severe rheumatic MS [4, 5].

2. Evaluation of severity

2.1. Echocardiography

Echocardiography is essential in the diagnosis and quantification of the severity of MS. Transthoracic echocardiography (TTE) provides sufficient data in most patients and should be performed in patients at initial presentation, in those with changing symptoms, and in asymptomatic patients periodically (**Figure 1**). It shows the restriction of the mitral valve opening caused by commissural fusion and the so-called doming of the mitral valve, thickness and calcification of the leaflets, and chordal thickening. A mitral valve area (MVA) ≤ 1.5 cm^2 and a pressure half-time (PHT) ≥ 150 ms correspond to severe MS. PHT is affected by left ventricular (LV) diastolic dysfunction and the severity of mitral and aortic regurgitation, while planimetry-derived MVA is more accurate and should be used for decision-making in most patients [6]. Mitral valve resistance might be a better predictor of hemodynamic burden of MS and can be used to determine the need for BMV in borderline cases [7]. The other parameters that are evaluated include transmitral valve gradient, MR severity, concomitant valvular involvement, atrial size, left and right ventricular functions, and pulmonary arterial pressure. Transesophageal echocardiography (TEE) is valuable when the images derived from TTE are not satisfactory or when the patient is candidate for BMV to rule out clots in the left atrium (LA) and the left atrial appendage (LAA) as well as for a detailed evaluation of MR severity.

2.2. Hemodynamic study

Cardiac catheterization, aside from guiding the procedure, is indicated when echocardiography is nondiagnostic. It is not routinely indicated; however, it is necessary when the results from echocardiography are ambiguous, when the severity of other valvular lesions is evaluated, and when there is a suspicion of coronary artery disease. Before BMV, measurement of the mitral valve gradient, pulmonary arterial pressure, and MVA using the Gorlin equation can be helpful in borderline cases and for confirming the severity of MS.

http://dx.doi.org/10.5772/67757

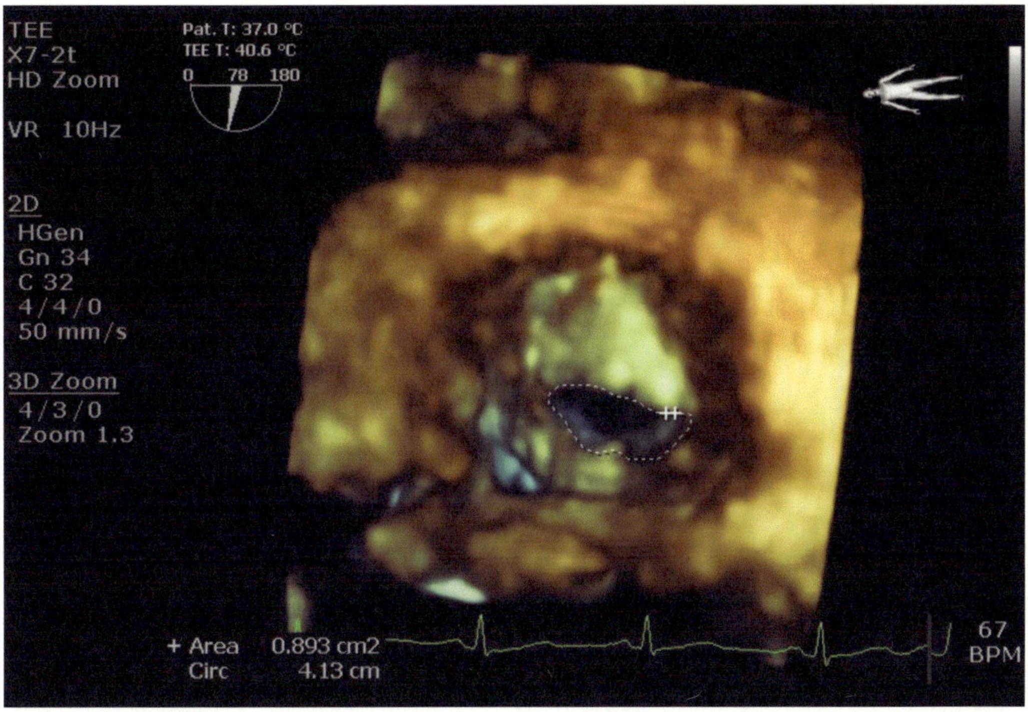

Figure 1. 3D echocardiography revealing bicommissural fusion, fish-mouth appearance of the mitral valve, and planimetry-derived mitral valve area of 0.89 cm^2.

3. Patient selection

3.1. Indications

BMV causes the splitting of the fused commissures and increases the MVA. Patients with symptomatic severe rheumatic MS with an MVA ≤ 1.5 cm^2 should be thoroughly evaluated and subjected to BMV if the valvular morphology is suitable [8] (**Figure 2**). Dyspnea is the most common symptom but it is not prominent in some patients. Additional attributable symptoms are exercise intolerance, fatigue, and chest pain. Given the proved long-term efficacy of BMV, even minimal symptoms should be regarded as the indication for intervention considering that this procedure is relatively safe in experienced hands. Patients with less severe obstruction (MVA > 1.5 cm^2) remain asymptomatic for many years and do not need non-pharmacologic intervention [9]. In addition, asymptomatic patients with very severe MS (MVA ≤ 1 cm^2) are reasonable candidates for BMV. In patients with asymptomatic severe MS (MVA ≤ 1.5 cm^2), BMV can be performed if pulmonary hypertension is present (pulmonary artery systolic pressure ≥ 50 mm Hg at rest and ≥ 60 mm Hg with exercise). Atrial fibrillation (AF) worsens the prognosis in patients with severe MS through deteriorating functional status, progressing structural damage, and increasing thromboembolic risk [10, 11]. Meanwhile, AF can be an indicator of progressive MS [12]. As a result, new AF in a

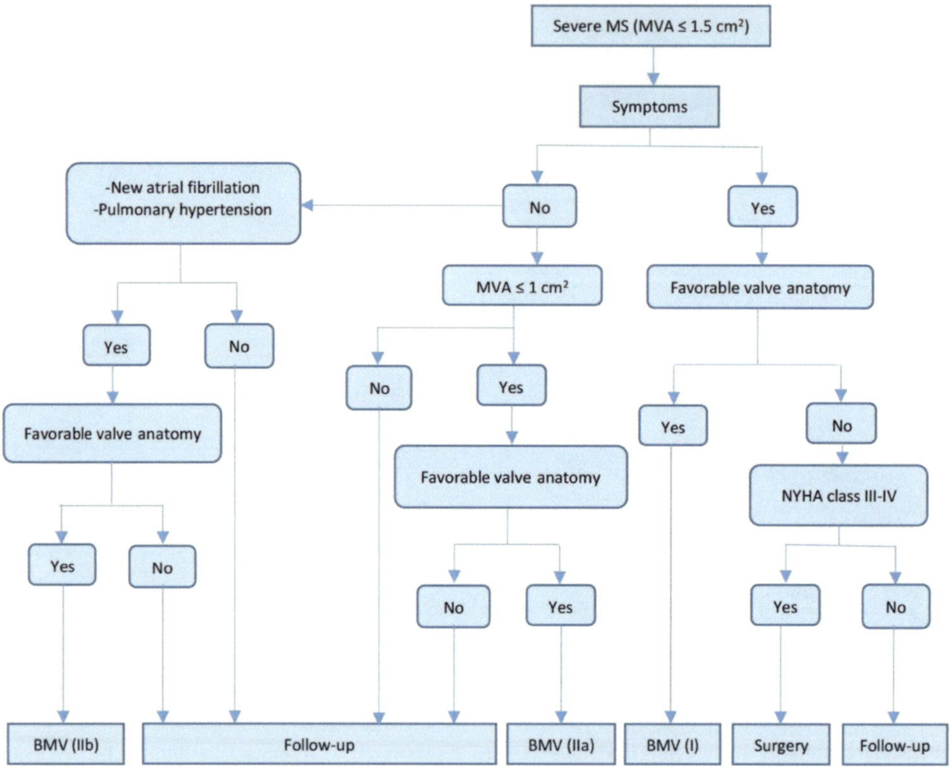

BMV: balloon mitral valvuloplasty; NYHA: New York Heart Association; MS: mitral stenosis; MVA: mitral valve area

Figure 2. Management of patients with severe mitral stenosis.

patient with severe MS mandates special consideration and might be an indication for BMV [8, 13]. The other potential indication for BMV is the presence of symptoms in a patient with mild MS (MVA > 1.5 cm^2) with the evidence of significant obstruction (pulmonary capillary wedge pressure >25 mm Hg) during exercise. BMV as a therapeutic option in a patient with the latter scenario should be only considered after a comprehensive hemodynamic study and the exclusion of other potential causes. In recent practice, we encounter a subset of very symptomatic old patients with severe MS and unfavorable valve anatomy who were not candidated for mitral valve replacement (MVR) because of their comorbidities. BMV might be considered in these patients, although the immediate result is suboptimal, complications are more frequent, and long-term efficacy is limited [8, 14].

3.1.1. Anatomic eligibility

When the patient is considered a likely candidate for BMV, morphologic characteristics should be evaluated using echocardiography. The Wilkins score comprises four echocardiographic characteristics of the mitral valve, including leaflet mobility, leaflet thickness, leaflet calcification, and subvalvular apparatus, each given a 1- to 4-point value according to the predefined definitions [15]. Patients with Wilkins scores ≤ 8 are particularly suitable for BMV. This means that the mitral valve is sufficiently pliable and most often does well in response to balloon dilatation. In our practice, most patients have Wilkins scores between 8 and 10. BMV in these relatively fibrotic, rigid, and calcified valves often results in unpredictable and somehow suboptimal acute and late final MVAs, but many patients still experience acceptable and durable functional recovery, deferring eventual surgery. The ideal patients do not have MR more than moderate in severity, and the LA and LAA are free from thrombi. Significant concomitant valvular involvement including more-than-moderate aortic stenosis and regurgitation and tricuspid stenosis should not be presented. Secondary tricuspid regurgitation, even if it is significant, is not a limiting factor and most patients experience reduction in its severity after successful BMV.

3.2. Contraindications

When the Wilkins score is >10, BMV is generally ineffective and is, instead, associated with a higher incidence of severe MR and should, therefore, be avoided. The severity of preprocedural MR predicts the possibility of severe MR after the procedure that is associated with a poor long-term outcome of BMV. Moderate-to-severe MR (≥3+) is regarded a contraindication for BMV considering that the procedure itself aggravates MR in many cases. LA thrombi or thrombi on the interatrial septum are the absolute contraindications of transseptal puncture and BMV, whereas LAA thrombi are considered a relative contraindication. Bicommissural and fluoroscopic valve calcification are associated with a poor outcome following BMV [16]. When the commissural fusion is absent, BMV is ineffective and should not be used. Many patients with MS receive oral anticoagulation because of AF. Transseptal puncture should be avoided in the presence of an International Normalized Ratio (INR) >1.5 or within 4 hours after the administration of intravenous heparin. The contraindications for BMV are outlined in **Table 1**.

Wilkins score > 10
Concomitant mitral regurgitation ≥ 3+
Concomitant aortic regurgitation ≥ 3+
Left atrial thrombus
Left atrial appendage thrombus (relative)
Severe or bicommissural calcification
Fluroscopic valve calcification
Absence of commissural fusion
Bleeding diastasis, INR > 1.5
Other cardiac disease (coronary, valvular, congenital) necessitating cardiac surgery

BMV, balloon mitral valvuloplasty; INR, International Normalized Ratio.

Table 1. Contraindications to BMV.

4. Procedure

4.1. Patient preparation

General considerations resemble those of the other interventional procedures. Fasting is needed for at least 8 hours for solid foods and 3 hours for liquids. The patient should be hydrated according to the standard protocols for the prevention of contrast-induced acute kidney injury. BMV and even transseptal catheterization can be performed with no or minimal contrast media; accordingly, contrast-induced nephropathy is not a major issue. Rapid heart rate in patients with AF might interfere in stable balloon dilatation and should be controlled. No specific pharmacologic pretreatment is needed before BMV, but most medications (beta-blockers, calcium channel blockers, digoxin, etc.) are routinely continued. Warfarin should be withheld for 3 days before the procedure. Instead, heparin is needed to be infused while the patient is under therapeutic INR levels (INR < 2). Heparin infusion is stopped 4 hours before the patient arrives at the catheterization laboratory. Preprocedural TEE is of paramount importance to exclude LA/LAA thrombi in all patients and should be performed preferably just before but not more than 2 weeks before BMV because the possibility of LA/LAA clot cannot be completely ruled out even with sinus rhythm. Antibiotic prophylaxis is not routinely prescribed before or during the procedure, but it might be needed if the aseptic barrier has been disrupted.

4.2. Anesthesia

Most BMV procedures can be performed under mild conscious sedation. Rarely, the patient has a tender septum and experiences discomfort during the transseptal puncture and might need analgesia and more sedation and exceptionally, general anesthesia. General anesthesia is also needed in uncooperative or unstable patients or when TEE is used to guide transseptal catheterization and BMV in difficult cases.

4.3. Approaches

The antegrade transvenous transseptal approach is most commonly used. The right femoral vein is preferred because appropriate alignment of the transseptal needle with the interatrial septum facilitates septostomy. The left femoral and rarely jugular veins also can be used [17, 18]. The femoral or radial arteries are used for hemodynamic monitoring, performing catheterization, and guiding the transseptal puncture. The retrograde non-transseptal approach from the femoral artery has been utilized with acceptable results; nonetheless, higher risks of arterial damage and more hemodynamic burden arising from the trans-aortic passage of the balloon catheter have limited its use [19].

4.4. Transseptal puncture

It is the first and very important step in performing a successful BMV. The transseptal puncture is the source of complexity and complications in many patients undergoing BMV. Although the puncture site is less important than that in the MitraClip and LAA occlusion, a central or slightly low puncture is recommended. An appropriate puncture site facilitates the crossing of the mitral valve by the balloon catheter. A low puncture is especially important when the double balloon or metallic commissurotome is used. Fluoroscopy is the fundamental imaging tool used to guide the transseptal puncture but TEE and intracardiac echocardiography (ICE) can help in difficult cases or for performing a site-specific puncture.

4.5. Techniques

Thus far, several techniques have been introduced. Of those, the Inoue balloon technique has gained the most popularity because of its safety and effectiveness.

4.5.1. Metallic commissurotome

A reusable metallic dilator has been developed to decrease the cost of the procedure. It has been reported that the procedure is safe, with good acute and long-term results comparable to the Inoue technique [20]. The risk of LV perforation and subsequent tamponade with the metallic device should be considered. The more demanding nature of the procedure and concerns about the reused devices have limited this technique in many countries.

4.5.2. Double balloon technique

In this antegrade transseptal technique, a balloon-tipped catheter is used to cross the mitral valve followed by introducing an exchange-length (260 cm) wire through the catheter lumen securing its end in the LV or the descending aorta. A second wire should be introduced by the same way or using a dual-lumen catheter. Two balloons (15–20 mm in diameter) are introduced over the wires and positioned across the mitral valve and inflated simultaneously [21]. In theory, two balloons side-by-side can exert a more focused pressure on the commissures than a single balloon. This technique is relatively safe and effective but is not widely used because of being more time-consuming than the Inoue technique and more hazardous because of the risk of wire-induced LV perforation. The multi-track system is a newer variant of double-balloon valvuloplasty that provides effectiveness of double-balloon inflation using a single wire.

4.5.3. Inoue balloon technique

The Inoue balloon catheter is a dumbbell-shaped balloon that self-positions in the mitral valve because of its unique physical properties and mode of inflation. It has been made from two latex layers and a middle nylon layer, giving the balloon its specialized shape and inflation characteristics. The balloon inflates in three sequential stages. The distal end of the balloon inflates at the first stage, followed by the proximal half, to facilitate positioning across the mitral valve. Finally, inflation of the waist portion of the balloon separates commissures [22]. Several balloon sizes are available (24, 26, 28, and 30 mm in diameter), and each can be inflated in a 4-mm diameter zone. The reference balloon size (RS) is calculated based on the height of the patient (patient's height in cm rounded to the nearest 0, divided by 10, and 10 added to the ratio) or the newly introduced method of inter-commissural diameter [23–25]. In patients with pliable valves, an RS-matched balloon is selected but in patients with pre-existing MR, severe commissural calcification, significant subvalvular involvement, or very severe MS (MVA ≤ 0.5 cm^2), as well as in patients with special situations where they do not need very large valve areas or in patients whose complications are more common and difficult to manage (i.e., old patients, pregnancy, etc.), a balloon 1 size smaller than the RS is chosen [23].

Immediately after the transseptal puncture, confirming the position of the needle tip in the LA and septal dilation, 70–100 IU/kg of heparin is administered intravenously to achieve an activated clotting time (ACT) of 250–300 s. A spring pigtail-like stiff wire is placed in the LA and a 14-French dilator is used to dilate both the femoral subcutaneous track and the atrial septum. A previously vented, de-aired, and calibrated slenderized balloon is sent to the LA over the wire and then reshaped to its original deflated configuration by removing the stretching tube and the wire and pulling back the gold tube. If there is any resistance when crossing the inguinal area, redilating the area using a larger dilator definitely helps. To overcome the resistance across the septum, the operator turns the balloon catheter in one or other directions or dilates the septum with a peripheral balloon (6–8 mm in diameter). By changing the projection from the anteroposterior (AP) to the right-anterior oblique (RAO), the operator introduces the stylet and while the balloon is partially inflated at its distal end acting as a floating balloon, the operator directs the balloon catheter toward and across the mitral valve with a combination of rotating anticlockwise and pulling the stylet and pushing the balloon. Free movement of the balloon in the LV toward the apex shows that the balloon has not been entrapped in the subvalvular apparatus and papillary muscles. In the final step, the distal half is fully inflated and the balloon is retracted to catch the mitral valve, followed by the inflation of the proximal and central part of the balloon until the disappearance of the waist (**Figure 3**). If any kind of distortion in the contour of the balloon is seen, the inflation should not be continued because of the possibility of balloon entrapment and subsequent severe MR. The balloon should be inflated with a diluted contrast medium (contrast-saline ratio of 1:5) to minimize the inflation-deflation period (2–4 s). It is recommended that the balloon be inflated in a stepwise fashion started 2–4 mm below the calculated RS. The balloon size is then increased 1 mm in each step, and the procedure should be stopped if any of the following criteria is met: (1) final MVA >1.5 cm^2 or an increase in the valve area of 50%, (2) a fall in the mean gradient by 50% or from >10 to <5 mm Hg, (3) complete opening of at least one commissure, and (4) appearance or aggravation of MR >1+ (**Table 2**).

4.6. Surveillance of the procedure

Imaging modalities combined with fluoroscopy can help to guide the procedure, assess the results, and diagnose complications. Evaluation of the mean LA pressure, transmitral valve gradient, and the contours of LA pressure between the inflations might help but they are subjected to variations and are not reliable markers of the success or occurrence of the complications. In addition, the MVA, estimated by the Gorlin formula, is affected by atrial shunt and MR. TTE is integral to guiding the procedure and should be performed between the inflations and at the end of BMV. The planimetry-derived MVA, splitting of the commissures, and the severity of MR can be readily and reliably assessed in many patients

http://dx.doi.org/10.5772/67757

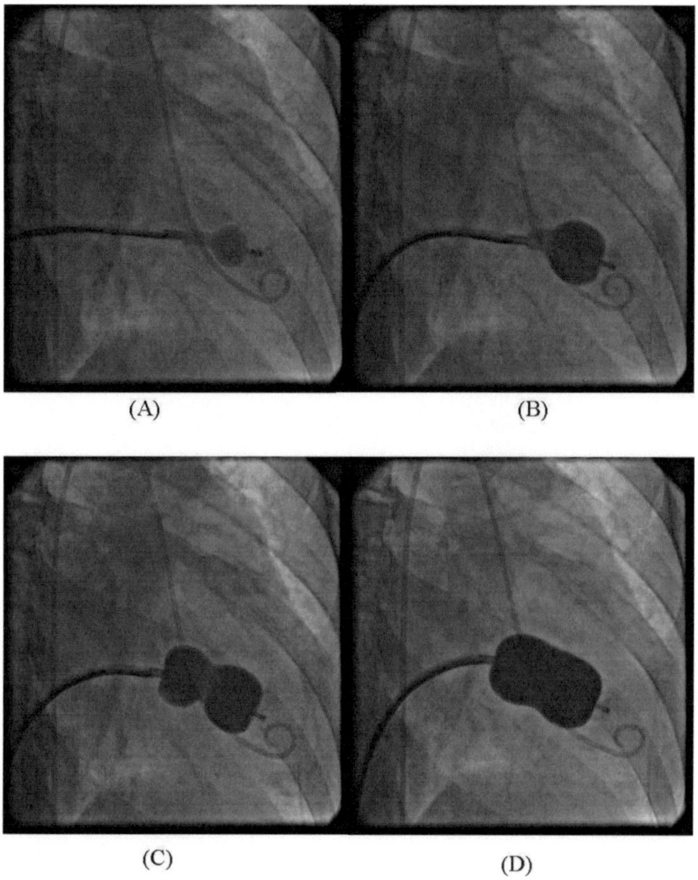

Figure 3. Inoue technique. Inflation of distal end of the balloon, retracted toward mitral valve (A–B). Inflation of proximal half catching the commissures in between (C). Full inflation of the balloon disappearing the waist (D).

using TTE. TEE needs general anesthesia and is difficult to perform in the catheterization laboratory but is helpful in patients with poor echo window and in pregnant women in whom fluoroscopy is of concern. The TEE also provides superior views to verify the positioning of the balloon in the mitral valve in difficult cases (**Figure 4**).

4.7. Postprocedural considerations

After the removal of the balloon catheter, the venous access site should be compressed to achieve hemostasis. The arterial access is managed depending on the site (femoral or radial). The patient should be monitored overnight in a step-down unit to detect complications. Most patients can be discharged within 1–2 days. In patients with AF, heparin can be restarted 3–4 hours after sheath removal, followed by warfarin. Bedside TTE can detect late accumulation of pericardial effusion. The patients who have developed complications need to be closely monitored in the intensive care unit. The PHT is affected by the change in compliance immediately after BMV; therefore, it is recommended to calculate the MVA by the PHT 2–3

Balloon reference size (RS)

- 0.1 × height (cm) + 10 (after rounding the patient's height to the nearest zero) or
- 30 for height >180 cm, 28 for 160–180 cm, 26 for <160 cm or
- Inter-commissural diameter measured on parasternal short-axis echocardiogram view

Balloon size selection

- RS-matched if the patient is young, valve is pliable, and MR is absent or less than 1+
- 1 size smaller than the RS if the valve is rigid, MR is >1+ and in high risk subjects (i.e., pregnancy, old age)

Inflation mode

- Start 2 mm below the RS in low risk patients, 4 mm in high risk patients
- Inflate in 1 mm increments under echocardiographic guidance

Closing criteria

- MVA > 1.5 cm^2
- 50% increase in the MVA
- 50% fall in mean gradient
- Fall in mean gradient from >10 mm Hg to <5 mm Hg
- Appearance or aggravation of MR > 1+
- Complete opening of at least one commissure

MR, mitral regurgitation; MVA, mitral valve area; RS, reference size.

Table 2. Inoue balloon selection and inflation protocol.

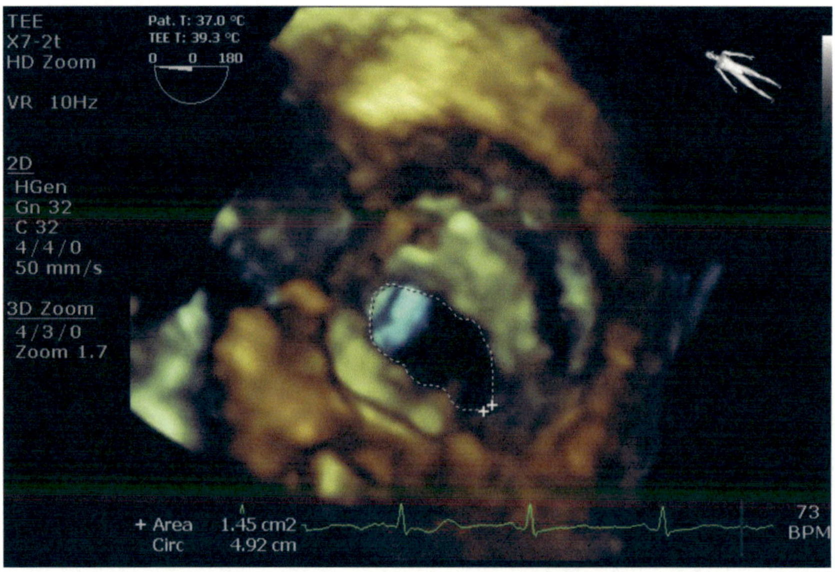

Figure 4. Postprocedural 3D imaging of the mitral valve revealing final mitral valve area of 1.45 cm^2.

http://dx.doi.org/10.5772/67757

days later. Direct planimetry yields the most accurate estimate of postprocedural MVA, but it might overestimate the MVA in the first day after the procedure and should be performed 1–2 days later allowing for the early loss [26]. TEE is not routinely recommended after successful BMV. If there is severe MR, TEE is essential for detecting its exact mechanism, which is important for further decision regarding conservative or invasive intervention.

5. Complications

General complications (i.e., vascular injury, arrhythmias, and contrast allergy) might occur and should be managed accordingly. Mortality has been reported in 1–2% and is mainly due to cardiac tamponade or the poor underlying condition of the patients [27].

5.1. Cardiac perforation and tamponade

Hemopericardium is the main complication of BMV and is seen in 1% of patients. The transseptal puncture is the source of most cardiac perforations during BMV. The anatomic factors of patients such as atrial enlargement and chest deformities increase the risk. TEE and ICE can guide the transseptal puncture, especially when the operator is inexperienced or in difficult cases, and reduce the risk of hemopericardium. Double-balloon mitral valvuloplasty and metallic commissurotome are associated with the risk of LV perforation because the wires are handled in the LV cavity. The management depends on the severity of pericardial effusion and the mechanism and consists of closed observation, reversal of heparin, pericardiocentesis, and emergent surgery. When the hemopericardium happens after septal dilation or LV perforation, especially if it is retractable despite prompt drainage, surgery is necessary to be proceeded.

5.2. Systemic embolism and stroke

While BMV might decrease the long-term risk of systemic embolism in patients with MS, the procedure itself can be associated with embolic stroke in about 1–1.5% of patients [28]. Meticulous anticoagulation and de-airing of the equipment and preprocedural TEE to rule out LA thrombi will reduce the chance of systemic embolism. An undiagnosed pre-existing LA/LAA clot and thrombus formation during the procedure are the main mechanisms, but calcium or air embolism also has a role.

5.3. Severe MR

Commissural opening, which is the main mechanism of increasing the MVA, is associated with aggravating MR after BMV in many patients but most are not significant and usually do not worsen functional status and long-term prognosis of the affected patients. Severe MR occurs in 2–15% of patients mainly because of non-commissural valve tearing and chordal rupture but exaggerated commissural splitting and rarely papillary muscle rupture are responsible [27, 29–31]. The incidence of severe MR does not change with different techniques

(Inoue vs. double balloon and metallic commissurotomy) [20, 32]. Unfavorable valve anatomy and inappropriate balloon sizing and inflation protocol predict the occurrence of severe MR after BMV, but their predictive value is not high and it can occur unpredictably in some patients with good morphologic features. Most patients need subsequent mitral valve surgery (mostly MVR) because severe MR is associated with the deterioration of functional status and poor outcomes. The timing of the surgery is determined by clinical tolerance, hemodynamic stability, mechanism of MR, and surgical risk. Most patients with severe MR can be managed conservatively and are subjected to mitral valve surgery on a scheduled basis. In a small number of patients who remain severely symptomatic despite initial medical therapy or who experience hemodynamic instability, or when the mechanical background of MR is severe and irreversible, urgent MVR should be planned. Patients with moderate MR can be often followed-up for a long period of time and some even experience a reduction in the severity of MR over time [33, 34].

5.4. Atrial septal defect

A wide range of frequency has been reported (10–90%) depending on modality that has been used for detection [35, 36]. Most defects decrease in size or disappear over time and have no adverse effects [37]. Infrequently, the defect is large enough to cause significant left-to-right shunting, especially when there is a significant residual mitral valve gradient and, therefore, surgical repair should be performed along with mitral valve surgery. Percutaneous closure of post-BMV residual atrial septal defects has not been reported and seems to be unsuccessful. In rare circumstances, right-to-left shunting and subsequent paradoxical embolism might happen in patients with significant pulmonary hypertension.

5.5. Emergent surgery

Rarely, patients need emergent surgery because of the complications. The most frequent cause is hemopericardium unresponsive to pericardiocentesis, especially when it happens after septal dilation and LV perforation. In most patients, the surgery includes repair of the tearing and MVR. Severe MR can also necessitate urgent surgery in some patients.

6. Special considerations

6.1. LAA/LAA thrombus

If the patient is clinically stable, BMV can be postponed for 3–6 months, while the patient receives intensive anticoagulation with an INR of 3–3.5. If repeated TEE shows that the clot has been completely resolved, BMV can be safely performed. If the thrombus persists, the patient should be referred for open mitral valvulotomy or MVR. If surgery is not a feasible option, BMV is not possible to be deferred, and the thrombus is small, fixed, and confined to the LAA, experienced operators might do BMV ensuing that the wire and balloon catheter are kept away from the LAA.

http://dx.doi.org/10.5772/67757

6.2. Previous valvulotomy

Restenosis is not infrequent after percutaneous or surgical commissurotomy. As a growing population, these patients account for one-third of all MS patients in developed countries. Depending on the mechanism, commissural fusion is not predominant in some cases, which limits the role of BMV as an effective intervention. BMV is a feasible option in patients with significant restenosis after percutaneous, closed, or open valvulotomy as long as the commissural fusion is present and valve anatomy is favorable [38]. Immediate and mid-term results are encouraging but might be slightly less satisfactory than with *de novo* MS.

6.3. Pregnancy

Significant hemodynamic burden caused by pregnancy, labor, and delivery might be not well-tolerated by patients with severe MS. Patients with severe MS often experience worsening of the symptoms or become symptomatic for the first time during pregnancy. Not surprisingly, MS is detected for the first time in many patients during pregnancy. If left untreated, severe MS is associated with a high maternal and perinatal mortality, not least in those who are highly symptomatic or have AF. The intrapartum and postpartum period carries the highest risk in these patients [39]. In patients who remain symptomatic, despite medical therapy, BMV should be performed because the surgery is associated with very high risk of fetal death [40]. BMV is an effective and safe method for relieving MS in pregnant women when performed by highly experienced operators. It has been reported that BMV during pregnancy has a high success rate and excellent short-term results and provides normal eventless deliveries in the majority of patients. In addition, stillbirth is infrequent and most babies have normal growth and developmental patterns [41, 42]. From a practical point of view, to avoid radiation during organogenesis, the procedure should be performed after the 12th week or ideally after the 20th week. The lead shields should cover the abdomen and pelvis and behind the patient. Fluoroscopy time should be minimized as much as possible. The Inoue balloon technique seems to be the preferred method considering shorter fluoroscopy time and inflation-deflation cycle of the balloon. Special care should be taken about the gravid uterus, possible difficulties in the passage of the equipment through the compressed inferior vena cava, and the chance of hypotension and subsequent fetal distress when the mother lies for a long period of time. The balloon size should be selected with great caution. A balloon 1 size smaller than the RS-matched is preferable in borderline cases. The more conservative method of measuring the inter-commissural diameter can be used for balloon sizing in these patients. The stepwise balloon dilatation of 0.5 mm is advisable, and aggressive balloon dilatation is necessarily avoided because it might result in severe MR and subsequently needs urgent surgery, which is unacceptably hazardous to mother and child. TEE can assist in the transseptal puncture, balloon positioning, and stepwise inflations and can limit fluoroscopy time. However, it needs general anesthesia in many cases, requiring that the position of the patient be changed to lateral decubitus to prevent hypotension in prolonged procedures.

6.4. Inoperable patients

BMV might be an option in patients who are old and have significant comorbidities. Given the suboptimal results and the higher incidence of complications arising from unfavorable morphologic characteristics of the mitral valve and poor condition of patients, BMV should be only used in highly symptomatic patients. In these patients, a more conservative BMV strategy is suggested. The Inoue technique is more appropriate because it is less demanding and provides a faster and smoother procedure. A balloon 1 size smaller than the RS is chosen, followed by a further stepwise dilatation of 0.5 mm. The final result should be judged on an individualized basis. Definitely, a smaller MVA is sufficient in most patients in exchange for severe MR and the difficulty in its management.

7. Results

7.1. Immediate results

A good immediate result is defined as an MVA > 1.5 cm^2 without MR more than moderate and is most probably achieved in patients with favorable morphologic features; nonetheless, other factors including age, history of previous commissurotomy, smaller baseline MVA, pre-existing MR, pulmonary artery pressure, sinus rhythm, functional status, and technical issues are also determining [43, 44].

7.2. Long-term results

When BMV has a good acute result, the long-term survival rate is high and the need for reintervention is infrequent. Anatomical characteristics and age are important predictors of long-term outcomes. Midterm outcomes (3–7 y) are favorable and comparable with open mitral valvulotomy and better than closed mitral valvulotomy [5].

Restenosis can occur after successful BMV, but its incidence is difficult to determine due to the absence of a uniform definition and different follow-up periods in the studies. An MVA < 1.5 cm^2 or a 50% loss in the initial MVA is generally defined as restenosis. The possible mechanisms include suboptimal initial results, recurrent rheumatic attacks, and a hemodynamic-related degenerative process. In patients with symptomatic severe restenosis, repeat BMV or mitral valve surgery should be selected according to the guidelines.

8. Conclusions

MS as the long-standing sequel of RHD is rare in developed countries, whereas it is still seen frequently in many areas of the world. BMV as a minimally invasive transcatheter technique is the method of choice in the treatment of these patients. In successful cases, BMV results in a very high survival rate and freedom from symptoms. Appropriate patient selection and a competent technique are the key factors for achieving an excellent result.

http://dx.doi.org/10.5772/67757

Acknowledgements

The authors like to thank Farshad Amouzadeh for his great assistance in the linguistic editing of this chapter.

Author details

Hamidreza Sanati* and Ata Firoozi

*Address all correspondence to: sanati56@yahoo.com

Cardiovascular Intervention Research Center, Rajaie Cardiovascular Medical and Research Center, Tehran, Iran

References

[1] Carapetis, J.R., M. McDonald, and N.J. Wilson, *Acute rheumatic fever.* The Lancet, 2005. **366**(9480): pp. 155-168.

[2] Iung, B. and A. Vahanian, *Epidemiology of valvular heart disease in the adult.* Nature Reviews Cardiology, 2011. **8**(3): pp. 162-172.

[3] Rahimtoola, S.H., et al., *Current evaluation and management of patients with mitral stenosis.* Circulation, 2002. **106**(10): pp. 1183-1188.

[4] Iung, B., et al., *Late results of percutaneous mitral commissurotomy in a series of 1024 patients analysis of late clinical deterioration: frequency, anatomic findings, and predictive factors.* Circulation, 1999. **99**(25): pp. 3272-3278.

[5] Cruz-Gonzalez, I., et al., *Predicting success and long-term outcomes of percutaneous mitral valvuloplasty: a multifactorial score.* The American Journal of Medicine, 2009. **122**(6): pp. 581. e11-581. e19.

[6] Mohan, J.C., et al., *Does chronic mitral regurgitation influence Doppler pressure half-time–derived calculation of the mitral valve area in patients with mitral stenosis?* American Heart Journal, 2004. **148**(4): pp. 703-709.

[7] Sanati, H., et al., *Mitral valve resistance determines hemodynamic consequences of severe rheumatic mitral stenosis and immediate outcomes of percutaneous valvuloplasty*. Echocardiography. 2017;34:162-168.

[8] Nishimura, R.A., et al., *2014 AHA/ACC guideline for the management of patients with valvular heart disease: a report of the American College of Cardiology/American Heart Association Task Force on Practice Guidelines.* Journal of the American College of Cardiology, 2014. **63**(22): pp. e57-e185.

[9] Horstkotte, D., R. Niehues, and B. Strauer, *Pathomorphological aspects, aetiology and natural history of acquired mitral valve stenosis.* European Heart Journal, 1991. **12**(suppl B): pp. 55-60.

[10] Moretti, M., et al., *Prognostic significance of atrial fibrillation and severity of symptoms of heart failure in patients with low gradient aortic stenosis and preserved left ventricular ejection fraction.* The American Journal of Cardiology, 2014. **114**(11): pp. 1722-1728.

[11] Halperin, J.L. and R.G. Hart, *Atrial fibrillation and stroke: new ideas, persisting dilemmas.* Stroke, 1988. **19**(8): pp. 937-941.

[12] Vahanian, A., et al., *Guidelines on the management of valvular heart disease (version 2012). The Joint Task Force on the Management of Valvular Heart Disease of the European Society of Cardiology (ESC) and the European Association for Cardio-Thoracic Surgery (EACTS).* Giornale Italiano di Cardiologia, 2013. **14**(3): pp. 167-214.

[13] Kirchhof, P., et al., *2016 ESC Guidelines for the management of atrial fibrillation developed in collaboration with EACTS. The Task Force for the management of atrial fibrillation of the European Society of Cardiology (ESC). Developed with the special contribution of the European Heart Rhythm Association (EHRA) of the ESC. Endorsed by the European Stroke Organisation (ESO).* European Journal of Cardio-Thoracic Surgery, 2016. p. ezw313.

[14] Ramondo, A., et al., *Relation of patient age to outcome of percutaneous mitral valvuloplasty.* The American Journal of Cardiology, 2006. **98**(11): pp. 1493-1500.

[15] Wilkins, G., et al., *Percutaneous balloon dilatation of the mitral valve: an analysis of echocardiographic variables related to outcome and the mechanism of dilatation.* British Heart Journal, 1988. **60**(4): pp. 299-308.

[16] Ribeiro, P.A., et al., *Mechanism of mitral valve area increase by in vitro single and double balloon mitral valvotomy.* The American Journal of Cardiology, 1988. **62**(4): pp. 264-269.

[17] Nath, R.K. and D.K. Soni, *Retrograde non trans-septal balloon mitral valvotomy in mitral stenosis with interrupted inferior vena cava, left superior vena cava, and hugely dilated coronary sinus.* Catheterization and Cardiovascular Interventions, 2015. **86**(7): pp. 1289-1293.

[18] Saejueng, B., et al., *Transjugular approach as a challenging access in PTMC: case report.* Journal of the Medical Association of Thailand, 2005. **88**(7): pp. 997-1002.

[19] Bahl, V., et al., *Balloon mitral valvotomy: comparison between antegrade Inoue and retrograde non-transseptal techniques.* European Heart Journal, 1997. **18**(11): pp. 1765-1770.

[20] Bhat, A., et al., *Comparison of percutaneous transmitral commissurotomy with Inoue balloon technique and metallic commissurotomy: immediate and short-term follow-up results of a randomized study.* American Heart Journal, 2002. **144**(6): pp. 1074-1080.

[21] Treviño, A.J., et al., *Immediate and long-term results of balloon mitral commissurotomy for rheumatic mitral stenosis: comparison between Inoue and double-balloon techniques.* American Heart Journal, 1996. **131**(3): pp. 530-536.

[22] Harikrishnan, S., M. Krishnakumar, and K. Suji, *22 inoue and accura balloons—the single balloon mitral valvotomy catheters.* Percutaneous Mitral Valvotomy. 2012. p. 215.

[23] Hung, J.S. and K.W. Lau, *Pitfalls and tips in Inoue balloon mitral commissurotomy.* Catheterization and Cardiovascular Diagnosis, 1996. **37**(2): pp. 188-199.

[24] Sanati, H.R., et al., *Percutaneous mitral valvuloplasty using echocardiographic intercommissural diameter as reference for balloon sizing: a randomized controlled trial.* Clinical Cardiology, 2012. **35**(12): pp. 749-754.

[25] Sanati, H.R., et al., *Percutaneous mitral valvuloplasty—a new method for balloon sizing based on maximal commissural diameter to improve procedural results.* The American Heart Hospital Journal, 2010. **8**: pp. 29-32.

[26] Harikrishnan, S., *Percutaneous Mitral Valvotomy.* 2012: Jaypee Brothers Medical Publishers Pvt. Ltd.

[27] Jneid, H., et al., *Impact of pre-and postprocedural mitral regurgitation on outcomes after percutaneous mitral valvuloplasty for mitral stenosis.* The American Journal of Cardiology, 2009. **104**(8): pp. 1122-1127.

[28] Liu, T.-J., et al., *Percutaneous balloon commissurotomy reduces incidence of ischemic cerebral stroke in patients with symptomatic rheumatic mitral stenosis.* International Journal of Cardiology, 2008. **123**(2): pp. 189-190.

[29] Essop, M.R., et al., *Mitral regurgitation following mitral balloon valvotomy. Differing mechanisms for severe versus mild-to-moderate lesions.* Circulation, 1991. **84**(4): pp. 1669-1679.

[30] Kim, M.-J., et al., *Long-term outcomes of significant mitral regurgitation after percutaneous mitral valvuloplasty.* Circulation, 2006. **114**(25): pp. 2815-2822.

[31] Kaul, U., et al., *Mitral regurgitation following percutaneous transvenous mitral commissurotomy: a single-center experience.* The Journal of Heart Valve Disease, 2000. **9**(2): pp. 262-266, discussion 266-268.

[32] Kang, D.-H., et al., *Long-term clinical and echocardiographic outcome of percutaneous mitral valvuloplasty: randomized comparison of Inoue and double-balloon techniques.* Journal of the American College of Cardiology, 2000. **35**(1): pp. 169-175.

[33] Krishnamoorthy, K., S. Radhakrishnan, and S. Shrivastava, *Natural history and predictors of moderate mitral regurgitation following balloon mitral valvuloplasty using Inoue balloon.* International Journal of Cardiology, 2003. **87**(1): pp. 31-36.

[34] Cheng, T.O., *Mechanism of spontaneous diminution of mitral regurgitation following percutaneous mitral valvuloplasty with the Inoue balloon.* International Journal of Cardiology, 2004. **93**(2): p. 329.

[35] Casale, P., et al., *Atrial septal defect after percutaneous mitral balloon valvuloplasty: immediate results and follow-up.* Journal of the American College of Cardiology, 1990. **15**(6): pp. 1300-1304.

[36] Arora, R., et al., *Atrial septal defect after balloon mitral valvuloplasty: a transesophageal echocardiographic study.* Angiology, 1993. **44**(3): pp. 217-221.

[37] Cequier, A., et al., *Left-to-right atrial shunting after percutaneous mitral valvuloplasty. Incidence and long-term hemodynamic follow-up.* Circulation, 1990. **81**(4): pp. 1190-1197.

[38] Fawzy, M.E., et al., *Immediate and long-term results of mitral balloon valvotomy for restenosis following previous surgical or balloon mitral commissurotomy.* The American Journal of Cardiology, 2005. **96**(7): pp. 971-975.

[39] McFaul, P., et al., *Pregnancy complicated by maternal heart disease. A review of 519 women.* BJOG: An International Journal of Obstetrics & Gynaecology, 1988. **95**(9): pp. 861-867.

[40] Zitnik, R.S., et al., *Pregnancy and open-heart surgery.* Circulation, 1969. **39**(5S1): pp. I-257–I-262.

[41] Nercolini, D.C., et al., *Percutaneous mitral balloon valvuloplasty in pregnant women with mitral stenosis.* Catheterization and Cardiovascular Interventions, 2002. **57**(3): pp. 318-322.

[42] Esteves, C.A., et al., *Immediate and long-term follow-up of percutaneous balloon mitral valvuloplasty in pregnant patients with rheumatic mitral stenosis.* The American Journal of Cardiology, 2006. **98**(6): pp. 812-816.

[43] Nobuyoshi, M., et al., *Indications, complications, and short-term clinical outcome of percutaneous transvenous mitral commissurotomy.* Circulation, 1989. **80**(4): pp. 782-792.

[44] Iung, B., et al., *Immediate results of percutaneous mitral commissurotomy a predictive model on a series of 1514 patients.* Circulation, 1996. **94**(9): pp. 2124-2130.

Chapter 6

Percutaneous Treatment of Mitral and Tricuspid Regurgitation in Heart Failure

Tomás Benito-González, Rodrigo Estévez-Loureiro, Javier Gualis Cardona, Armando Pérez de Prado, Mario Castaño Ruiz and Felipe Fernández-Vázquez

Additional information is available at the end of the chapter

http://dx.doi.org/10.5772/intechopen.68493

Abstract

Heart failure has become a real epidemic condition related to poor outcomes despite advances in medical therapies. Prevalence of significant mitral and/or tricuspid regurgitation is high in patients with advanced heart failure. Novel transcatheter techniques have recently emerged as a minimally invasive alternative in patients deemed high-risk for surgery or inoperable. Among them, MitraClip® system is thus far the first device that received regulatory approval and gained widespread clinical application, especially in patients with functional mitral regurgitation. Furthermore, first experiences with new devices for percutaneous mitral and tricuspid valves repair, and transcatheter mitral valve prosthesis have been increasingly reported. Percutaneous therapies for valvular heart disease have therefore become one of the most promising fields in the present and future of interventional cardiology and heart failure.

Keywords: mitral valve, tricuspid valve, advanced heart failure, MitraClip®, percutaneous edge-to-edge mitral valve repair, Cardioband®, Mitralign®, Carillon®, percutaneous tricuspid valve repair, transcatheter mitral valve prosthesis

1. Introduction

Heart failure (HF) is one of the most important causes of morbidity and mortality in developed countries [1]. The improvement in care of cardiac diseases has significantly reduced acute mortality of this condition, in turn, increasing chronic HF prevalence [2]. Hospitalizations for

HF are similarly increasing, resulting in very high costs for national health systems [3]. Despite developments in drug therapies and the widespread use of implantable cardiac devices, outcomes remain poor [4]. Several transcatheter implantable devices have recently emerged in an attempt to improve the prognosis and quality of life of such patients. In this chapter, we will review the percutaneous treatment alternatives for mitral and tricuspid regurgitation (TR) associated with advanced HF.

2. Transcatheter mitral valve intervention in mitral regurgitation

2.1. Functional mitral regurgitation and heart failure. Why a percutaneous approach?

Mitral regurgitation (MR) is one of the most common valvular disease worldwide [5] and its frequency is increasing with the age of the population. Functional MR (FMR) is a consequence of left ventricular (LV) remodeling with structurally preserved mitral valve (MV) leaflets. Significant MR may be present in half of the patients with congestive HF [6] and the development of MR after an acute myocardial infarction or in patients with dilated cardiomyopathy is associated with an increased risk of developing cardiac adverse events [7–11].

Surgery is the treatment of choice for patients with severe MR who refer symptoms or present LV dysfunction (LVD) [12]. However, up to 50% of patients cannot undergo MV surgery due to prohibitive surgical risk, usually related to advanced age, LVD or comorbidities [13]. Moreover, the proportion of patients with FMR undergoing surgical treatment is even lower [14]. Interestingly, open-heart surgery has yielded conflicting results in this sort of patients, with a lack of clear survival benefit and high recurrence rates even with modern techniques [15–18]. On the other hand, conservatively managed unoperated patients have poor clinical outcomes, especially those with FMR, whose mortality can exceed 50% at 5-years follow-up [19]. Large series from Duke University has proved that isolated medical management in patients with ischemic MR is associated with the highest rates of death after 20 years [20]. Thus, patients with FMR managed medically represent a high-risk population with high rates of death and readmission for HF [21]. Percutaneous MV therapies are emerging as an alternative for this population in order to fill a large unmet need.

2.2. Percutaneous mitral valve repair

The MV has a complex structure and its competence depends on the preservation of the MV leaflets, the subvalvular apparatus, the mitral annulus (MA) and the LV normal shape. Dysfunction of any of these different components may lead to the development of MR [22]. In the last few years, several percutaneous devices have been under investigation, addressing different anatomical and pathophysiological targets involved in MR [23, 24]. Percutaneous ongoing therapies have somehow tried to reproduce any of the already contrasted open-surgery techniques, such as edge-to-edge MV repair (MitraClip®), undersized annuloplasty (Carillon®, Cardioband®, Mitralign®) or chordal implantation (Neochord®). Some of them have gained approval for human use and have been tested in small clinical trials (**Table 1**).

http://dx.doi.org/10.5772/intechopen.68493

Device	Target of therapy	Year of CE mark	Current number of patients treated	Surgical background	Vascular access
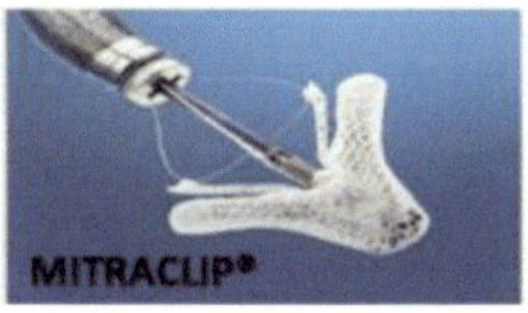	Leaflet coaptation	2008	>40,000	Edge-to-edge repair	Transfemoral
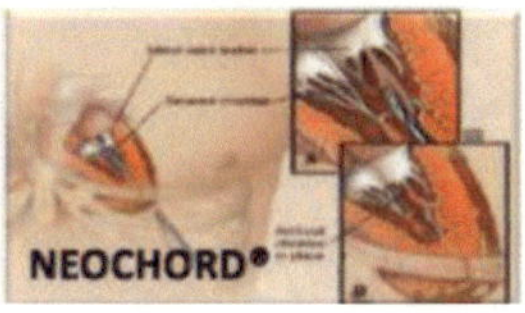	Chordae implantation	2013	>300	Chordae implantation	Transapical
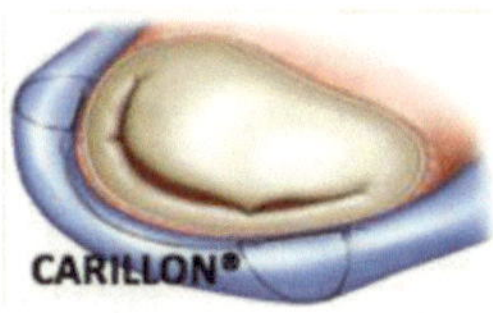	Indirect annuloplasty	2009	>100	No	Transjugular
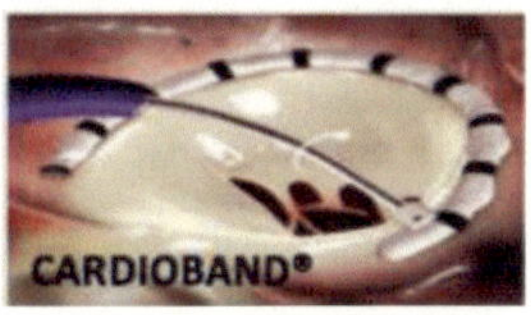	Direct annuloplasty	2015	>100	Flexible ring	Transfemoral
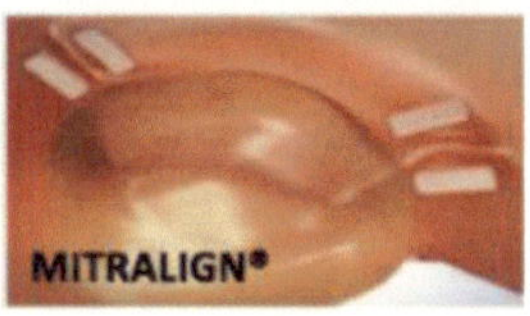	Direct annuloplasty	2016	>100	Commissuroplasty	Transarterial retrograde

Table 1. Summary of commercially available catheter-based therapies for PMVR.

2.2.1. Percutaneous edge-to-edge mitral valve repair (PMVR): MitraClip®

The MitraClip® system (Abbott Vascular, IL, USA) is thus far the first device that received regulatory approval and gained widespread clinical application. This device consists of two clip arms and opposing grippers, which can be opened and closed against each other in order to grasp and gain cooptation of MV leaflets at the origin of the regurgitant jet. The procedure is carried out under general anesthesia and using fluoroscopic and transesophageal echo guidance. Once the transseptal access is obtained, the system is advanced across the MV into the LV. Once the device is below the leaflets the two arms are opened and the device is retracted to capture and subsequently closed to increase the coaptation surface of the MV leaflets. The clip can be reopened and repositioned if the obtained result is not acceptable. Further clips can be placed as needed for optimal MR reduction. The amount of remainder MV tissue and resulting increase in transmitral pressure gradient are the main procedural limitations for further clip deployment. A second-generation device with improved maneuverability is now available.

Transcatheter edge-to-edge MV repair has proven to be a safe and effective technique in selected patients with either functional or degenerative MR. Feasibility of the therapy with MitraClip® was first demonstrated in the Endovascular Valve Edge-to-Edge Repair Study (EVEREST) I trial [25] and subsequently compared with conventional surgery in the randomized controlled trial (RCT) EVEREST II [26]. In these studies, stringent echo criteria were used to guide the feasibility of device insertion and deployment. However, with increasing experience more complex valve pathologies can be treated with excellent results [27].

The vast majority of clinical evidence in PMVR is related to MitraClip® and it is currently the most advanced available technology for clinical use. In the EVEREST II trial, 184 patients were randomized (2:1) to receive MitraClip® therapy and 95 patients to undergo surgical MV repair or replacement. Included study population was older than reported surgical series of MV repair (mean age 67 years old) and presented higher rates of comorbidities. The device proved to be safer than surgery with a significant reduction of major adverse events (9.6% versus 57% with surgery, $p < 0.0001$), although this difference was mainly driven by a greater need for blood transfusion with surgery. Conversely, in the intent to treat analysis, survival free from the primary endpoint (death, MV surgery and MR > 2+) was lower with MitraClip® as compared with surgery (55% vs 73%, $p = 0.0007$) [26]. Results of this trial at 5 years follow-up confirmed the initial results of the study. In those patients with an initial successful repair, no differences in mortality or reoperation were found in the PMVR arm compared to surgery. The proportion of patients with MR grade 3+ or 4+ at 5-year follow-up was 19%, just the same observed at 1 year, reassuring the durability of the PMVR [28].

2.2.1.1. Real-world candidates for percutaneous edge-to-edge mitral repair

Although most patients included in the EVEREST II trial had degenerative MR, in the subgroup of patients with LVD and/or FMR, no differences in outcomes were observed between MV surgery and MitraClip®, opening a new niche for PMVR. In fact, subsequent observational studies, have mainly recruited patients with FMR, especially in Europe (**Table 2**) [29–36]. Beyond the learning curve, real-world reported results showed increasing rates of procedural success over 90–95%, compared to initial experience in the EVEREST I and II trials. Furthermore, observational published registries have reported very low short-term adverse events and consistent improvements in symptoms, quality of life and MR reduction. Cohorts included in the main European registries may draw the profile of the current prototype of patient candidate for PMVR: advanced age, high-surgical risk, FMR and frequent history of ischemic heart disease, LVD and implantable stimulation device therapies (**Table 3**).

http://dx.doi.org/10.5772/intechopen.68493

Study	Type of study	Number of patients treated with MitraClip®	Location (number of sites)	Enrollment years	Functional MR (%)	Procedural success (MR ≤ 2+) (%)
EVEREST I [26]	Feasibility trial	24	USA (11)	2003–2005	21	74
EVEREST II [28]	RCT	184	USA (37)	2005–2008	49	77
EVEREST II HR [55]	Registry	351	USA (38)	2007–2014	70.1	85.8
ACESS-EU [29]	Registry	567	Europe (11)	2009–2011	77	91.2
MitraSwiss [30]	Registry	100	Switzerland (4)	2009–2011	62	85
Armoiry et al. [31]	Registry	62	France (7)	2010–2012	74	88.2
SENTINEL [32]	Registry	628	Europe (25)	2011–2012	72	95.4
TRAMI [33, 34, 52]	Registry	1064	Germany (20)	2010–2013	71	95.2
MARS [35]	Registry	145	Asia (8)	2011–2013	54	94
STS/ACC TVT [36]	Registry	564	USA (61)	2013–2014	14	93

Table 2. Main multicenter trials and registries of PMVR.

2.2.1.2. Special subsects of patients candidates for MitraClip

2.2.1.2.1. Non-responders to cardiac resynchronization therapy

MitraClip® has also been proved to be a useful tool for those patients with HF not responding to cardiac resynchronization therapy (CRT) [37]. Auricchio et al. reported their experience with 51 patients who were severely symptomatic despite CRT therapy. In this cohort, PMVR was associated with a significant reduction in MR, clinical improvement and favorable remodeling echocardiographic parameters during a median follow-up of 14 months.

Appropriate candidates	Other potential candidates
Functional mitral regurgitation	Acute ischemic mitral regurgitation
Severe left ventricular dysfunction	Hemodynamically unstable
High-risk for conventional surgery or inoperable	Low probability of successful surgical repair
Prior cardiac surgery (CABG)	Falling surgical ring
Non-responders to cardiac resynchronization therapy	Advanced heart failure

Table 3. Profile of patients that should be considered for PMVR.

2.2.1.2.2. End-stage heart failure

The effect of MitraClip® in patients with end-stage HF was reported by Franzen et al., analyzing the treatment of 50 patients with LV ejection fraction (LVEF) ≤ 25%, MR ≥ 3+ and severely symptomatic (NYHA III–IV) [38]. The acute procedural success was 94%, and 92% of patients were discharged with MR ≤ 2+. One month mortality was 6% (predicted by EuroScore 34%). At 6-month follow-up, 72% patients were in functional class NYHA I or II; there was inverse remodeling on echo follow-up and a relevant reduction in BNP levels. Several reasons may account for these results: first, the positive hemodynamic changes observed after treatment with reductions in pulmonary pressure, capillary wedge pressure and increase in cardiac output (CO). Second, the avoidance of the low CO post MV surgery; and third, the favorable remodeling in LV [39–41]. However, patients with very poor LVEF are at high-risk of mortality even with this thearpy. Careful selection of these candidates based on operators' experience, probability of success and expected benefits is strongly advisable [34].

2.2.1.2.3. Acute ischemic mitral regurgitation

Acute ischemic MR is a severe complication associated with high rates of morbimortality even when surgically corrected [42]. MitraClip® has proved to be a safe and effective alternative to surgical intervention in these unstable patients [43, 44]. Acute MR usually develops in a previously normal MV and therefore anatomical features are optimal for PMVR. Rapid improvement in patient's hemodynamics and the avoidance of the systemic inflammatory response associated with cardiopulmonary bypass are potential advantages of transcatheter approach [45]. MitraClip® implantation could be considered as an urgent therapy during admission in patients with recurrent pulmonary edema and/or cardiogenic shock in which MR is deemed to be the main cause of decompensation [46].

2.2.1.2.4. Failing annuloplasty rings

Undersized annuloplasty is currently the standard approach for MV surgical repair [47]. Even with the modern prosthetic mitral rings, long-term durability is a major concern in patients with FMR, in which the risk for recurrence can be over 50% at 2 years [48]. These patients are frequently symptomatic, with an increased number of hospitalizations, and present often significant LVD. Series from Italy and Spain have proved that the use of the device is safe and produces a persistent reduction in MR, hemodynamic improvement and symptom relief [49, 50]. Therefore, MitraClip® should be considered as an alternative therapy in this sort of patients, given the unacceptable high-risk that may carry reoperation.

2.2.1.3. Expected benefits from percutaneous edge-to-edge repair

2.2.1.3.1. Persistent reduction in mitral regurgitation

Persistent MR reduction is one of the main goals of PMVR. The target proposed since the EVEREST trials is to achieve a reduction of mitral insufficiency to a degree ≤2+ and this has been considered as a definition for procedural success (PS) and an acceptable result during follow-up [25]. Interestingly, the EVERST II trial was the one with the lower PS reported (77%)

[26]. The use of a single clip in almost all the patients and the fact that the trial was conducted in the beginning of the learning curve of most centers may explain the lower efficacy of the device compared to surgery. With increasing following experience, PS has raised to over 90% of cases in most series, highly impacting the prognosis of patients [29, 32–34, 51, 52]. A persistent MR reduction is linked to better outcomes and "the less MR possible" should be the target of all procedures [53]. Conversely, inability to reduce MR is an independent marker of adverse prognosis [32, 34]. The mechanisms supporting this observation are likely to be related to the hemodynamic changes observed after MR correction [39, 40]. Recurrence of significant MR is around 6–21.1% at 1 year [29, 32]; notably similar figures are reported with surgical repair for ischemic FMR [18].

2.2.1.3.2. *Symptoms improvement*

Symptomatic improvement is one of the most reported benefits of this therapy. Preprocedure patients are usually highly symptomatic with proportions of NYHA functional class III–IV over 85% in published series. After treatment with MitraClip®, there is a significant recovery in the functional capacity with patients presenting on NYHA functional class I–II in a range of 63.3–86% [29, 32, 34, 54, 55]. Furthermore, patients as well experience improvement in 6 minutes-walk test [29] and quality of life [54, 56], and a significant reduction in serum BNP levels [38]. Clinical improvement does also lead to a significant reduction in readmissions for HF, which reduces costs of patients' health care and might probably turn into better prognosis [55].

2.2.1.3.3. *Survival advantage*

Survival of patients with FMR treated with MitraClip® is in the range of 15.3–20.3% within the first year [29, 32, 34]. The largest follow-up reported showed an actuarial survival at 3 years of 74.5% [55].

The available evidence to date regarding this issue relies mainly on retrospective studies. The first published was the EVEREST high-risk study [57], where 78 patients with high-surgical risk (STS ≥ 12%) were treated with MitraClip® and compared with a cohort of 36 patients managed medically. At 1 year, MitraClip® patients have significant higher survival rates (76% PMVR vs. 55% medical therapy, $p = 0.045$). In a study by Swaans et al. [58], 139 patients treated percutaneously were compared to 59 patients medically treated. After controlling by propensity score matching, MitraClip® was associated with a relative reduction in the risk of mortality of 59%. In another paper, Velazquez et al. [59] compared the outcomes of 351 patients included in the EVEREST high-risk registry with a historic comparator cohort. Two-hundred and thirty-nine propensity-matched patients in each group were analyzed and MitraClip® was associated with a 1 year improved survival (mortality 22.4% MitraClip® vs. 32% medical therapy, $p = 0.043$). The relative risk reduction in mortality associated with the device was 34%. Finally, Giannini et al. [60] included 60 patients treated with MitraClip® and propensity matched with 60 patients with OMT. After a median follow-up of 515 days, patients treated with PMVR showed less mortality, less cardiac mortality and less readmissions due to heart failure (log-rank test $p = 0.007$, $p = 0.002$ and $p = 0.04$, respectively). While we wait for the final confirmation of these results in currently ongoing RCTs, this information encourages the application of the therapy.

2.2.1.3.4. *Effect on heart remodeling: mitral annulus and left ventricle*

Reverse LV remodeling is the 'holy grail' of PMVR. Reported results from surgical series of primary MR have been linked to better prognosis [61]. Echo reports from EVEREST trial have demonstrated that there is an inverse remodeling after a successful MitraClip® procedure involving both the left chambers (ventricle and atrium) [62]. Interestingly, the magnitude of the reverse remodeling is greater with greater reduction in MR and this positive effect is maintained at 5 years follow-up [28]. Similar findings were reported in the EVEREST high-risk cohort [55, 57], although, in these series, patients with LVEF below 25% and severe LV dilation (LV end-systolic diameter > 55 mm) were excluded. By contrast, real-world FMR patients treated with MitraClip® tend to exhibit poor or no remodeling at all [32]. One possible explanation for these conflicting results is that real-world patients are treated too late in the natural history of the chronic HF disease, when the LV is largely dilated and LVEF is severely depressed. These patients are less likely to show reverse remodeling and this is a hint for the best timing for PMVR.

Although PMVR with MitraClip® reproduces somehow the Alfieri procedure, traction forces within MV may also favor MA remodeling. Recent studies have demonstrated that in FMR, the MA size (anteroposterior diameter), the MA area and the tenting area are significantly reduced after device implantation [63]. Furthermore, this reduction is associated with an improved functional status at 6 month after the procedure [64]. Conversely, in primary MR, MA parameters remain stable after clipping. Therefore, the potential association of an indirect annuloplasty-like effect may improve mid-term results of this therapy in patients with FMR.

2.2.2. *Percutaneous chordal replacement: Neochord®*

Neochord® (Neochord, Minnesota, MN) are the first ePTFE chordal loops conceived to be implanted on the MV leaflets to correct flail or prolapse [65]. Colli et al. reported the results of transapical off-pump mitral valve implantation of Neochord in 62 patients with MV prolapse [66]. Thirty-day major adverse events included one acute myocardial infarction (2%) and two cases of sepsis (3%). MR at 30 days was grade 1+ or 2+ in 55 patients (88.7%).

2.2.3. *Transcatheter mitral valve annuloplasty (TMVA): Carillon®, Cardioband®, Mitralign®*

Annuloplasty is the most common surgical repair performed to treat MR [47]. This technique is widely used as a stand-alone procedure to enhance MV coaptation in FMR or added to leaflet repair in degenerative MR in order to improve durability [67]. Based on prior large surgical experience, some percutaneous novel devices have tried to reproduce undersized MV annuloplasty to address dilatation of the MA. A reliable TMVA has the potential to improve outcomes in combination with edge-to-edge repair in selected patients and to increase therapeutic alternatives in patients with anatomic ineligibility for MitraClip®. As a further potential advantage, unlike the MitraClip®, this approach preserves the native valve anatomy, thus keeping the option for future valve implantation open. In fact, some of the annuloplasty rings may actually serve as a dock for the anchoring of available transcatheter aortic valves ("valve-in-ring" procedure).

2.2.3.1. *Carillon®*

The coronary sinus (CS) encircles approximately two-thirds of the MA, in close relation to the posterior and anterior MV leaflets. This was the rationale for the first catheter-based devices that aim to achieve an indirect annuloplasty through the cannulation of the CS. The Carillon® Mitral Contour System (Cardiac Dimension, Inc., Kirkland, WA, USA) obtained the CE mark in 2011. This deformable annular system is implanted in the CS and can reduce the septolateral diameter of the MA by postimplant cinching [68]. The procedure can be easily performed under fluoroscopic guidance through a jugular vein access and without general anesthesia. Nevertheless, some limitations have hampered the development of this technique. Advance imaging studies have demonstrated that the location of the CS is no coplanar to the MA, but basally displaced into the LA [69]. Moreover, potentially serious complications have also been reported, including compression of the circumflex artery or damage of the septal conduction system [70]. Finally, the lack of prior surgical background for the CS approach may be a concern as regards the long-term outcomes of this procedure.

To date, published evidence is limited to a couple observational studies. In the Titan trial, only 36 of 53 (67.9%) patients underwent permanent system implantation due to transient coronary compromise or reduction of MR < 1+ (recapture of the device was carried out in those cases) [71]. Rates of death at 1 and 12 months in this study were 1.9 and 22.6%. In the TITAN II trial, the system was successfully implanted in 30 of 36 (83.3%) patients, and 30-day and 1-year reported mortality were 2.8 and 23%, respectively. Both trials showed that device implantation was related to a significant reduction in MR, and to clinical improvement and reverse LV remodeling in patients with FMR and HF during up to 24-month follow-up. Ongoing REDUCE trial will compare the device to OMT in HF subjects with FMR, thus, providing further evidence of the potential benefits of this technology.

2.2.3.2. *Cardioband®*

Cardioband® (Valtech, Inc, Or Yehuda, Israel) is the transcatheter device that most closely resembles surgical direct annuloplasty technique. The system consists of a flexible annuloplasty band that is delivered from a transseptal approach and implanted onto the atrial side of the MA. This incomplete Dacron ring is attached in a supraannular position with multiple spiral anchors from commissure to commissure under transesophageal echo and fluoroscopic guidance. After implantation, the Cardioband® length can be shortened in order to improve leaflet coaptation and reduce MR.

Although flexible partial rings have failed in this sort of patients when implanted surgically [72], initial clinical experiences with Cardioband® are promising, confirming the feasibility and safety of the device implantation [73]. The CE Mark Trial has enrolled high-risk subjects with symptomatic FMR despite OMT. Early outcomes of this trial in 31 patients at 1 month showed a significant reduction in the septolateral dimension of the MA in all but two patients (36.8 ± 4.8 vs. 29 ± 5.5 mm, $p < 0.01$) and an increased leaflet coaptation surface [74]. Following Cardioband® adjustment (29 of 31 patients), MR was none or trace in 6 (21%), mild in 21 (72%) and moderate in 2 (7%) cases. Procedural mortality was zero and in-hospital mortality was 6.5%

(2 of 31 patients, neither procedure nor device-related). At 30 days, 22 of the 25 patients (88%) had MR grade ≤ 2+. Following results of this trial showed persistent reduction in MR (92% MR ≤ 2+) and improvement in functional class (77% NYHA I–II) at 24-month follow up. Reported procedural success rate (reduction in at least one grade in MR at discharge) was 86%. In 2017, an RCT comparing Cardioband® versus stand-alone OMT will start recruiting in the USA.

2.2.3.3. Mitralign®

The Mitralign® (Mitralign, Inc., Tewksbury, MA, USA) is a transcatheter direct annuloplasty system that mimics the Kay-Wooler commissuroplasty [75]. The device allows selective plication of the medial and lateral aspects of the MA by deploying pairs of transannular "pledgets". The procedure is carried out from a transfemoral retrograde approach under live echo and fluoroscopic guidance. Each pledget pair can be pulled together resulting in a segmental posterior annuloplasty [76]. In the CE Mark Trial, the system was successfully implanted in 70.4% of 71 high-risk subjects with FMR [77]. No intraprocedural death occurred, but four (8.9%) patients experienced cardiac tamponade. 30-days and 6-month reported all-cause mortality were 4.4 and 12.2%, respectively. Significant improvements in MR and clinical functional class, reduction in MA dimensions and LV remodeling were demonstrated at 6 months.

2.2.4. Transcatheter multimodal approach for mitral regurgitation

One of the lessons learned from heart valve surgery is that a combination of diverse techniques addressing different mechanisms of MR may improve long-term outcomes [67]. Recently, first experiences of direct and indirect TMVA after failure of PMVR with MitraClip® have been published [78, 79]. MitraClip® is currently the most widespread technique that focus on MV leaflets, with contrasted effective results. Nevertheless, reported recurrence of significant MR can surpass 20% at 1 year [29]. Notably, transcatheter mitral rings may play a role as valuable adjunct catheter-based procedures to Mitraclip® (or percutaneous chordal replacement) in selected patients (such as very dilated LA and MA).

2.3. Transcatheter mitral valve replacement (TMVR)

The simpler structure of the aortic valve (AV) has probably facilitated the success of a stent-like transcatheter approach for the treatment of AV disease. On the contrary, the much more complex structure of the MV may explain the slower way to find a safe and effective alternative for TMVR. Many companies have completed first-in-human cases; however, no devices are currently approved beyond compassionate use, and several others remain in preclinical development. These percutaneous MV prostheses vary either in the access site, the design and the anchoring technology within the MA or the subvalvular apparatus [80] (**Figure 1**). Currently, eight different devices have been already implanted in-human since 2012 (CardiAQ®, Neovasc Tiara®, Edwards Fortis®, Tendyne®, Twelve®, Navigate®, Highlife®, Caisson®) [81–84]. These initial experiences showed heterogeneous rates of morbidity and mortality across different platforms and pointed out some important challenging issues that might be determinant in the development of this technique: the LV outflow obstruction, the delivery profile and the access route (transapical vs transeptal). Interestingly, patients with

http://dx.doi.org/10.5772/intechopen.68493

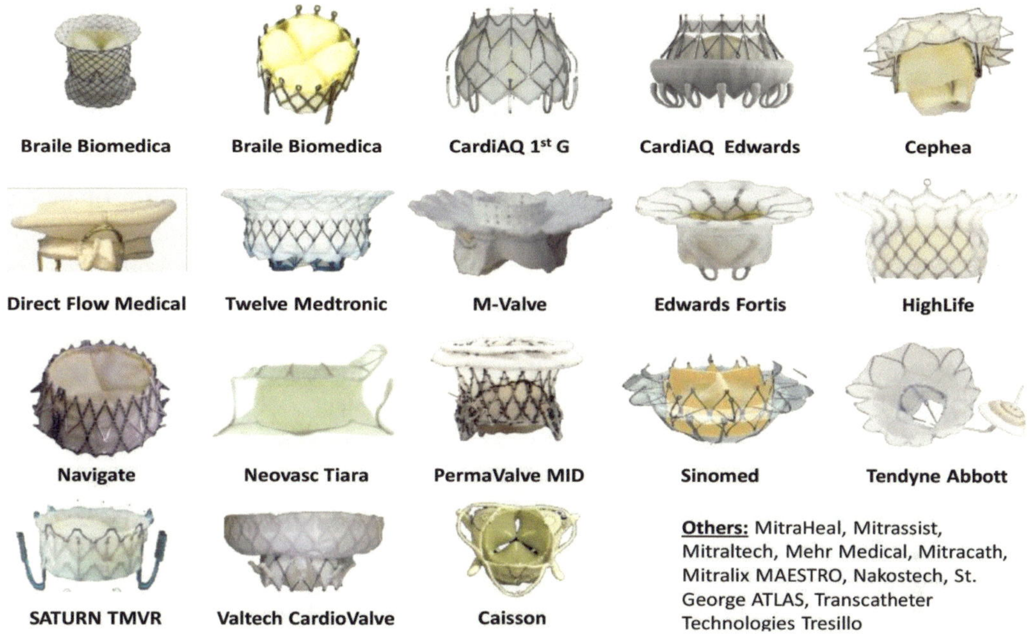

Figure 1. Current mitral valve platforms under development.

poor ejection fraction presented the higher rates of adverse outcomes and might not benefit from this procedure.

Recently, promising results from the Tendyne® feasibility trial have been published [85]. In this study 30 high-risk patients (mean age 75.6 years) with predominantly FMR (76.6%) grade 3 or 4 underwent TMVR. Successful device implantation was achieved in 28 patients (93.3%). No acute major cardiovascular adverse events were reported. One patient died 13 days after TMVR from hospital-acquired pneumonia and prosthetic leaflet thrombosis was detected in one patient at follow-up. At 30 days, transthoracic echocardiography showed mild central MR in 1 patient, and no residual MR in the remaining 26 patients with valves *in situ*. A significant decrease in LV dimensions was documented. Seventy-five percent of the patients reported mild or no symptoms at follow-up. Successful device implantation free of cardiovascular mortality, stroke and device malfunction at 30 days was 86.6%.

3. Percutaneous therapies for tricuspid regurgitation in heart failure

3.1. Functional tricuspid regurgitation

Functional tricuspid regurgitation (TR) represents over 90% of cases of TR and it is typically due to tricuspid annular dilatation (mainly in anteroposterior diameter) and right ventricular (RV) enlargement (leading to leaflet tethering) secondary to progressive left heart disease (LHD) [86]. The tricuspid valve (TV) has been considered for years the "forgotten" valve. This issue may be explained by the fact that TR was believed to be well tolerated and reduced after treating LHD. On the contrary, patients with significant TR and HF tend to be highly symptomatic due to decrease in CO and abdominal and peripheral congestion [87]. Furthermore, the presence of moderate or severe TR is independently associated with an increased mortality (over 25% at 1 year) regardless of biventricular function or pulmonary pressures [88, 89].

Despite surgical treatment of LHD, significant TR can be found in over two-thirds of patients in long-term follow-up, suggesting that a lower threshold for TV repair should be considered when MV surgery is carried out [87, 90–92]. Current data support that TV repair at the time of MV surgery is safe, whereas reoperation for persistent TR is related to high morbidity and mortality rates [93–95]. Notwithstanding, few patients undergo TR surgery and the vast majority are managed medically. Data from the STS database suggest that moderate to severe TR is present in almost 2 million of patients in the United States, but not even 10,000 undergo TV surgery each year. Progressive RV dysfunction may lead to an irreversible RV damage, which is thought to be the reason for the poor outcomes of late surgery in this scenario. Therefore, there is a large unmet clinical need for patients with significant TR who are not referred for conventional surgery, mainly due to expected high-surgical risk. Percutaneous therapies for functional TR are emerging as an alternative to surgery in this scenario. Patients with symptomatic severe TR and prior open-heart surgery and those with significant TR and progressive RV dysfunction and failure despite OMT may benefit from transcatheter TV interventions. Initial experiences include the off-label use MV devices and first-in-human cases of dedicated new technologies [96] (**Table 4**). Among different therapies that have been tested in preclinical setting, transcatheter TV annuloplasty, resembling different successful surgical techniques, might be one of the most promising approaches [97, 98].

3.2. Transcatheter tricuspid valve interventions

3.2.1. Percutaneous tricuspid valve repair with mitral valve dedicated devices

The acquired experience in catheter-based therapies for MV with satisfactory results has emerged the appealing concept of using some of these devices in tricuspid position. Recently, Braun et al. have reported first series of edge-to-edge TV repair in 18 patients with moderate to severe functional TR and right-sided heart failure [99]. Six patients were treated for isolated severe TR, whereas 12 patients were treated concomitantly to PMVR. A reduction of at least one TR grade was achieved in all patients and no in-hospital major events were reported. A significant improvement in TR was observed (TR ≥ 3+ 94% vs. 33%, $p < 0.001$) and sixteen patients (89%) referred an improvement in NYHA functional class at 30-day follow-up. In 2015, the first-in-human transcatheter TV repair with Mitralign® system was published, reproducing Kay posterior annuloplasty [100]. Recently, acute results of Trialign® early human use were reported. A single pair of pledgets was successfully implanted in 14 of the 16 patients (87.5%), with an average postprocedural reduction of 37% in TA and 59% in TV regurgitant orifice area. No procedural mortality occurred. Potential advantage of additional pledgets will be assessed. Cardioband® has been also successfully implanted in TA in humans [101] and European CE mark study (TRI-REPAIR) is currently initiated.

http://dx.doi.org/10.5772/intechopen.68493

Device	Features	Strengths	Challenges
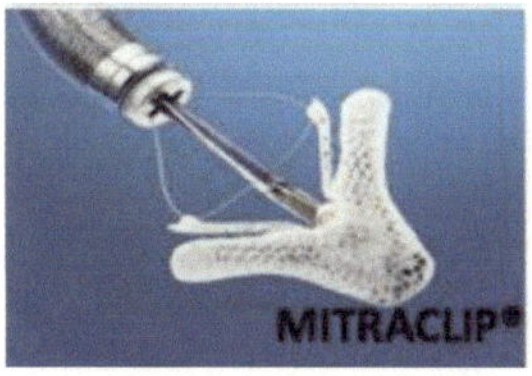	Bicuspidization of the tricuspid valve First series reported	Large experience in mitral valve Friendly to operators	Vascular access route Modified clipping technique Three-leaflets configuration of the valve Annular dilatation not addressed
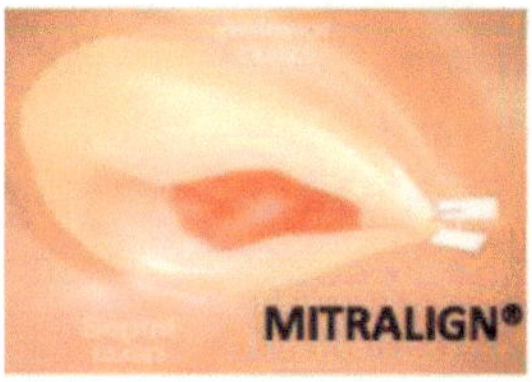	Bicuspidization of the tricuspid valve (posterior commissure) First series reported Ongoing CE mark trial	Surgical background High safety profile	Risk of leaflet or right coronary artery injury Technically demanding Transesophageal echo guidance Valvular tissue properties
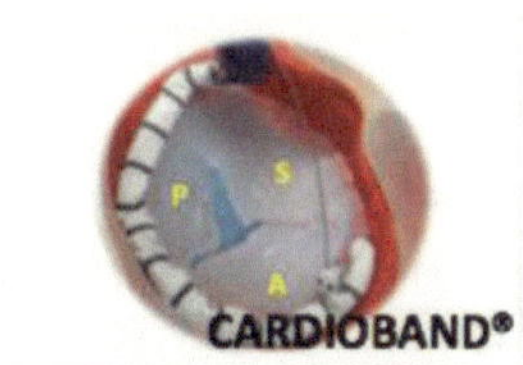	Flexible-ring annuloplasty First in-human cases reported Ongoing CE mark trial	Surgical background	Little experience in mitral valve Risk of right coronary artery injury
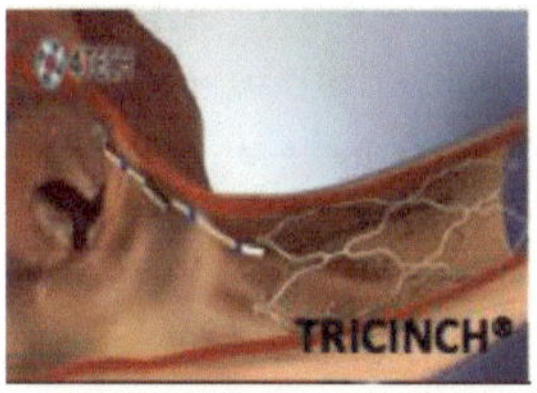	Simple indirect annuloplasty Ongoing CE mark trial	Surgical background High safety profile Fully retrievable before stenting	Risk of leaflet or right coronary artery injury Inferior vena cava dilatation
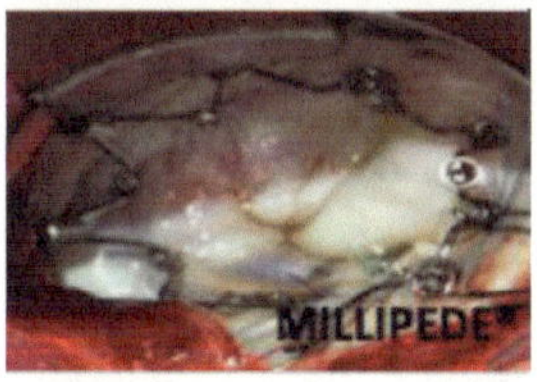	Semi-rigid complete ring implanted in the atrial side of the tricuspid annulus First in-human cases reported	Surgical background Repositionable & retrievable	Risk of atrioventricular block
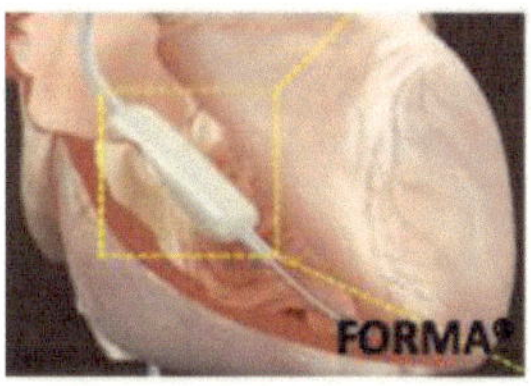	Valve spacer to fulfil regurgitant orifice First in-human cases reported Ongoing CE mark trial	Good preliminary clinical results	Surgical pocket Large devices needed to fill coaptation gap No surgical background

Table 4. Catheter-based therapies for TR that have been already tested in humans.

3.2.2. Transcatheter tricuspid valve repair therapies

TriCinch® (4Tech Cardio, Galway, Ireland) consists of a steerable catheter with a corkscrew at the tip. Under echocardiographic and fluoroscopic guidance, supraannular fixation of the device is carried out in the mid part of the anterior TA. Afterwards, the catheter is tensioned in order to produce TA cinching, therefore reducing the anteroseptal dimension of the TA and improving leaflet coaptation. Finally, a self-expandable nitinol stent is positioned at the inferior vena cava in order to secure the system and maintain the tension applied. TriCinch® implantation preserves the native anatomy, allowing potential future treatment options. First in-human cases [102, 103] and early results from the PREVENT CE trial have been reported. The system was successfully implanted in 13 of 18 patients (72%). Two patients developed periprocedural hemopericardium and device TA detachment was observed in two patients. No mortality events occurred during up to 29 months follow-up. A significant improvement in 6-minute walk test and quality of life were documented, although only 37.5% remain in NYHA class I–II during this period.

3.2.3. Other percutaneous approaches for tricuspid regurgitation

The FORMA® Repair System (Edwards Lifescience, Irvine, USA) is a valve spacer created to increase coaptation surface by occupying space in the regurgitant orifice of the TV. The device is usually delivered through a transsubclavian venous route and anchored to the RV apex distally and proximally fixed within a small surgically prepared pocket. Preliminary results in seven high-risk patients with severe TR and advanced NYHA functional class III–IV were recently available [104]. The device was successfully implanted in all patients without major complications, obtaining at least one grade acute reduction in TR. 30-day results showed clinical improvements (100% NYHA class II) and stable TR reduction (100% moderate TR) without significant tricuspid stenosis.

Author details

Tomás Benito-González[1], Rodrigo Estévez-Loureiro[1]*, Javier Gualis Cardona[2], Armando Pérez de Prado[1], Mario Castaño Ruiz[2] and Felipe Fernández-Vázquez[1]

*Address all correspondence to: roiestevez@hotmail.com

1 Department of Cardiology, Interventional Cardiology Unit, University Hospital of León, León, Spain

2 Department of Cardiovascular Surgery, University Hospital of León, León, Spain

References

[1] Go AS, Mozaffarian D, Roger VL, et al. Heart Disease and Stroke Statistics—2014 Update: A Report from the American Heart Association. 2014. Epub ahead of print 2014. DOI: 10.1161/01.cir.0000441139.02102.80

[2] Roger VL. Epidemiology of heart failure. Circulation Research. 2013;**113**:646-659

[3] Braunschweig F, Cowie MR, Auricchio A. What are the costs of heart failure? Europace. 2011;**13**:13-17

[4] Metra M, Carubelli V, Ravera A, et al. Heart failure 2016: Still more questions than answers. International Journal of Cardiology. 2016;**227**:766-777

[5] Nkomo VT, Gardin JM, Skelton TN, et al. Burden of valvular heart diseases: A population-based study. Lancet. 2006;**368**:1005-1011

[6] Bursi F, Barbieri A, Grigioni F, et al. Prognostic implications of functional mitral regurgitation according to the severity of the underlying chronic heart failure: A long-term outcome study. European Journal of Heart Failure. 2010;**12**:382-388

[7] Bursi F, Enriquez-Sarano M, Nkomo VT, et al. Heart failure and death after myocardial infarction in the community: The emerging role of mitral regurgitation. Circulation. 2005;**111**:295-301

[8] Robbins JD, Maniar PB, Cotts W, et al. Prevalence and severity of mitral regurgitation in chronic systolic heart failure. American Journal of Cardiology. 2003;**91**:360-362

[9] Trichon BH, Felker GM, Shaw LK, et al. Relation of frequency and severity of mitral regurgitation to survival among patients with left ventricular systolic dysfunction and heart failure. American Journal of Cardiology. 2003;**91**:538-543

[10] Grigioni F, Enriquez-Sarano M, Zehr KJ, et al. Ischemic mitral regurgitation: Long-term outcome and prognostic implications with quantitative Doppler assessment. Circulation. 2001;**103**:1759-1764

[11] López-Pérez M, Estévez-Loureiro R, López-Sainz A, et al. Long-term prognostic value of mitral regurgitation in patients with ST-segment elevation myocardial infarction treated by primary percutaneous coronary intervention. American Journal of Cardiology. 2014;**113**:907-912

[12] Nishimura RA, Otto CM, Bonow RO, et al. 2014 AHA/ACC guideline for the management of patients with valvular heart disease: Executive summary: A report of the American college of cardiology/American heart association task force on practice guidelines. Journal of the American College of Cardiology. 2014;**63**:2438-2488

[13] Mirabel M, Iung B, Baron G, et al. What are the characteristics of patients with severe, symptomatic, mitral regurgitation who are denied surgery? European Heart Journal. 2007;**28**:1358-1365

[14] Borger MA, Alam A, Murphy PM, et al. Chronic ischemic mitral regurgitation: Repair, replace or rethink? Annals of Thoracic Surgery. 2006;**81**:1153-1161

[15] Wu AH, Aaronson KD, Bolling SF, et al. Impact of mitral valve annuloplasty on mortality risk in patients with mitral regurgitation and left ventricular systolic dysfunction. Journal of the American College of Cardiology. 2005;**45**:381-387

[16] Hung J, Papakostas L, Tahta SA, et al. Mechanism of recurrent ischemic mitral regurgitation after annuloplasty: Continued LV remodeling as a moving target. Circulation. 2004;**110**:II85-II90

[17] McGee EC, Gillinov AM, Blackstone EH, et al. Recurrent mitral regurgitation after annuloplasty for functional ischemic mitral regurgitation. Journal of Thoracic and Cardiovascular Surgery. 2004;**128**:916-924

[18] Acker MA, Parides MK, Perrault LP, et al. Mitral-Valve repair versus replacement for severe ischemic mitral regurgitation. The New England Journal of Medicine. 2014;**370**: 23-32

[19] Agricola E, Ielasi A, Oppizzi M, et al. Long-term prognosis of medically treated patients with functional mitral regurgitation and left ventricular dysfunction. European Journal of Heart Failure. 2009;**11**:581-587

[20] Castleberry AW, Williams JB, Daneshmand MA, et al. Surgical revascularization is associated with maximal survival in patients with ischemic mitral regurgitation: A 20-year experience. Circulation. 2014;**129**:2547-2556

[21] Goel SS, Bajaj N, Aggarwal B, et al. Prevalence and outcomes of unoperated patients with severe symptomatic mitral regurgitation and heart failure: Comprehensive analysis to determine the potential role of mitraclip for this unmet need. Journal of the American College of Cardiology. 2014;**63**:185-186

[22] Dal-Bianco JP, Beaudoin J, Handschumacher MD, et al. Basic mechanisms of mitral regurgitation. Canadian Journal of Cardiology. 2014;**30**:971-981

[23] Estevez-Loureiro R, Franzen O. Current state of percutaneous transcatheter mitral valve therapies. Panminerva Medica. 2013;**55**:327-337

[24] Herrmann HC, Maisano F. Transcatheter therapy of mitral regurgitation. Circulation. 2014;**130**:1712-1722

[25] Feldman T, Wasserman HS, Herrmann HC, et al. Percutaneous mitral valve repair using the edge-to-edge technique: Six-month results of the EVEREST phase I clinical trial. Journal of The American College of Cardiology. 2005;**46**:2134-2140

[26] Feldman T, Foster E, Glower DD, Kar S, Rinaldi MJ, Fail PS, Smalling RW, Siegel R, Rose GA, Engeron E, Loghin C, Trento A, Skipper ER, Fudge T, Letsou GVL. Percutaneous repair or surgery for mitral regurgitation. The New England Journal of Medicine. 2011;**364**:1395-1406

[27] Boekstegers P, Hausleiter J, Baldus S, et al. Percutaneous interventional mitral regurgitation treatment using the Mitra-Clip system. Clinical Research in Cardiology. 2014;**103**:85-96

[28] Feldman T, Kar S, Elmariah S, et al. Randomized comparison of percutaneous repair and surgery for mitral regurgitation 5-Year results of EVEREST II. Journal of the American College of Cardiology. 2015;**66**:2844-2854

[29] Maisano F, Franzen O, Baldus S, et al. Percutaneous mitral valve interventions in the real world: Early and 1-year results from the ACCESS-EU, A prospective, multicenter, nonrandomized post-approval study of the Mitraclip therapy in Europe. Journal of the American College of Cardiology. 2013;**62**:1052-1061

[30] Sürder D, Pedrazzini G, Gaemperli O, et al. Predictors for efficacy of percutaneous mitral valve repair using the MitraClip system: The results of the MitraSwiss registry. Heart. 2013;**99**:1034-1040

[31] Armoiry X, Brochet É, Lefevre T, et al. Initial French experience of percutaneous mitral valve repair with the MitraClip: A multicentre national registry. Archives of Cardiovascular Diseases. 2013;**106**:287-294

[32] Nickenig G, Estevez-Loureiro R, Franzen O, et al. Percutaneous mitral valve edge-to-edge Repair: In-hospital results and 1-year follow-up of 628 patients of the 2011-2012 pilot European Sentinel Registry. Journal of the American College of Cardiology. 2014;**64**:875-884

[33] Schillinger W, Hünlich M, Baldus S, et al. Acute outcomes after MitraClip® therapy in highly aged patients: Results from the German TRAnscatheter Mitral valve Interventions (TRAMI) Registry. EuroIntervention. 2013;**9**:84-90

[34] Puls M, Lubos E, Boekstegers P, et al. One-year outcomes and predictors of mortality after MitraClip therapy in contemporary clinical practice: Results from the German transcatheter mitral valve interventions registry. European Heart Journal. 2016;**37**:703-712

[35] Yeo KK, Yap J, Yamen E, et al. Percutaneous mitral valve repair with the MitraClip: Early results from the MitraClip Asia-Pacific Registry (MARS). EuroIntervention. 2014;**10**:620-625

[36] Sorajja P, Mack M, Vemulapalli S, et al. Initial experience with commercial transcatheter mitral valve repair in the United States. Journal of the American College of Cardiology. 2016;**67**:1129-1140

[37] Auricchio A, Schillinger W, Meyer S, et al. Correction of mitral regurgitation in nonresponders to cardiac resynchronization therapy by MitraClip improves symptoms and promotes reverse remodeling. Journal of the American College of Cardiology. 2011;**58** 2283-2289

[38] Franzen O, Van Der Heyden J, Baldus S, et al. MitraClip® therapy in patients with end-stage systolic heart failure. European Journal of Heart Failure. 2011;**13**:569-576

[39] Siegel RJ, Biner S, Rafique AM, et al. The acute hemodynamic effects of mitraclip therapy. Journal of the American College of Cardiology. 2011;**57**:1658-1665

[40] Biner S, Siegel RJ, Feldman T, et al. Acute effect of percutaneous MitraClip therapy in patients with haemodynamic decompensation. European Journal of Heart Failure. 2012;**14**:939-945

[41] Gaemperli O, Biaggi P, Gugelmann R, et al. Real-time left ventricular pressure-volume loops during percutaneous mitral valve repair with the mitraclip system. Circulation. 2013;**127**:1018-1027

[42] Chevalier P, Burri H, Fahrat F, et al. Perioperative outcome and long-term survival of surgery for acute post-infarction mitral regurgitation. European Journal of Cardio-Thoracic Surgery. 2004;**26**:330-335

[43] Bilge M, Alemdar R, Yasar AS. Successful percutaneous mitral valve repair with the mitraclip system of acute mitral regurgitation due to papillary muscle rupture as complication of acute myocardial infarction. Catheterization and Cardiovascular Interventions. 2014;**83**:E137-E140

[44] Estévez-Loureiro R, Arzamendi D, Freixa X, et al. Percutaneous mitral valve repair for acute mitral regurgitation after an acute myocardial infarction. Journal of the American College of Cardiology. 2015;**66**:91-92

[45] van Boven W-JP, Gerritsen WB, Driessen AH, et al. Myocardial oxidative stress, and cell injury comparing three different techniques for coronary artery bypass grafting. European Journal of Cardio-Thoracic Surgery. 2008;**34**:969-975

[46] Leurent G, Corbineau H, Donal E. Uncontrolled daily pulmonary oedema due to severe mitral regurgitation emergently and effectively corrected by Mitraclip(R) implantation. European Heart Journal: Acute Cardiovascular Care. 2015;**5**:1-2

[47] Maisano F, Skantharaja R, Denti P, et al. Mitral annuloplasty. Multimedia Manual of Cardiothoracic Surgery MMCTS/European Association for Cardiothoracic Surgery 2009; 2009: mmcts.2008.003640

[48] Goldstein D, Moskowitz AJ, Gelijns AC, et al. Two-Year outcomes of surgical treatment of severe ischemic mitral regurgitation. The New England Journal of Medicine 2016;**374**:344-353

[49] Grasso C, Ohno Y, Attizzani GF, et al. Percutaneous mitral valve repair with the MitraClip system for severe mitral regurgitation in patients with surgical mitral valve repair failure. Journal of the American College of Cardiology. 2014;**63**:836-838

[50] Estévez-Loureiro R, Arzamendi D, Carrasco-Chinchilla F, et al. Usefulness of MitraClip for the treatment of mitral regurgitation secondary to failed surgical annuloplasty. Revista Española de Cardiología (English Edition) 2016;**69**:446-448

[51] Grasso C, Capodanno D, Scandura S, et al. One- and twelve-month safety and efficacy outcomes of patients undergoing edge-to-edge percutaneous mitral valve repair (from the grasp registry). American Journal of Cardiology. 2013;**111**:1482-1487

[52] Franzen O, Baldus S, Rudolph V, et al. Acute outcomes of MitraClip therapy for mitral regurgitation in high-surgical-risk patients: Emphasis on adverse valve morphology and severe left ventricular dysfunction. European Heart Journal. 2010;**31**:1373-1381

[53] Paranskaya L, D'Ancona G, Bozdag-Turan I, et al. Residual mitral valve regurgitation after percutaneous mitral valve repair with the MitraClip?? system is a risk factor for adverse one-year outcome. Catheterization and Cardiovascular Interventions. 2013;**81**:609-617

[54] Taramasso M, Maisano F, Latib A, et al. Clinical outcomes of MitraClip for the treatment of functional mitral regurgitation. EuroIntervention. 2014;**10**:746-752

[55] Glower DD, Kar S, Trento A, et al. Percutaneous mitral valve repair for mitral regurgitation in high-risk patients: Results of the EVEREST II study. Journal of the American College of Cardiology. 2014;**64**:172-181

[56] Ussia GP, Cammalleri V, Sarkar K, et al. Quality of life following percutaneous mitral valve repair with the MitraClip System. International Journal of Cardiology. 2012;**155**: 194-200

[57] Whitlow PL, Feldman T, Pedersen WR, et al. Acute and 12-month results with catheter-based mitral valve leaflet repair: The EVEREST II (Endovascular Valve Edge-to-Edge Repair) High Risk Study. Journal of the American College of Cardiology. 2012;**59**:130-139

[58] Swaans MJ, Bakker ALM, Alipour A, et al. Survival of transcatheter mitral valve repair compared with surgical and conservative treatment in high-surgical-risk patients. JACC: Cardiovascular Interventions. 2014;**7**:875-881

[59] Velazquez EJ, Samad Z, Al-Khalidi HR, et al. The MitraClip and survival in patients with mitral regurgitation at high risk for surgery: A propensity-matched comparison. American Heart Journal. 2015;**170**:1050-1059

[60] Giannini C, Fiorelli F, De Carlo M, et al. Comparison of percutaneous mitral valve repair versus conservative treatment in severe functional mitral regurgitation. American Journal of Cardiology. 2016;**117**:271-277

[61] Enriquez-Sarano M, Akins CW, Vahanian A. Mitral regurgitation. Lancet. 2009;**373**: 1382-1394

[62] Grayburn PA, Foster E, Sangli C, et al. Relationship between the magnitude of reduction in mitral regurgitation severity and left ventricular and left atrial reverse remodeling after mitraclip therapy. Circulation. 2013;**128**:1667-1674

[63] Schmidt FP, Von Bardeleben RS, Nikolai P, et al. Immediate effect of the MitraClip® procedure on mitral ring geometry in primary and secondary mitral regurgitation. European Heart Journal Cardiovascular Imaging. 2013;**14**:851-857

[64] Schueler R, Momcilovic D, Weber M, et al. Acute changes of mitral valve geometry during interventional edge-to-edge repair with the MitraClip system are associated with mid-term outcomes in patients with functional valve disease: Preliminary results from a prospective single-center study. Circulation: Cardiovascular Interventions. 2014;**7**:390-399

[65] Seeburger J, Rinaldi M, Nielsen SL, et al. Off-pump transapical implantation of artificial neo-chordae to correct mitral regurgitation: The tact trial (transapical artificial chordae tendinae) proof of concept. Journal of the American College of Cardiology. 2014;**63**:914-919

[66] Colli A, Manzan E, Rucinskas K, et al. Acute safety and efficacy of the NeoChord procedure. Interactive CardioVascular and Thoracic Surgery. 2015;**20**:575-581

[67] De Bonis M, Lapenna E, Maisano F, et al. Long-Term results (≤18 years) of the edge-To-edge mitral valve repair without annuloplasty in degenerative mitral regurgitation implications for the percutaneous approach. Circulation. 2014;**130**:S19-S24

[68] Schofer J, Siminiak T, Haude M, et al. Percutaneous mitral annuloplasty for functional mitral regurgitation: Results of the CARILLON mitral annuloplasty device european union study. Circulation. 2009;**120**:326-333

[69] Maselli D, Guarracino F, Chiaramonti F, et al. Percutaneous mitral annuloplasty: An anatomic study of human coronary sinus and its relation with mitral valve annulus and coronary arteries. Circulation. 2006;**114**:377-380

[70] Degen H, Schneider T, Wilke J, et al. Coronary sinus devices for treatment of functional mitral valve regurgitation. Solution or dead end? Herz. 2013;**38**:490-500

[71] Siminiak T, Wu JC, Haude M, et al. Treatment of functional mitral regurgitation by percutaneous annuloplasty: Results of the TITAN Trial. European Journal of Heart Failure. 2012;**14**:931-938

[72] Spoor MT, Geltz A, Bolling SF. Flexible versus nonflexible mitral valve rings for congestive heart failure: Differential durability of repair. Circulation. 2006;**114**:I67-71

[73] Maisano F, La Canna G, Latib A, et al. First-in-man transseptal implantation of a surgical-like mitral valve annuloplasty device for functional mitral regurgitation. JACC: Cardiovascular Interventions. 2014;**7**:1326-1328

[74] Maisano F, Taramasso M, Nickenig G, et al. Cardioband, a transcatheter surgical-like direct mitral valve annuloplasty system: Early results of the feasibility trial. European Heart Journal. 2016;**37**:817-825

[75] Kay JH, Magidson O, Meihaus JE. The surgical treatment of mitral insufficiency and combined mitral stenosis and insufficiency using the heart-lung machine. American Journal of Cardiology. 1962;**9**:300-306

[76] Siminiak T, Dankowski R, Baszko A, et al. Percutaneous direct mitral annuloplasty using the Mitralign Bident system: Description of the method and a case report. Kardiologia Polska 2013;**71**:1287-1292

[77] Nickenig G, Schueler R, Dager A, et al. Treatment of chronic functional mitral valve regurgitation with a percutaneous annuloplasty system. Journal of the American College of Cardiology. 2016;**67**:2927-2936

[78] Latib A, Ancona MB, Ferri L, et al. Percutaneous direct annuloplasty with cardioband to treat recurrent mitral regurgitation after MitraClip implantation. JACC: Cardiovascular Interventions. 2016;**9**:e191-e192

[79] Abdelrahman N, Chowdhury MA, Al Nooryani A, et al. A case of dilated cardiomyopathy and severe mitral regurgitation treated using a combined percutaneous approach of MitraClip followed by CARILLON ® mitral contour system. Cardiovascular Revascularization Medicine. 2016;**17**:578-581

[80] Krishnaswamy A, Mick S, Navia J, et al. Transcatheter mitral valve replacement: A frontier in cardiac intervention. Cleveland Clinic Journal of Medicine. 2016;**83**:S10-S17

[81] Ussia GP, Quadri A, Cammalleri V, et al. Percutaneous transfemoral-transseptal implantation of a second-generation CardiAQ™ mitral valve bioprosthesis: First procedure description and 30-day follow-up. EuroIntervention. 2016;**11**:1126-1131

[82] Cheung A, Webb J, Verheye S, et al. Short-term results of transapical transcatheter mitral valve implantation for mitral regurgitation. Journal of the American College of Cardiology. 2014;**64**:1814-1819

[83] Abdul-Jawad Altisent O, Dumont E, Dagenais F, et al. Initial Experience of transcatheter mitral valve replacement with a novel transcatheter mitral valve procedural and 6-Month Follow-Up results. Journal of the American College of Cardiology. 2015;**66**:1011-1019

[84] Quarto C, Davies S, Duncan A, et al. Transcatheter mitral valve implantation. Innovations: Technology & Techniques in Cardiothoracic & Vascular Surgery 2016;**11**:174-178

[85] Muller DWM, Farivar RS, Jansz P, et al. Transcatheter mitral valve replacement for patients with symptomatic mitral regurgitation. Journal of the American College of Cardiology. 2016;**69**:381-391

[86] Dreyfus GD, Martin RP, Chan KMJ, et al. Functional tricuspid regurgitation: A need to revise our understanding. Journal of the American College of Cardiology. 2015;**65**:2331-2336

[87] Taramasso M, Vanermen H, Maisano F, et al. The growing clinical importance of secondary tricuspid regurgitation. Journal of the American College of Cardiology. 2012;**59**: 703-710

[88] Nath J, Foster E, Heidenreich PA. Impact of tricuspid regurgitation on Long-Term survival. Journal of the American College of Cardiology. 2004;**43**:405-409

[89] Topilsky Y, Nkomo VT, Vatury O, et al. Clinical outcome of isolated tricuspid regurgitation. JACC: Cardiovascular Imaging 2014;**7**:1185-1194

[90] Porter A, Shapira Y, Wurzel M, et al. Tricuspid regurgitation late after mitral valve replacement: Clinical and echocardiographic evaluation. Journal of Heart Valve Disease. 1999;**8**:57-62

[91] Kwak JJ, Kim YJ, Kim MK, et al. Development of tricuspid regurgitation late after left-sided valve surgery: A single-center experience with long-term echocardiographic examinations. American Heart Journal. 2008;**155**:732-737

[92] Dreyfus GD, Corbi PJ, Chan KMJ, et al. Secondary tricuspid regurgitation or dilatation: Which should be the criteria for surgical repair? Annals of Thoracic Surgery. 2005;**79**:127-132

[93] Rogers JH, Bolling SF. Surgical approach to functional tricuspid regurgitation: Should we be more aggressive? Current Opinion in Cardiology. 2014;**29**:1-7

[94] Teman NR, Huffman LC, Krajacic M, et al. 'Prophylactic' tricuspid repair for functional tricuspid regurgitation. Annals of Thoracic Surgery. 2014;**97**:1520-1524

[95] Kim Y-J, Kwon D-A, Kim H-K, et al. Determinants of surgical outcome in patients with isolated tricuspid regurgitation. Circulation. 2009;**120**:1672-1678

[96] Taramasso M, Pozzoli A, Guidotti A, et al. Percutaneous tricuspid valve therapies: The new frontier. European Heart Journal. 2017; **38**:639-647

[97] Rogers JH, Bolling SF. The tricuspid valve: Current perspective and evolving management of tricuspid regurgitation. Circulation. 2009;**119**:2718-2725

[98] Navia JL, Nowicki ER, Blackstone EH, et al. Surgical management of secondary tricuspid valve regurgitation: Annulus, commissure, or leaflet procedure? The Journal of Thoracic and Cardiovascular Surgery. 2010;**139**:1473-1482.e5

[99] Braun D, Nabauer M, Orban M, et al. Transcatheter treatment of severe tricuspid regurgitation using the edge-to-edge repair technique. EuroIntervention. 2017;12:e1837-e1844

[100] Schofer J, Bijuklic K, Tiburtius C, et al. First-in-human transcatheter tricuspid valve repair in a patient with severely regurgitant tricuspid valve. Journal of the American College of Cardiology. 2015;**65**:1190-1195

[101] Kuwata S, Taramasso M, Nietlispach F, et al. Transcatheter tricuspid valve repair toward a surgical standard: First-in-man report of direct annuloplasty with a cardioband device to treat severe functional tricuspid regurgitation. European Heart Journal. 2017 Jan 10. pii: ehw660. doi: 10.1093/eurheartj/ehw660. [Epub ahead of print]

[102] Schofer J. Transcatheter interventions for tricuspid regurgitation: Trialign and Mitralign. EuroIntervention. 2016;**12**:Y119-Y120

[103] Taramasso M, Nietlispach F, Zuber M, et al. Transcatheter repair of persistent tricuspid regurgitation after MitraClip with the TriCinch system: Interventional valve treatment toward the surgical standard. European Heart Journal. 2016 Dec 9. pii: ehw541. [Epub ahead of print]

[104] Puri R, Rodés-cabau J, Heart Q, et al. Transcatheter interventions for tricuspid regurgitation: The FORMA Repair System. Eurointervention 2016;12:Y113-Y115

Section 4

Cardiogenic Shock

Chapter 7

Cardiogenic Shock

Abdulwahab Hritani, Suhail Allaqaband and
M. Fuad Jan

Additional information is available at the end of the chapter

http://dx.doi.org/10.5772/intechopen.69059

Abstract

Cardiogenic shock is the second most common cause of circulatory shock, occurs secondary to myocardial infarction, which accounts for 80% of the cases, and remains one of the leading causes of death in patients with acute myocardial infarction. Cardiogenic shock carries a high morbidity and mortality despite recent advances in medical and mechanical therapies. Cardiogenic shock also occurs in non-acute coronary syndrome conditions, such as Takotsubo cardiomyopathy, fulminant myocarditis, end stage heart failure, and others. In this chapter, we provide a brief review on the pathophysiology, diagnosis, and acute management of cardiogenic shock patients. We will focus more on the management of acute coronary syndrome related cardiogenic shock, given that it is the most common etiology.

Keywords: cardiogenic shock, acute coronary syndrome, hemodynamic support, mechanical circulatory support devices, vasopressors, inotropes

1. Definition

Circulatory shock is defined as the failure to meet the body's cellular oxygen demands. It typically occurs when the systolic blood pressure falls below 90 mmHg or the mean arterial blood pressure falls below 65 mmHg for 30 min. In circulatory shock there are signs of tissue hypoperfusion such as altered mental status, decreased urine output (<0.5 ml/kg/h), cold and clammy skin, and elevated serum lactic acid level (>1.5 mmol/l) [1].

Cardiogenic shock (CS) is the shock that results from cardiac causes and can be defined as a circulatory failure in addition to severely reduced cardiac index (<1.8 L/min/m^2 without support or <2.0–2.2 L/min/m with support) in the presence of adequate filling pressures (left ventricular end diastolic pressure (LVEDP) > 18 mmHg or right ventricular end diastolic pressure >10–15 mmHg) [2].

To differentiate CS from other types of shock, the following general hemodynamic measures can be used with the help of echocardiography or pulmonary artery catheterization (**Table 1**).

	Cardiogenic	Distributive (e.g. septic shock)	Hypovolemic	Obstructive	
				PE	Tamponade
PCWP/LVEDP	↑	Unchanged or ↓	↓	Usually unchanged	↑
SVR	↑ or unchanged	↓	↑	↑	↑
CI/CO	↓	↑ But might be ↓	↓	↓	↓

PCWP, pulmonary capillary wedge pressure, LVEDP, left ventricular end diastolic pressure; SVR, systematic vascular resistance; CI, cardiac index; CO, cardiac output.

Table 1. General hemodynamic measures to differentiate between cardiogenic shock and other types of shock.

2. Epidemiology

CS is the second most common type of circulatory shock representing 16% of patients presenting with shock [3]. CS complicates up to 8.6% of patients with ST segment elevation myocardial infarction (STEMI) and about 2.5% of patients with non-ST segment elevation myocardial infarction (NSTEMI), and remains one of the leading causes of death in patients presenting with acute myocardial infarction (AMI) [4]. Despite the advancement in the medical and technological management, CS carries a poor prognosis with high morbidity and mortality (40–60% of patients with CS will die within 6 months) [5–7].

AMI is the most common cause of CS, and patients with AMI older than 75 years tend to present more frequently with CS than patients younger than 75 [2–4, 8].

3. Etiology and pathophysiology

Acute coronary syndrome (ACS) leading to ischemia and left ventricular (or right ventricular) failure is the leading cause of CS and represents around 80% of CS cases (8% of those are caused by mechanical complications of AMI such as ventricular septal rupture, free wall rupture, papillary muscle rupture and acute mitral regurgitations) [7].

The pathophysiology of ischemia leading to CS is illustrated as a vicious cycle in **Figure 1**. AMI may lead to severe left ventricular (LV) dysfunction and pump failure. The hypotension that accompanies CS leads to the release of inflammatory cytokines and catecholamines leading to increased contractility, which in turn leads to increased myocardial oxygen demand that

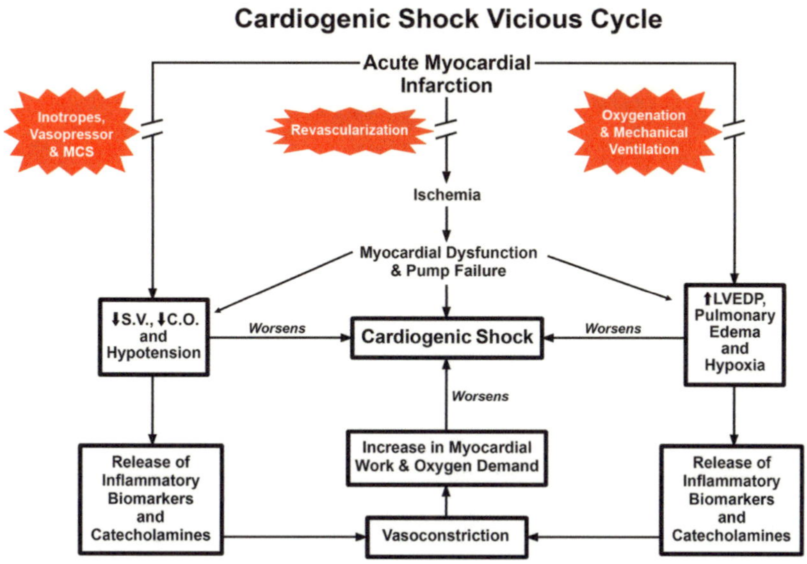

Figure 1. The vicious cycle of cardiogenic shock. SV, stroke volume; CO, cardiac output; LVEDP, left ventricular end diastolic pressure; MCS, mechanical circulatory support.

causes worsening of the ischemia and shock state. The increase in catecholamines also causes peripheral vasoconstriction that in turn leads to an increase in the afterload, worsening the ischemia and the shock state [2].

CS also occurs in the absence of coronary artery disease; those etiologies represent around 20% of CS cases. The non-ACS-related CS patients tend to do slightly better than those with ACS [7]. Those conditions may include hypertrophic cardiomyopathy, end stage heart failure, acute fulminant myocarditis, severe valvular stenosis, and acute valvular regurgitation secondary to trauma or infection. CS complicates about 10% of patients presenting with Takotsubo cardiomyopathy and carries a poorer prognosis than the rest of Takotsubo cardiomyopathy population [1, 9, 10].

CS could also occur secondary to right ventricular (RV) dysfunction and failure secondary to RV ischemia, acute pulmonary embolism, pulmonary hypertension (PH) and others [2, 11, 12].

The right ventricle is affected in nearly 50% of inferior STEMI patients, however, RV infarction leading to CS occurs in approximately 5% of CS cases caused by AMI; despite that, it carries high mortality similar to that of LV failure. RV failure leads to decreased transpulmonary delivery of LV preload and intraventricular dependence, which in turn may lead to decreased LV filling. The RV end diastolic pressure in CS secondary to RV failure is usually very high, exceeding 20 mmHg [2, 11–13].

Figure 2 summarizes the most common causes of CS.

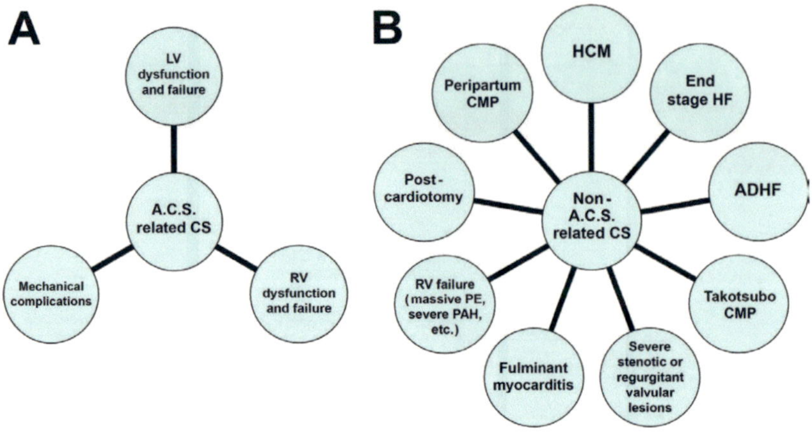

Figure 2. The most common causes of cardiogenic shock. (A) ACS represents 80% of CS cases, (B) non-ACS etiologies, which represent 20% of CS causes. ACS, acute coronary syndrome; LV, left ventricle; RV, right ventricle; HCM, hypertrophic cardiomyopathy; ADHF, acute decompensated heart failure; CMP, cardiomyopathy; PE, pulmonary embolism; PAH, pulmonary arterial hypertension.

4. Diagnosis and clinical presentation

The diagnosis of CS requires a high index of suspicion due to its high morbidity and mortality. It should be noted that up to 70% of patients with CS will develop shock later during their hospital stay [4].

Most patients with CS are critically ill and might complain of chest pain and/or dyspnea. There are physical exam findings that are more specific to CS than other types of shock, such as elevated jugular venous pressure (JVP), S3 gallop and the presence of pulmonary rales. In fact, the presence of elevated JVP > 8 cmH_2O and rales more than one-third of the lung bases predicted CS with very high sensitivity and specificity [14]. The risk factors that are associated with a higher risk of CS in ACS patients are female gender, diabetes mellitus, anterior wall MI, prior history of MI and older age [14, 15].

Other signs and symptoms of CS are generally those of tissue hypoperfusion, such as the presence of hypotension (SBP < 90 mmHg or MAP < 65 mmHg) in addition to tachycardia, altered mentation, decreased urine output and cold and clammy skin.

Electrocardiogram (ECG) and chest X-ray (CXR) should be obtained in all patients presenting with shock. CXR in CS may show pulmonary edema, pleural effusion, pulmonary vascular congestion or enlarged cardiac silhouette. Cardiac troponin is also mandatory for all patients with suspicion of shock from cardiac causes at the time of presentation and then repeated within 3–6 h [16].

ECG can help diagnose acute STEMI, Q waves or any active cardiac ischemia; although in a routine general practice only about 50% of patients with suspected NSTEMI will have ECG changes that are diagnostic of myocardial infarction at the time of presentation [17].

http://dx.doi.org/10.5772/intechopen.69059

The presentation ECG carries prognostic information, as well, and can identify high-risk patients. In an analysis from the SHOCK trial [17], which included CS patients caused by AMI, a higher baseline heart rate was associated with a higher one-year mortality. Also, in CS patients secondary to inferior MI who received medical management, a longer QRS duration and a higher sum of ST segment depression in all leads were associated with a higher one-year mortality [17].

Echocardiography is of utmost importance in the evaluation of shock patients especially when the etiology of shock is not well established. It is noninvasive and readily available at bedside. It helps identify severe valvular regurgitant or stenotic lesions, evaluate for ventricular or septal rupture post-AMI and check for cardiac tamponade.

Two-dimensional echocardiography allows for the identification of LV ejection fraction, assessment of segmental wall motion abnormalities and RV function. Doppler echocardiography allows for the assessment of early mitral filling velocity (E) and the mitral annulus tissue velocity (e') which greatly helps the clinician identifying elevated LV filling pressures with excellent sensitivity and specificity. E:e' > 15 correlates with LVEDP > 14 mmHg and E/e' < 8 correlates with normal LVEDP [18, 19].

Pulmonary artery (PA) catheterization—Swan-Ganz catheter—is an excellent tool for confirming the diagnosis and guiding the medical and mechanical management. In CS, there is an increase in the right atrial (RA) pressure, RV systolic and diastolic pressures and pulmonary capillary wedge pressure (PCWP), and a decrease in the cardiac output and index (**Figure 3**). SVR can also be calculated using the PA catheter and is frequently elevated in CS patients. Currently, the main indication for PA catheter use is to establish the diagnosis of CS when the

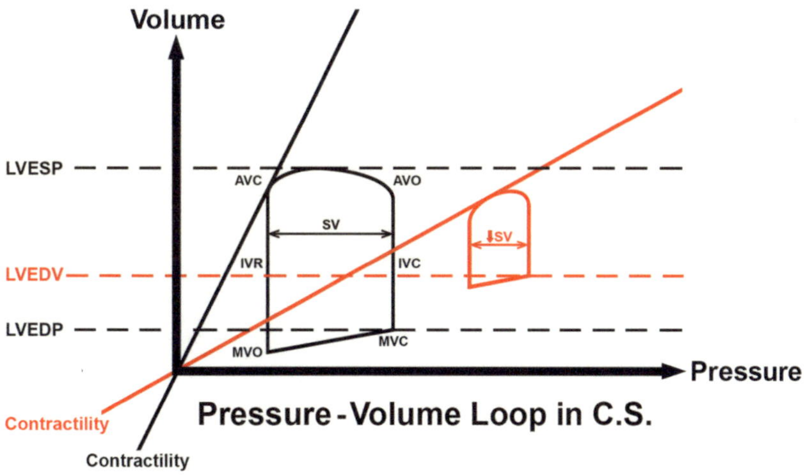

Figure 3. The pressure volume loop in cardiogenic shock. The left loop is that of a normal individual while the right one is the CS loop. In CS, there is an increase in LVEDP and LVDEV; there is a decrease in contractility and SV. LVEDP, left ventricular end diastolic pressure; LVESP, left ventricular end systolic pressure; LVEDV, left ventricular end diastolic volume; SV, stroke volume; AVO, aortic valve opens; AVC, aortic valve closes; MVO, mitral valve opens; MVC, mitral valve closes; IVC, isovolumetric contraction; IVR, isovolumetric relaxation.

clinical picture is not clear, or when hemodynamic stabilization is not achieved despite escalating doses of vasopressors and inotropes. PA catheter is also recommended when mechanical circulatory support devices are considered. It should be noted that the routine use of PA catheter is discouraged in patients with a confirmed diagnosis and those who stabilize rather quickly [20].

5. Treatment

Since the most common etiology behind CS is ACS, the mainstay of therapy is coronary revascularization to relieve the vicious cycle of ischemia-shock state. Treatment also involves general supportive measures, pharmacotherapy, vasopressors, inotropes and mechanical circulatory support (MCS) in the setting of refractory shock (**Figure 4**).

5.1. General measures and pharmacotherapy used in acute coronary syndrome

All patients with suspected AMI—STEMI or NSTEMI—should receive a loading dose of aspirin (162–325 mg) as a chew non-enteric coated capsule and a maintenance dose of aspirin should be continued indefinitely after that. A high dose statin (atorvastatin 80 mg) is also indicated in all patients presenting with AMI without contraindications and should be continued indefinitely. Treatment with high dose statins for ACS patients reduced the risk of death, recurrent myocardial infarction, stroke and the need for coronary revascularization. Oxygen therapy is indicated for all patients with hypoxemia (O_2 saturation < 90%) [16, 21].

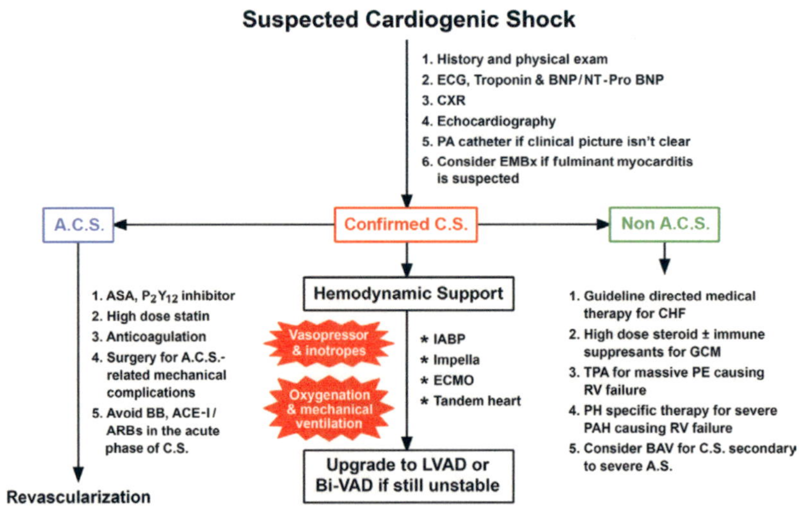

Figure 4. Cardiogenic shock treatment flow chart. CXR , chest X-ray; PA, pulmonary artery; EMBx, endomyocardial biopsy; A.C.S, acute coronary syndrome; BB, beta blockers; ACE-I, angiotensin converting enzyme inhibitors; ARB, angiotensin receptor blockers; LVAD, left ventricular assist device; Bi-VAD, biventricular assist device; CHF, congestive heart failure; GCM, giant cell myocarditis; TPA , tissue plasminogen activator; PE, pulmonary embolism; PH, pulmonary hypertension; PAH, pulmonary artery hypertension; BAV, balloon aortic valvuloplasty.

http://dx.doi.org/10.5772/intechopen.69059

Beta blockers (BB), angiotensin converting enzyme inhibitors (ACE-I) or angiotensin receptor blockers (ARB) should be avoided in patients at risk for CS [16, 21].

In patients with STEMI, a loading dose of a P2Y12 inhibitor should be administered as early as possible or at the time of primary coronary intervention (PCI) (clopidogrel 600 mg, ticagrelor 180 mg or prasugrel 60 mg). Patients with NSTEMI who are undergoing early revascularization should also receive a loading dose of a P2Y12 inhibitor as soon as possible. It should be noted that prasugrel is contraindicated in patients with prior history of stroke or transient ischemic attack (TIA) [16, 21–23].

All patients with STEMI undergoing PCI should receive anticoagulation unless they have contra-indications. Unfractionated heparin (UFH) can be used with or without glycoprotein (GP) IIb/IIIA inhibitors. The recommended dose of UFH is 50–70 units/kg as IV bolus if used with GP IIb/IIIa inhibitors to achieve a therapeutic activated clotting time (ACT) of 200–250 s, or 70–100 u/kg as a bolus if used without GP IIb/IIIa inhibitors to achieve therapeutic ACT of (250–300 s). Bivalirudin can be used in STEMI patients as well, and is preferred as a monotherapy over the combination of UFH-GP IIb/IIIa inhibitor in patients at high risk for bleeding [21].

In patients with NSTEMI the anticoagulation regimen differs slightly from patients with STEMI, UFH can be used with a loading dose of 60 u/kg (maximum dose of 4000 units) followed by infusion of 12 u/kg/h with (maximum dose of 1000 u/h) adjusted to keep therapeutic activated partial thromboplastin time (PTT) during the period of treatment. Enoxaparin is another option for anticoagulation at a dose of 1 mg/kg every 12 h. Most NSTEMI patients presenting with CS will undergo early revascularization, which makes bivalirudin another good option for anticoagulation as bivalirudin is only indicated in NSTEMI patients who undergo early invasive strategy [16].

Most clinicians prefer to use UFH in the setting of CS complicating an NSTEMI given that most of these patients will undergo early invasive strategy, and UFH has the advantage to turn on and off, or even reverse rather easily.

GP IIb/IIIa inhibitors might be considered for NSTEMI patients undergoing early invasive strategy and are treated with dual antiplatelet therapy (DAPT) [16].

5.2. Revascularization

Early revascularization is the cornerstone of treatment in AMI patients presenting with CS. The randomized SHOCK trial proved a statistically significant mortality benefit at 6 months in AMI patients complicated by CS treated with emergency revascularization as opposed to medical stabilization [5]. The non-randomized SHOCK registry also showed the same mortality benefit of early revascularization in patients older than 75 [24].

The goal in STEMI patients is first medical contact (FMC) to device time of less than 90 min, and revascularization can still be done even up to 12 h after ischemic symptoms onset. But, in patients with CS complicating a STEMI, revascularization should be performed regardless of the time of symptoms onset. It is also reasonable to intervene on non-infarct arteries in STEMI patients complicated by CS at the time of PCI [21].

Early revascularization within 2 h of presentation should be done in all NSTEMI patients with CS, as well as those with high-risk features (such as refractory angina, electrical instability, signs of heart failure or worsening mitral regurgitation, as well as sustained ventricular tachycardia or fibrillation) [16].

PCI is not the only option for revascularization; coronary artery bypass grafting (CABG) should be considered especially if successful PCI is not feasible, there are mechanical complications such as ventricular septal or papillary muscle rupture, and in those with left main disease or three vessels, CAD. Emergent CABG can be done within 2–4 h in capable facilities [16, 25].

Thirty-six percent of patients undergoing revascularization in the SHOCK trial underwent CABG; those patients were more likely to be diabetic and have left main or three vessels CAD. The survival rate at 30 days and at 1 year was similar between those who underwent PCI or CABG in the SHOCK trial [26].

Compared to patients without CS undergoing CABG, those with CS were more likely to have had suffered AMI within 24 h prior to CABG, were more likely to have left main disease, have lower ejection fraction and were more likely to have intra-aortic balloon pump (IABP) used preoperatively [25].

It should be noted that patients with CS undergoing CABG have worse morbidity and mortality and longer intensive care unit (ICU) stay than those without CS. And even though older age was associated with higher morbidity and mortality, around 70% of patients with CS above the age of 75 survived this major surgery making CABG suitable for carefully selected elderly CS patients [25].

5.3. Fibrinolysis

If PCI cannot be performed within 120 min of FMC in STEMI patients, fibrinolytics can be used in those without contraindications and even up to 12 h after symptoms onset, and up to 24 h in those with large areas of ischemia, hemodynamic instability, or have clinical or ECG signs of continuous ischemia. **Table 2** summarizes the absolute contraindications to fibrinolysis [21].

Any prior intracranial hemorrhage	Any active bleeding or bleeding diathesis (not including menses)
Known malignant intracranial neoplasm	Suspected aortic dissection
Known cerebral structural vascular lesion	Ischemic stroke within the past 3 months (except for those with ischemic stroke in the past 4.5 h)
Severe uncontrolled refractory hypertension	Any significant closed head or facial trauma in the past 3 months
Intracranial or intraspinal surgery in the past 2 months	If streptokinase is used, prior treatment within the previous 6 months (streptokinase is antigenic)

Table 2. Absolute contraindications to fibrinolytics [21].

Patients with RV infarction secondary to proximal right coronary artery (RCA) occlusion with extensive clot burden might be resistant to fibrinolytic therapy; there is also a higher rate of re-occlusion after thrombolysis of the RCA [13, 27, 28].

Patients with CS secondary to STEMI who are treated with fibrinolytics should be transferred immediately to a PCI-capable facility after receiving fibrinolysis.

In patients with NSTEMI, fibrinolytics are contraindicated; those patients should be stabilized and transferred immediately to a PCI-capable facility for coronary angiography and revascularization [16].

5.4. Vasopressors and inotropes

There is no optimal vasopressor or inotrope in the setting of CS, but catecholamines are the most frequently used vasopressors, with norepinephrine and dopamine being the most widely used. Catecholamines exhibit their effects through the stimulation of A1, B1, B2, and dopaminergic receptors (D1 and D2) [9, 29].

Norepinephrine is a potent A1 agonist; it induces an increase in systolic blood pressure (SBP), diastolic blood pressure (DBP), and the pulse pressure. Norepinephrine has minimal effect on myocardial contractility and HR [29].

Dopamine produces a multitude of effects at different doses: at lower doses (<3 ug/kg/min), it works primarily on the D1 receptors and causes coronary and renal vasodilatation; at intermediate doses (3–10 ug/kg/min), dopamine stimulates the B receptors and causes an increase in inotropy and HR; and at higher doses (10–20 ug/kg/min), dopamine works primarily on A1 receptors and causes vasoconstriction. The renal vasodilatory effect—so-called renal dose—of low dose dopamine remains controversial, and glomerular filtration rate (GFR) does not change with use of those renal doses of dopamine [30, 31].

Epinephrine has high affinity towards A1, B1 and B2 receptors, with B effects more pronounced at lower doses and Alpha effects at higher doses. Prolonged use of epinephrine is associated with direct cardiac toxicity through damage to the arterial wall that results in myocardial necrosis and stimulation of myocyte apoptosis [29, 32].

Vasopressin or "antidiuretic hormone" is a non-adrenergic vasopressor; it stimulates the V1 and V2 receptors. The stimulation of the V1 receptors causes vasoconstriction while the stimulation of the V2 receptors enhances water reabsorption in the renal collecting ducts. It augments the pressor effect of norepinephrine and has no effect on cardiac output (CO). Vasopressin's pressor effect is relatively preserved during the acidotic state that develops in most shock patients [29, 33].

Dobutamine is a B1 and B2 agonist; it primarily induces an inotropic effect, exhibits a modest increase in HR and causes peripheral vasodilatation through the stimulation of B2 receptors. Dobutamine induces an increase in the cardiac output and a reduction in the LVEDP. Pharmacologic tolerance to dobutamine usually develops after 72 h of use. Dobutamine could induce arrhythmias, myocardial ischemia and tachycardia, especially at higher doses (>15 ug/kg/min), but these effects are reversed rather rapidly due to the short half-life of the drug (2.3 min).

The prolonged use of dobutamine (7–52 days) is associated with much higher 6-month mortality [29, 30, 34–36].

Milrinone is a noncatecholamine inotrope and peripheral vasodilator, has lusitropic effect and has less effect on HR than dobutamine. Milrinone works through the inhibition of phosphodiesterase enzymes (PDE), which in turn, leads to an increase in intracellular cyclic adenosine monophosphate (cAMP), which leads to an increase in the rate of entry and removal of calcium from the cardiac myocytes thus increasing myocardial contractility. Milrinone has been mainly used in the treatment of advanced severe heart failure patients, and—to date—there have been head-to-head trials comparing dobutamine to milrinone. Milrinone should be avoided in advanced kidney disease patients as it is cleared renally [30, 37, 38].

Levosimendan is a calcium-sensitizing agent that enhances myocardial inotropy and lusitropy and causes peripheral vasodilation, and it is not yet approved for use in the USA. Levosimendan is associated with similar mortality rates as compared to dobutamine but it tends to cause more peripheral vasodilation and hypotension than dobutamine [30, 39, 40].

Norepinephrine is preferred over dopamine as dopamine has been associated with a higher incidence of arrhythmias and a higher rate of death at 28 days in the CS patient subgroup [3].

In CS secondary to RV infarction, IV fluids are always the first line, but the excessive administration of IV fluids beyond an RA pressure of 15 mmHg could result in the deterioration of LV performance, and the use of dobutamine in this scenario can be particularly helpful in improving myocardial performance. Despite the severe hemodynamic compromise, arrhythmias, and increased in-hospital mortality, many patients with severe RV infarction recover within 3–10 days and typically, global RV function recovers within 3–12 months [13, 29, 41].

Vasopressors and inotropes are essential in stabilizing CS patients but caution should always be taken with their use. The use of these agents causes an increase in the myocardial oxygen demand and can induce arrhythmias, and thus their use should always be individualized and guided by hemodynamic monitoring. The long-term use of inotropes is strongly discouraged, and should only be considered as a bridge to heart transplantation or ventricular assist devices (VAD) or as a palliative therapy in advanced heart failure patients [20, 29].

It is recommended to combine two small doses of vasopressors and inotropes than the use of a maximal dose of a single agent to avoid dose-related adverse events, also, the addition of vasopressin can help with "catecholamine sparing" [29]. The use of epinephrine in CS patients is associated with higher 90-day mortality independent of a prior cardiac arrest, and, thus, its use is discouraged unless it is a last resort medication [42].

Our experience with these vasoactive agents in CS has been to initiate norepinephrine followed by an inotrope and then a stepwise approach in the addition of further vasopressors and/or inotropes in the setting of refractory shock. A concomitant shock etiology, such as septic shock, should always be investigated as the choice of these agents might differ.

References [20, 29] provide further information about inotropes and their mechanism of action.

http://dx.doi.org/10.5772/intechopen.69059

6. Mechanical circulatory support devices

In certain patients with CS, hemodynamic stabilization might not be achieved despite aggressive pharmacotherapy and revascularization, as a result, percutaneous mechanical circulatory support (MCS) devices might be considered for temporary stabilization [43]. The optimal MCS device offers rapid hemodynamic stabilization along with a low complication rate. To date, no trial has shown mortality benefit with the use of these devices in CS patients.

6.1. Intra-aortic balloon pump counterpulsation

IABP counterpulsation is the most common form of percutaneous LV support. The original idea of counterpulsation started in the 1960s as an external counterpulsation device stimulating the hemidiaphragm around the distal thoracic aorta with each diastole. IABP is implanted percutaneously through either of the femoral arteries using a double lumen catheter that is 7.5–8 Fr and is placed in the thoracic aorta with its tip distal to the left subclavian artery take off, and its proximal portion above the renal vessels (**Figure 5**) [43, 44].

IABP is a form of internal counterpulsation and acts as an assisting circulatory support device that inflates during diastole and deflates during systole. Its main mechanism is by diastolic augmentation during inflation that contributes to the coronary, cerebral, and systemic circulation. The presystolic deflation lowers the impedance to systolic ejection and subsequently lowers the myocardial work and oxygen demand. IABP usually causes between 0.5 and 1.0

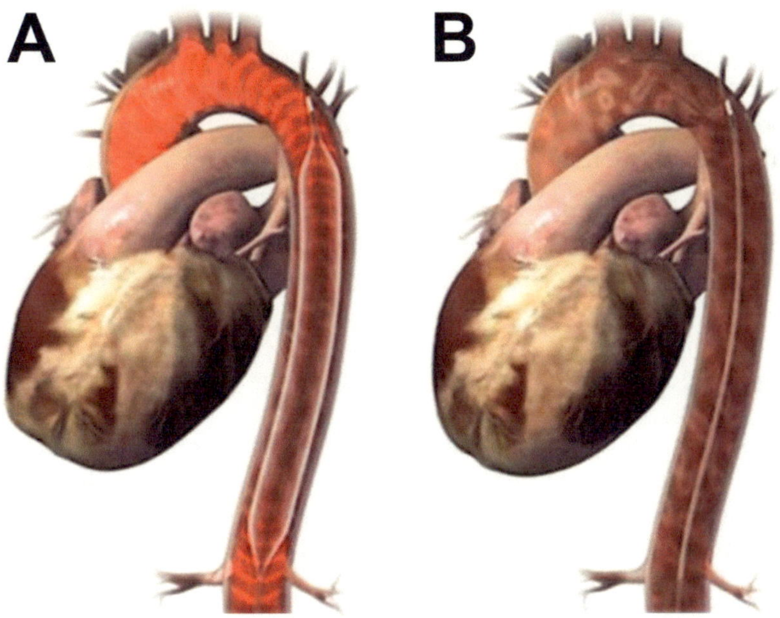

Figure 5. Intra-aortic balloon pump. The left panel shows the balloon inflation during diastole and the right panel shows the balloon deflation during systole. Reproduced with permission from Getinge.

L/min increase in the CO. IABP induces around 10% drop in SBP indicating proper systolic unloading, causes an increase in DBP which in turn improves the coronary perfusion and leads to a net increase in the mean arterial pressure (MAP). There is also an increase in the LV ejection fraction with IABP and a decrease in the LV end diastolic volume and pressure [44–47].

Despite all the hemodynamic advantages with IABP, studies have failed to show any mortality benefit with its use. The SHOCK II trial, which compared IABP vs. medical stabilization, showed no difference in mortality along with other variables such as time to hemodynamic stabilization, length of ICU stay, the dose and duration of catecholamines, and changes in renal function [6, 48].

Currently the main indication for IABP counterpulsation is CS refractory to pharmacotherapy; IABP is currently a class IIa indication for the treatment of CS complicating a STEMI in the American Heart Association/American College of Cardiology guidelines (AHA/ACC), while its routine use in CS is discouraged by the European Society of Cardiology [21, 49].

Other indications where IABP can help stabilize the patient include refractory heart failure, papillary muscle rupture or acute mitral regurgitation, ventricular septal rupture, refractory unstable angina, high-risk PCI or the inability to wean from cardiopulmonary bypass [44, 49, 50].

The absolute contraindications to IABP are significant aortic regurgitation and aortic dissection. Other relative exclusion criteria include: significant peripheral arterial disease (PAD) that precludes placement, severe coagulopathy, active infection, and cancer with metastasis [44].

The complication rate with IABP is rather rare with thrombocytopenia and fever being the most common (about 50% and 40% of patients, respectively). Other major complications include: major limb ischemia (0.9% of patients); severe access site bleeding (0.8%); amputation (0.1%); balloon leak (1%); and IABP-related mortality (0.05%). The main risk factors associated with IABP complications are female gender, PAD, small body surface area (BSA) (BSA < 1.65 m^2), and advanced age (>75 years) [51, 52].

Due to the lack of data, the use of anticoagulation with IABP is variable among different centers. Most centers, like ours, use anticoagulation, but some will not, especially with 1:1 pumping [43].

6.2. Impella devices

The Impella device is a nonpulsatile, axial flow device that is implanted inside the LV percutaneously, commonly through the femoral artery for the 2.5 Impella or with surgical cutdown, commonly through the axillary artery for the 5.0 Impella. The Impella acts as a pump that propels blood from the LV into the ascending aorta (**Figure 6**) [43].

The Impella device has three versions; 2.5 Impella, which is a 12 Fr system that provides a maximal flow of 2.5 L/min, the 5.0 Impella which is a 21 Fr system and provides a maximal flow of 5 L/min, and the CP Impella, which is a 14 Fr system that provides between 3 and 4 L/min of flow [43, 53].

http://dx.doi.org/10.5772/intechopen.69059

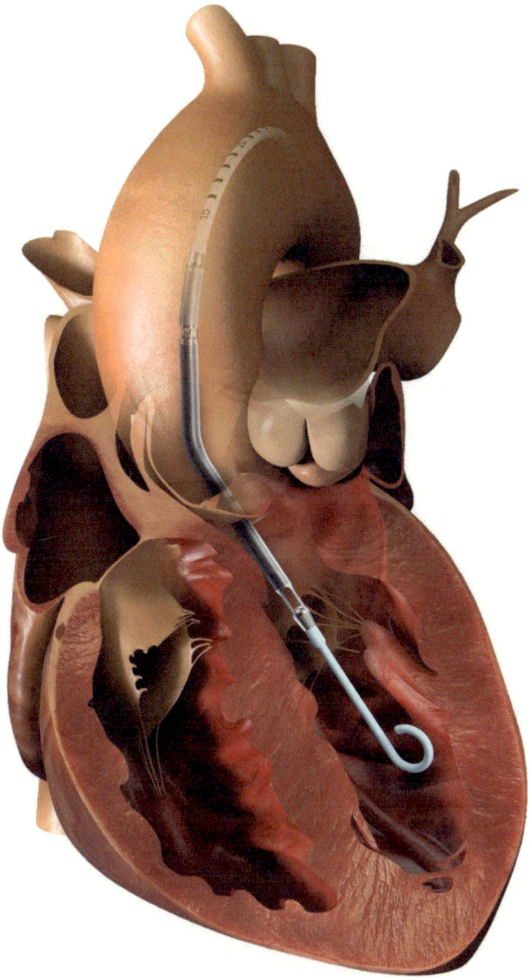

Figure 6. The Impella device with the pump inside the left ventricle and the outer catheter inside the aorta. Reproduced with permission from Abiomed.

The Impella unloads the LV, reduces the left ventricular end diastolic volume (LVEDV) and the LV wall tension and improves the systemic and coronary perfusion through an increase in the mean arterial pressure. The Impella device requires an adequate RV function (or an RV assist device) to maintain adequate LV preload, and unlike the IABP, the Impella devices can work properly through transient arrhythmias.

The main indications of the Impella devices are similar to those of the IABP counterpulsation with slight differences, for example, the Impella may worsen right-left shunting in patients with ventricular septal defect (VSD).

The main contraindications to Impella are mechanical aortic valve and LV thrombus. Other relative exclusion criteria are severe aortic regurgitation and severe PAD. The most common complications are those of vascular nature such as access site bleeding, retroperitoneal hematoma, limb ischemia and vascular injury. Hemolysis is also common with the Impella device due to the mechanical shear stress of the device on the red blood cells. In addition, anticoagulation is generally required during treatment with Impella [43, 53].

Compared to the IABP, Impella does provide greater hemodynamic support but it has not been shown to change the mortality [54]. In the largest most recent randomized controlled trial (the IMPRESS trial) comparing Impella to IABP in CS complicating AMI; 48 patients with severe CS complicating STEMI were randomized to the Impella device (24 patients) and to IABP (24 patients), the mortality at 30 days and at 6 months was similar between the two groups (50% in both groups at 6 months). Of note: those were extremely ill patients with 92% of the entire group having cardiac arrest prior to randomization, and half the mortality at 6 months was attributed to brain damage in both groups [55].

And although not commonly done, the successful use of Impella in combination with IABP has been reported [56].

A brief comparison between the Impella and the IABP is summarized in **Table 3**.

6.3. Other percutaneous mechanical circulatory support devices

The IABP and the Impella are not the only circulatory support devices used in CS, there are other—less commonly used—devices such as the Tandemheart, the extracorporeal membrane oxygenation (ECMO) and others.

The TandemHeart is left atrial to aorta support device that is inserted percutaneously and requires a transseptal puncture to access the left atrium. It bypasses the LV and pumps blood—extracorporeally—from the left atrium into the iliofemoral arterial system (**Figure 7**) [43, 57].

	Impella	IABP
ECG	Unrelated to systole or diastole	Inflates with diastole and deflates with systole
CO	Up to 5 L/min of CO	Modest increase in CO (0.5–1 L increase CO)
LVEDV	Reduces LVEDV and LVEDP	Reduces LVEDV and LVEDP
Catheter size	Between 12 and 21 Fr	7.5–8 Fr
Rhythm	Does not require a stable rhythm (although asystole and VF are poorly tolerated)	Requires a stable rhythm
Absolute contraindications	Mechanical AV, LV thrombus	Severe AR, aortic dissection
Complications	Similar complication profile of vascular injury and access site bleeding, with these complications being slightly higher with the Impella	
Mortality	No difference in mortality between both devices in CS patients complicating AMI	

CO, cardiac output; LVEDV, left ventricular end diastolic volume; LV, left ventricle; AV, aortic valve; AR, aortic regurgitation.

Table 3. A brief comparison between intra-aortic balloon pump (IABP) and Impella.

http://dx.doi.org/10.5772/intechopen.69059

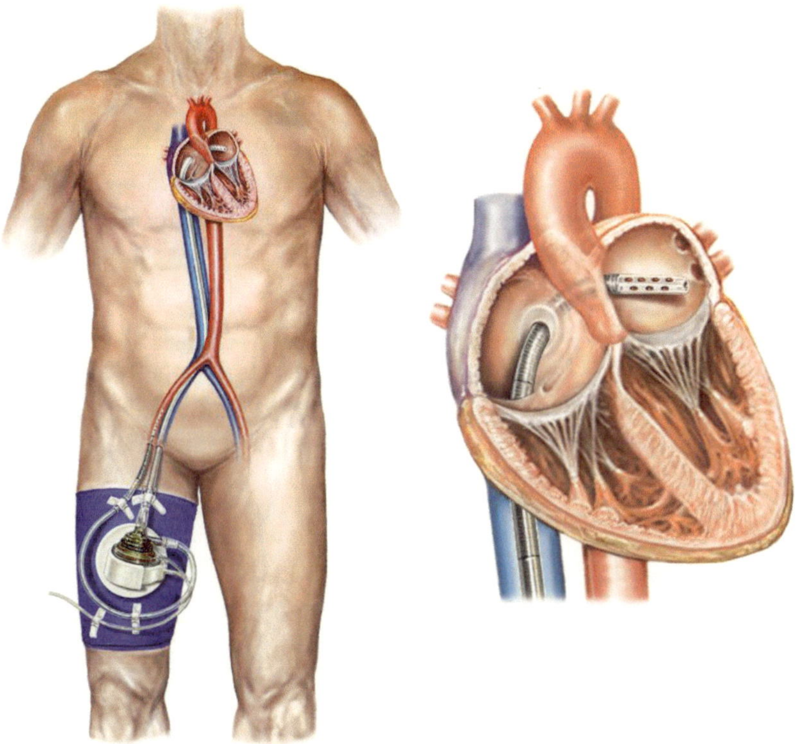

Figure 7. The TandemHeart. The left panel shows the entire system: there is a venous catheter and an arterial catheter, and the pump is situated extracorporeally. The right panel shows the transseptal puncture and how the venous catheter bypasses the left ventricle. Reproduced with permission from Tandemlife.

The TandemHeart device has two separate catheters, a 21 Fr venous catheter that goes transseptally and aspirates the LA blood and an arterial perfusion outflow cannula between 15 and 19 Fr. The TandemHeart pump can provide flow rates up to 4.5 L/min of assisted cardiac output [8, 43].

The TandemHeart has been studied in severe refractory CS patients not responding to vasopressors/inotropes in combination with IABP. The TandemHeart significantly improved the hemodynamics in this extremely ill population, along with PCWP, lactic acid levels and creatinine levels. This device can also be used as a bridge to a more definitive therapy such as left ventricular assist device (LVAD) or heart transplantation [28].

ECMO can provide a full pulmonary and/or cardiac support for those with failing hearts and/or lungs. The ECMO device can be either venoarterial (V-A ECMO) or venovenous (V-V ECMO); the V-A ECMO is ideal for those with CS and poor oxygenation while the V-V ECMO provides oxygenation only when the cardiac hemodynamics are stable. The venous catheter size is usually 20 Fr and the arterial catheter size is 17 Fr. ECMO can provide even more than 6 L/min of CO depending on catheter size and unlike other MCS devices, a trained perfusionist is required to manage the ECMO [43].

IABP, Impella, TandemHeart and ECMO can all be used in the setting of CS with slight differences in indications. They offer hemodynamic support, and it is recommended that one of these devices be inserted rapidly in CS if hemodynamic stability cannot be achieved with fluid resuscitation and/or pharmacotherapy. The experience with these devices in CS patients has been to start with an IABP along with vasopressors/inotropes, and if hemodynamic stability cannot be achieved, one may consider upgrading to one of the more powerful percutaneous MCS devices. Although these devices are FDA approved for the use of up to 6 h, they have been used successfully for days in patients with prolonged shock [43].

Our center's experience is to insert an IABP or an Impella—depending on operator's experience—rapidly in CS patients secondary to AMI prior to attempted revascularization. We recommend—as it is endorsed by the 2015 SCAI/ACC/HFSA/STS consensus document for the use of MCS devices—that one of these devices inserted rapidly if hemodynamic stability cannot be achieved rapidly with pharmacotherapy.

Other devices are being used such as the right ventricular assist devices (RVAD), which is used for the failing RV, and others. For further read on these devices and other MCS devices, refer to the 2015 SCAI/ACC/HFSA/STS expert consensus statement on the use of percutaneous MCS [43].

7. Treatment considerations in non-ACS related CS

The mechanical complications of AMI such as acute MR, papillary muscle rupture, ventricular septal rupture and LV free wall rupture are catastrophic, and carry very high mortality and are surgical emergencies. IABP helps stabilize these patients, especially acute MR patients, and the other MCS devices can be used in these situations as well.

RV failure resulting in CS also carries high mortality; ECMO or RVAD might be especially helpful in this situation. In CS secondary to massive pulmonary embolism, fibrinolysis (or mechanical thrombectomy) might be helpful, and in RV failure secondary to severe pulmonary arterial hypertension, the use of pulmonary hypertension (PH) specific therapy might provide improvement in the PA pressures and RV function.

The treatment considerations in acute decompensated heart failure (ADHF) and end stage cardiomyopathy are those of the heart failure guidelines [20], and the above-mentioned MCS devices can be used interchangeably.

In most patients with myocarditis, the course is usually self-limiting and presents with acute heart failure; on the other hand, fulminant myocarditis will present with acute severe heart failure and even CS. Close to 90% of patients with fulminant myocarditis will have full recovery with minimal long-term sequelae if recognized early. The treatment of CS secondary to fulminant myocarditis includes hemodynamic support with pharmacotherapy or MCS devices, along with high dose steroids with or without immunosuppressants if giant cell myocarditis is diagnosed [58].

8. Summary and conclusion

Cardiogenic shock still carries high morbidity and mortality and remains the leading cause of death in acute myocardial infarction patients. Early recognition and treatment is the key to improving survival, and early revascularization in CS secondary to myocardial infarction remains the cornerstone of therapy in these patients. The early use of vasopressors/inotropes is recommended in this population, and the early use of the mechanical circulatory support devices is encouraged if hemodynamic stability cannot be achieved rapidly with pharmacotherapy.

One should keep in mind the mechanical complications of myocardial infarction and the grave prognosis if not recognized early.

There is a multitude of etiologies for non-ACS related cardiogenic shock; those should be treated similarly with vasopressors/inotropes, and MCS devices, keeping in mind guidelines directed medical therapy for those with congestive heart failure.

Acknowledgements

We would like to thank Susan Nord and Jennifer Pfaff of Aurora Cardiovascular Services for their help with the manuscript and Brian Miller and Brian Schurrer of Aurora Research Institute for their help with the figures.

Author details

Abdulwahab Hritani[1], Suhail Allaqaband[1,2,3] and M. Fuad Jan[1,2*]

*Address all correspondence to: publishing18@aurora.org

1 Aurora Cardiovascular Services, Aurora Sinai/St. Luke's Medical Centers, Aurora Health Care, Milwaukee, WI, USA

2 Department of Medicine, University of Wisconsin School of Medicine and Public Health, Wisconsin, USA

3 Cardiac Catheterization Laboratory, Aurora St. Luke's Medical Center, Milwaukee, Wisconsin, USA

References

[1] Vincent JL, De Backer D. Circulatory shock. New England Journal of Medicine. 2013;**369** (18):1726-1734

[2] Reynolds HR, Hochman JS. Cardiogenic shock: Current concepts and improving outcomes. Circulation. 2008;**117**(5):686-697

[3] De Backer D, Biston P, Devriendt J, Madl C, Chochrad D, Aldecoa C, Brasseur A, Defrance P, Gottignies P, Vincent JL; SOAP II Investigators. Comparison of dopamine and norepinephrine in the treatment of shock. New England Journal of Medicine. 2010;**362**(9):779-789

[4] Babaev A, Frederick PD, Pasta DJ, Every N, Sichrovsky T, Hochman JS; NRMI Investigators. Trends in management and outcomes of patients with acute myocardial infarction complicated by cardiogenic shock. JAMA. 2005;**294**(4):448-454

[5] Hochman JS, Sleeper LA, Webb JG, Sanborn TA, White HD, Talley JD, Buller CE, Jacobs AK, Slater JN, Col J, McKinlay SM, LeJemtel TH. Early revascularization in acute myocardial infarction complicated by cardiogenic shock. SHOCK Investigators. Should We Emergently Revascularize Occluded Coronaries for Cardiogenic Shock. New England Journal of Medicine. 1999;**341**(9):625-634

[6] Thiele H, Zeymer U, Neumann FJ, Ferenc M, Olbrich HG, Hausleiter J, Richardt G, Hennersdorf M, Empen K, Fuernau G, Desch S, Eitel I, Hambrecht R, Fuhrmann J, Böhm M, Ebelt H, Schneider S, Schuler G, Werdan K; IABP-SHOCK II Trial Investigators. Intraaortic balloon support for myocardial infarction with cardiogenic shock. New England Journal of Medicine. 2012;**367**(14):1287-1296

[7] Harjola VP, Lassus J, Sionis A, Køber L, Tarvasmäki T, Spinar J, Parissis J, Banaszewski M, Silva-Cardoso J, Carubelli V, Di Somma S, Tolppanen H, Zeymer U, Thiele H, Nieminen MS, Mebazaa A; CardShock Study Investigators. GREAT network. Clinical picture and risk prediction of short-term mortality in cardiogenic shock. European Journal of Heart Failure. 2015;**17**(5):501-509. Erratum in: Eur J Heart Fail. 2015;17(9):984

[8] Jan MF, Allaqaband S. Cardiac emergencies in the intensive care unit: Coronary shock and acute coronary syndrome. In: Jindal SK, editor. Textbook of Pulmonary and Critical Care Medicine. New Delhi, India: Jaypee Brothers Medical Publishers; 2010. pp. 1746-1766

[9] Templin C, Ghadri JR, Diekmann J, Napp LC, Bataiosu DR, Jaguszewski M, Cammann VL, Sarcon A, Geyer V, Neumann CA, Seifert B, Hellermann J, Schwyzer M, Eisenhardt K, Jenewein J, Franke J, Katus HA, Burgdorf C, Schunkert H, Moeller C, Thiele H, Bauersachs J, Tschöpe C, Schultheiss HP, Laney CA, Rajan L, Michels G, Pfister R, Ukena C, Böhm M, Erbel R, Cuneo A, Kuck KH, Jacobshagen C, Hasenfuss G, Karakas M, Koenig W, Rottbauer W, Said SM, Braun-Dullaeus RC, Cuculi F, Banning A, Fischer TA, Vasankari T, Airaksinen KE, Fijalkowski M, Rynkiewicz A, Pawlak M, Opolski G, Dworakowski R, MacCarthy P, Kaiser C, Osswald S, Galiuto L, Crea F, Dichtl W, Franz WM, Empen K, Felix SB, Delmas C, Lairez O, Erne P, Bax JJ, Ford I, Ruschitzka F, Prasad A, Lüscher TF. Clinical features and outcomes of takotsubo (stress) cardiomyopathy. New England Journal of Medicine. 2015;**373**(10):929-938

[10] Wu AH. Management of patients with non-ischemic cardiomyopathy. Heart. 2007;**93**(3):403-408

[11] Lahm T, McCaslin CA, Wozniak TC, Ghumman W, Fadl YY, Obeidat OS, Schwab K, Meldrum DR. Medical and surgical treatment of acute right ventricular failure. Journal of the American College of Cardiology. 2010;**56**(18):1435-1446

[12] Jacobs AK, Leopold JA, Bates E, Mendes LA, Sleeper LA, White H, Davidoff R, Boland J, Modur S, Forman R, Hochman JS. Cardiogenic shock caused by right ventricular infarction: A report from the SHOCK registry. Journal of the American College of Cardiology. 2003;**41**(8):1273-1279

[13] Goldstein JA. Acute right ventricular infarction: Insights for the interventional era. Current Problems in Cardiology. 2012;**37**(12):533-557

[14] Vazquez R, Gheorghe C, Kaufman D, Manthous CA. Accuracy of bedside physical examination in distinguishing categories of shock: A pilot study. Journal of Hospital Medicine. 2010;**5**(8):471-474

[15] Hochman JS, Ingbar DH. Cardiogenic shock and pulmonary edema. In: Longo DL, Fauci AS, Kasper DL, Hauser SL, Jameson JL, Loscalzo J, editors. Harrison's Principles of Internal Medicine, 18e. New York: McGraw-Hill; 2012

[16] Amsterdam EA, Wenger NK, Brindis RG, Casey DE Jr, Ganiats TG, Holmes DR Jr, Jaffe AS, Jneid H, Kelly RF, Kontos MC, Levine GN, Liebson PR, Mukherjee D, Peterson ED, Sabatine MS, Smalling RW, Zieman SJ; American College of Cardiology; American Heart Association Task Force on Practice Guidelines; Society for Cardiovascular Angiography and Interventions; Society of Thoracic Surgeons; American Association for Clinical Chemistry. 2014 AHA/ACC guideline for the management of patients with non-ST-elevation acute coronary syndromes: A report of the American College of Cardiology/American Heart Association Task Force on Practice Guidelines. Journal of the American College of Cardiology. 2014;**64**(24):e139-e228. Erratum in: J Am Coll Cardiol. 2014 Dec 23;64(24):2713-4. Dosage error in article text

[17] White HD, Palmeri ST, Sleeper LA, French JK, Wong CK, Lowe AM, Crapo JW, Koller PT, Baran KW, Boland JL, HochyWagner GS; SHOCK Trial Investigators. Electrocardiographic findings in cardiogenic shock, risk prediction, and the effects of emergency revascularization: Results from the SHOCK trial. American Heart Journal. 2004;**148**(5):810-817

[18] McLean AS. Echocardiography in shock management. Critical Care. 2016;**20**:275

[19] Tajik AJ, Jan MF. The heart of the matter: Prime time E/e' prime! JACC. Cardiovascular Imaging. 2014;**7**(8):759-761

[20] Yancy CW, Jessup M, Bozkurt B, Butler J, Casey DE Jr, Drazner MH, Fonarow GC, Geraci SA, Horwich T, Januzzi JL, Johnson MR, Kasper EK, Levy WC, Masoudi FA, McBride PE, McMurray JJ, Mitchell JE, Peterson PN, Riegel B, Sam F, Stevenson LW, Tang WH, Tsai EJ, Wilkoff BL; American College of Cardiology Foundation; American Heart Association Task Force on Practice Guidelines. 2013 ACCF/AHA guideline for the management of heart failure: A report of the American College of Cardiology Foundation/American Heart Association Task Force on Practice Guidelines. Journal of the American College of Cardiology. 2013;**62**(16):e147-e239

[21] American College of Emergency Physicians; Society for Cardiovascular Angiography and Interventions, O'Gara PT, Kushner FG, Ascheim DD, Casey DE Jr, Chung MK, de Lemos JA, Ettinger SM, Fang JC, Fesmire FM, Franklin BA, Granger CB, Krumholz

HM, Linderbaum JA, Morrow DA, Newby LK, Ornato JP, OuN, RadfordMJ, Tamis-HollandJE, TommasoCL, TracyCM, WooYJ, ZhaoDX, AndersonJL, JacobsAK, HalperinJL, AlbertNM, BrindisRG, CreagerMA, DeMetsD, GuytonRA, HochmanJS, KovacsRJ, KushnerFG, OhmanEM, StevensonWG, YancyCW. 2013 ACCF/AHA guideline for the management of ST-elevation myocardial infarction: A report of the American College of Cardiology Foundation/American Heart Association Task Force on Practice Guidelines. Journal of the American College of Cardiology. 2013;**61**(4):e78-e140

[22] Wiviott SD, Braunwald E, McCabe CH, Montalescot G, Ruzyllo W, Gottlieb S, Neumann FJ, Ardissino D, De Servi S, Murphy SA, Riesmeyer J, Weerakkody G, Gibson CM, Antman EM; TRITON-TIMI 38 Investigators. Prasugrel versus clopidogrel in patients with acute coronary syndromes. New England Journal of Medicine. 2007;**357**(20):2001-2015

[23] Wallentin L, Becker RC, Budaj A, Cannon CP, Emanuelsson H, Held C, Horrow J, Husted S, James S, Katus H, Mahaffey KW, Scirica BM, Skene A, Steg PG, Storey RF, Harrington RA; PLATO Investigators, Freij A, Thorsén M. Ticagrelor versus clopidogrel in patients with acute coronary syndromes. New England Journal of Medicine. 2009;**361**(11):1045-1057

[24] Dzavik V, Sleeper LA, Cocke TP, Moscucci M, Saucedo J, Hosat S, Jiang X, Slater J, LeJemtel T, Hochman JS; SHOCK Investigators. Early revascularization is associated with improved survival in elderly patients with acute myocardial infarction complicated by cardiogenic shock: A report from the SHOCK Trial Registry. European Heart Journal. 2003;**24**(9):828-837

[25] Mehta RH, Grab JD, O'Brien SM, Glower DD, Haan CK, Gammie JS, Peterson ED; Society of Thoracic Surgeons National Cardiac Database Investigators. Clinical characteristics and in-hospital outcomes of patients with cardiogenic shock undergoing coronary artery bypass surgery: Insights from the Society of Thoracic Surgeons National Cardiac Database. Circulation. 2008;**117**(7):876-885

[26] White HD, Assmann SF, Sanborn TA, Jacobs AK, Webb JG, Sleeper LA, Wong CK, Stewart JT, Aylward PE, Wong SC, Hochman JS. Comparison of percutaneous coronary intervention and coronary artery bypass grafting after acute myocardial infarction complicated by cardiogenic shock: Results from the Should We Emergently Revascularize Occluded Coronaries for Cardiogenic Shock (SHOCK) trial. Circulation. 2005;**112**(13):1992-2001

[27] Kar B, Gregoric ID, Basra SS, Idelchik GM, Loyalka P. The percutaneous ventricular assist device in severe refractory cardiogenic shock. Journal of the American College of Cardiology. 2011;**57**(6):688-696

[28] Zeymer U, Neuhaus KL, Wegscheider K, Tebbe U, Molhoek P, Schröder R. Effects of thrombolytic therapy in acute inferior myocardial infarction with or without right ventricular involvement. HIT-4 Trial Group. Hirudin for Improvement of Thrombolysis. Journal of the American College of Cardiology. 1998;**32**(4):876-881

[29] Overgaard CB, Dzavík V. Inotropes and vasopressors: Review of physiology and clinical use in cardiovascular disease. Circulation. 2008;**118**(10):1047-1056

[30] Francis GS, Bartos JA, Adatya S. Inotropes. Journal of the American College of Cardiology. 2014;**63**(20):2069-2078

[31] Chen HH, Anstrom KJ, Givertz MM, Stevenson LW, Semigran MJ, Goldsmith SR, Bart BA, Bull DA, Stehlik J, LeWinter MM, Konstam MA, Huggins GS, Rouleau JL, O'Meara E, Tang WH, Starling RC, Butler J, Deswal A, Felker GM, O'Connor CM, Bonita RE, Margulies KB, Cappola TP, Ofili EO, Mann DL, Dávila-Román VG, McNulty SE, Borlaug BA, Velazquez EJ, Lee KL, Shah MR, Hernandez AF, Braunwald E, Redfield MM; NHLBI Heart Failure Clinical Research Network. Low-dose dopamine or low-dose nesiritide in acute heart failure with renal dysfunction: The ROSE acute heart failure randomized trial. JAMA. 2013;**310**(23):2533-2543

[32] Singh K, Xiao L, Remondino A, Sawyer DB, Colucci WS. Adrenergic regulation of cardiac myocyte apoptosis. Journal of Cellular Physiology. 2001;**189**(3):257-265

[33] Hamu Y, Kanmura Y, Tsuneyoshi I, Yoshimura N. The effects of vasopressin on endotoxin-induced attenuation of contractile responses in human gastroepiploic arteries in vitro. Anesthesia and Analgesia. 1999;**88**(3):542-548

[34] Sonnenblick EH, Frishman WH, LeJemtel TH. Dobutamine: A new synthetic cardioactive sympathetic amine. New England Journal of Medicine. 1979;**300**(1):17-22

[35] Unverferth DA, Blanford M, Kates RE, Leier CV. Tolerance to dobutamine after a 72 hour continuous infusion. American Journal of Medicine. 1980;**69**(2):262-266

[36] Leier CV, Unverferth DV. Drugs five years later. Dobutamine. Annals of Internal Medicine. 1983;**99**(4):490-496

[37] O'Connor CM, Gattis WA, Uretsky BF, Adams KF Jr, McNulty SE, Grossman SH, McKenna WJ, Zannad F, Swedberg K, Gheorghiade M, Califf RM. Continuous intravenous dobutamine is associated with an increased risk of death in patients with advanced heart failure: Insights from the Flolan International Randomized Survival Trial (FIRST). American Heart Journal. 1999;**138**(1 Pt 1):78-86

[38] Konstam MA, Cody RJ. Short-term use of intravenous milrinone for heart failure. American Journal of Cardiology. 1995;**75**(12):822-826

[39] Mebazaa A, Nieminen MS, Packer M, Cohen-Solal A, Kleber FX, Pocock SJ, Thakkar R, Padley RJ, Põder P, Kivikko M; SURVIVE Investigators. Levosimendan vs dobutamine for patients with acute decompensated heart failure: The SURVIVE Randomized Trial. JAMA. 2007;**297**(17):1883-1891

[40] Packer M, Colucci W, Fisher L, Massie BM, Teerlink JR, Young J, Padley RJ, Thakkar R, Delgado-Herrera L, Salon J, Garratt C, Huang B, Sarapohja T; REVIVE Heart Failure Study Group. Effect of levosimendan on the short-term clinical course of patients with acutely decompensated heart failure. JACC Heart Failure. 2013;**1**(2):103-111

[41] Ferrario M, Poli A, Previtali M, Lanzarini L, Fetiveau R, Diotallevi P, Mussini A, Montemartini C. Hemodynamics of volume loading compared with dobutamine in severe right ventricular infarction. American Journal of Cardiology. 1994;**74**(4):329-333

[42] Tarvasmäki T, Lassus J, Varpula M, Sionis A, Sund R, Køber L, Spinar J, Parissis J, Banaszewski M, Silva Cardoso J, Carubelli V, Di Somma S, Mebazaa A, Harjola VP; CardShock study investigators. Current real-life use of vasopressors and inotropes in cardiogenic shock—adrenaline use is associated with excess organ injury and mortality. Critical Care. 2016;**20**(1):208

[43] Rihal CS, Naidu SS, Givertz MM, Szeto WY, Burke JA, Kapur NK, Kern M, Garratt KN, Goldstein JA, Dimas V, Tu T; Society for Cardiovascular Angiography and Interventions (SCAI); Heart Failure Society of America (HFSA); Society for Thoracic Surgeons (STS); American Heart Association (AHA); American College of Cardiology (ACC). 2015 SCAI/ACC/HFSA/STS Clinical Expert Consensus Statement on the Use of Percutaneous Mechanical Circulatory Support Devices in Cardiovascular Care (Endorsed by the American Heart Association, the Cardiological Society of India, and Sociedad Latino Americana de Cardiologia Intervencion; Affirmation of Value by the Canadian Association of Interventional Cardiology-Association Canadienne de Cardiologie d'intervention). Journal of Cardiac Failure. 2015;**21**(6):499-518

[44] Parissis H, Graham V, Lampridis S, Lau M, Hooks G, Mhandu PC. IABP: History-evolution-pathophysiology-indications: What we need to know. Journal of Cardiothoracic Surgery. 2016;**11**(1):122

[45] Freedman RJ. The intra-aortic balloon pump system: Current roles and future directions. Journal of Applied Cardiology. 1991;**6**:313-318

[46] Koenig SC, Litwak KN, Giridharan GA, Pantalos GM, Dowling RD, Prabhu SD, Slaughter MS, Sobieski MA, Spence PA. Acute hemodynamic efficacy of a 32-ml subcutaneous counterpulsation device in a calf model of diminished cardiac function. ASAIO Journal. 2008;**54**(6):578-584

[47] Maddoux G, Pappas G, Jenkins M, Battock D, Trow R, Smith SC Jr, Steele P. Effect of pulsatile and nonpulsatile flow during cardiopulmonary bypass on left ventricular ejection fraction early after aortocoronary bypass surgery. American Journal of Cardiology. 1976;**37**(7):1000-1006

[48] Sjauw KD, Engström AE, Vis MM, van der Schaaf RJ, Baan J Jr, Koch KT, de Winter RJ, Piek JJ, Tijssen JG, Henriques JP. A systematic review and meta-analysis of intra-aortic balloon pump therapy in ST-elevation myocardial infarction: Should we change the guidelines? European Heart Journal. 2009;**30**(4):459-468

[49] Task Force on the management of ST-segment elevation acute myocardial infarction of the European Society of Cardiology (ESC), Steg PG, James SK, AtarD, BadanoLP, Blomstrom-LundqvistC, BorgerMA, Di MarioC, DicksteinK, DucrocqG, Fernandez-AvilesF, GershlickAH, GiannuzziP, HalvorsenS, HuberK, JuniP, KastratiA, KnuutiJ, LenzenMJ, MahaffeyKW, ValgimigliM, vant HofA, WidimskyP, ZahgerD. ESC Guidelines for the management of acute myocardial infarction in patients presenting with ST-segment elevation. Eur Heart J. 2012;**33**(20):2569-2619

[50] Jolly S, et al. Complications of intra-aortic balloon pump: Can we prevent them? Cardiology Rounds. 2005;**10**:1-6

[51] Parissis H, Soo A, Al-Alao B. Intra aortic balloon pump: Literature review of risk factors related to complications of the intraaortic balloon pump. Journal of Cardiothoracic Surgery. 2011;**6**:147

[52] Ferguson JJ 3rd, Cohen M, Freedman RJ Jr, Stone GW, Miller MF, Joseph DL, Ohman EM. The current practice of intra-aortic balloon counterpulsation: Results from the Benchmark Registry. Journal of the American College of Cardiology. 2001;**38**(5):1456-1462

[53] Burzotta F, Trani C, Doshi SN, Townend J, van Geuns RJ, Hunziker P, Schieffer B, Karatolios K, Møller JE, Ribichini FL, Schäfer A, Henriques JP. Impella ventricular support in clinical practice: Collaborative viewpoint from a European expert user group. International Journal of Cardiology. 2015;**201**:684-691

[54] Seyfarth M, Sibbing D, Bauer I, Fröhlich G, Bott-Flügel L, Byrne R, Dirschinger J, Kastrati A, Schömig A. A randomized clinical trial to evaluate the safety and efficacy of a percutaneous left ventricular assist device versus intra-aortic balloon pumping for treatment of cardiogenic shock caused by myocardial infarction. Journal of the American College of Cardiology. 2008;**52**(19):1584-1588

[55] Ouweneel DM, Eriksen E, Sjauw KD, van Dongen IM, Hirsch A, Packer EJ, Vis MM, Wykrzykowska JJ, Koch KT, Baan J, de Winter RJ, Piek JJ, Lagrand WK, de Mol BA, Tijssen JG, Henriques JP. Percutaneous mechanical circulatory support versus intra-aortic balloon pump in cardiogenic shock after acute myocardial infarction. Journal of the American College of Cardiology 2017;**69**(3):278-287

[56] Gupta A, Allaqaband S, Bajwa T. Combined use of Impella device and intra-aortic balloon pump to improve survival in a patient in profound cardiogenic shock post cardiac arrest. Catheterization and Cardiovascular Interventions. 2009;**74**(6):975-976

[57] Basra SS, Loyalka P, Kar B. Current status of percutaneous ventricular assist devices for cardiogenic shock. Current Opinion in Cardiology. 2011;**26**(6):548-554

[58] Gupta S, Markham DW, Drazner MH, Mammen PP. Fulminant myocarditis. Nature Clinical Practice. Cardiovascular Medicine. 2008;**5**(11):693-706

Chapter 8

Cardiogenic Shock Due to Coronary Artery Stent Thrombosis

Mustafa Yildiz, Dogac Oksen and Ibrahim Akin

Additional information is available at the end of the chapter

http://dx.doi.org/10.5772/intechopen.68362

Abstract

Stent thrombosis is an uncommon but serious complication that causes sudden death or myocardial infarction (MI). A large MI, especially with ST elevation, can cause cardiogenic shock and pose a significant incidence of morbidity and mortality. Largeness of ischemic territory is the main reason that causes cardiogenic shock. The fundamental treatment strategies are immediate coronary revascularization and perfusion support to avoid end organ damage with medically or mechanical in intensive care units. The prevention, incidences, mechanisms, management, and clinical impacts of cardiogenic shock discussed under this topic.

Keywords: cardiogenic shock, stent thrombosis, drug-eluting stent, bare-metal stent, bioabsorbable stent, treatment

1. Introduction

1.1. Stent thrombosis: incidence, pathophysiological mechanisms, technological developments

Percutaneous coronary interventions are the main treatment of coronary artery disease patients with target vessel stenting. In 1977, firstly, it was performed by Andreas Gruntzig; afterward in 1994, the Food and Drug Administration (FDA) approved the procedure. Nowadays, coronary stent use is more than 90% of the percutaneous coronary interventions. Since the start of revascularization of coronary arteries with percutaneous transluminal coronary angioplasty (PTCA), invasive cardiologists face with a fatal problem, stent thrombosis.

Today, invasive cardiologists have a lot of options between bare metal stents (BMSs), first and second generation of drug-eluting stents (DESs) and bioresorbable vascular stents (BVSs). The decision of which kind of stent is up to physicians and particular factors about patient and his/her clinics have an effect on the choice. Widespread use of stents for target vessel revascularization brings the problem of different rates of restenosis which has a percutaneous reintervention necessity [1]. The neo-endothelial coverage with proliferation and migration of vascular smooth muscle and proteoglycan deposition causes restenosis. Restenosis may occur mostly within the first 6–9 months after implantation, depending on type of strut and procedure. Drug released from DES inhibits the signal transduction pathways of proliferation of vascular smooth muscle cell and migration. DES delays reendothelialization and avoid from prothrombogenic events.

Bare metal stent implantation reduces the risk of restenosis more than 50% when compared to balloon angioplasty. However, BMS has still a risk of 20–30% restenosis in the following year after implantation. Restenosis mostly occurs in diabetic patients, small vessels, and long lesions. Currently, BMSs often used in shortening dual antiplatelet time after implantation. DES significantly reduces restenosis compared to BMS [2].

Stent thrombosis is the acute, completely thrombotic occlusion of the stented segment of coronary artery. The incidence has been reported in various studies about 0.5–2% for elective cases and up to 6% for the patients presented with acute coronary syndromes underwent PCI. Stent thrombosis causes ST elevation myocardial infarction (MI) in 70–80% cases. Major clinical impacts, high mortality rates, nearly 40%, make the issue nightmare of interventional cardiologists [3]. Stent thrombosis alters by the time event occurs with different mechanisms. Mostly, stent thrombosis occurs within 30 days after placement. Acute stent thrombosis becomes in 24 h, if any thrombosis occurs between 24 h and 30 days, defined as early stent thrombosis. These are arising from mechanical issues, failure of platelet adhesion aggregation suppression, persistence of slow coronary flow and prothrombotic constituents. Late stent thrombosis (up to 1 year) and very late stent thrombosis (after the first year) are results of delayed reendothelialization and neointimal coverage. Delay of neointimal restoration and ongoing vascular repair is particularly the effects of agents used in DES to prevent proliferation [4].

The first generation of DES, paclitaxel and sirolimus eluting stents, has an increased risk of late and very late stent thrombosis, as compared to BMS caused more delayed reendothelialization, impaired arterial healing and long lasting inflammation. However, in newer generation of DES, late stent thrombosis risks are similar with BMS, lower than first generation. Signalizations of inflammatory and thrombotic pathways are similar, and inflammation activates clotting cascade and enhances the platelet activation [5].

Binding of von Willebrand's factor with factor VIII, glycoproteins Ib and Ia/IIb and collagen assures platelet adhesion to stent struts. Platelets provide aggregation by glycoproteins Ib, IIb/IIIa, serotonin, and fibrinogen causes thrombosis. BMS thrombosis mostly occurs within the first 24 h after stent implantation, less often within 30 days. Similarly, DES thrombosis mostly occurs in 30 days, but in DES, stent thrombosis risk continues up to 5 years. Because of the delayed endothelialization and promoted inflammation, very late stent thrombosis more likely seen in DES rather than BMS. Despite all of these, the first generation of DES such as paclitaxel—eluting stent, sirolimus—eluting stent is effective and reliable in use compared with BMS.

In the Swedish Coronary Angiography and Angioplasty Registry (SCAAR), 42,150 individuals underwent PCI with either BMS or DES. During 661-day follow-up, the rate of described stent thrombosis was 1.2%, and half of this was acute and subacute. The rates after the following year decrease to 0.3–0.4% per year constantly up to 3 years. First 6 months after stent implantation and onward, the risk for stent thrombosis was higher in DES compared with BMS (adjusted risk ratio, 2.02; 99% CI, 1.30–3.14). DES compared with BMS, initially, BMS demonstrated a higher risk of stent thrombosis, after the first months, stent thrombosis risk was higher with DES [6]. In the Bern-Rotterdam registry, the annual rate of stent thrombosis was 0.4–0.6% for up to 4 years in an 8146 patients who underwent percutaneous coronary interventions with either sirolimus-eluting stent or paclitaxel-eluting stent. Diabetes is an independent predictor of early stent thrombosis, whereas acute coronary syndrome, younger age, and paclitaxel-eluting stent implantation are associated with late stent thrombosis [7]. Use of new generation DES has significantly lower risk of restenosis and stent thrombosis though; triggers chronic vessel inflammation, fibrin deposition and cause medial cell loss, delay stent strut endothelialization therefore increase the risk of very late stent thrombosis [8].

Second-generation DES developed with more bioabsorbable and biocompatible polymers and thinner strut stent platforms, which reduce chronic inflammation similar with BMS but more effective than BMS also safer than first-generation DES with lower risk of late and very late stent thrombosis. The most recent innovation in stent technology was third generation bioabsorbable stents that after implantation polymers gradually degraded. Bioabsorbable stents are expensive in comparison with DES. In a meta-analysis of Palmerini et al. [9], data from 89 trials including 85,490 patients were analyzed. Bioabsorbable polymer-based stents were associated with superior clinical outcomes compared with BMS and first-generation DES and similar outcomes of cardiac death/MI, target vessel revascularization compared with second-generation DES. Real-world studies suggested an increased risk of mortality, MI and late stent thrombosis with first-generation DES compared to BMS, especially after discontinuation of dual antiplatelet therapy [10].

Bioresorbable stents with completely absorbable materials have some benefits over BMS and DES. These novel stents resolve the shortcoming of DES by enabling re-stent implantation to same region and restoration of vasomotor activity. Bioresorbable stents are associated with low revascularization rates which also have better short-term outcomes when compared with metallic stent technology. As there is a complete bioabsorbtion without any remnant material, late and very late stent thrombosis will be significantly less seen. Bioresorbable scaffolds liberate vessel walls from metallic stent material, therefore decrease late remodeling and luminal enlargement and save the vessels biomechanics property. Earlier complete resorption allows shortening dual antiplatelet treatment duration [11].

In a meta-analysis, 3738 patients in six trials underwent percutaneous coronary intervention with either everolimus-eluting bioresorbable vascular scaffold (n = 2337) or everolimus-eluting metallic stent (n = 1401) were included. Patients receiving bioresorbable vascular scaffolds had a similar risk of target lesion revascularization (OR, 0.97 [95% CI, 0.66–1.43]; p = 0.87), target lesion failure (1.20 [0.90–1.60]; p = 0.21), MI (1.36 [0.98–1.89]; p = 0.06), and death (0.95 [0.45–2.00]; p = 0.89) when compared with metallic stent receivers. Bioresorbable vascular scaffold implanted group had a higher risk of stent thrombosis than metallic stent group (OR, 1.99 [95% CI, 1.00–3.98]; p = 0.05). The highest risk was between 1 and 30 days after implantation (3.11 [1.24–7.82]; p = 0.02). Bioresorbable scaffolds had similar rates necessity of revascularization; however, subacute stent thrombosis risk had increased [12].

Stent thrombosis is a main problem as a completely risk of MI and high fatality rates that has been stated almost 45%. After a stent implantation, dual antiplatelet therapy is prescribed as a routine in the following year. With the use of dual antiplatelet therapy, stent thrombosis declined approximately 1% but can be higher after stenting emergency cases or complex lesions [3]. Clinical, procedural, and lesion specific factors induce the development of stent thrombosis. Premature withdrawal of dual antiplatelet therapy still constitutes the majority [13]. Beside patients noncompliance, clopidogrel or acetylsalicylic acid resistance and hypercoagulation disorders predispose to its development. Further risk factors about clinical contain diabetes mellitus, congestive heart failure, renal failure, implantation during acute MI, previous brachytherapy. Lesion specific factors are long lesions, smaller vessels, multivessel disease, and bifurcation lesions. Persistent dissection, stent underexpansion, incomplete wall apposition, multiple stenting, overlapping stents, crush technique, residual flow defect, and sort of polymer materials are described as procedure-related risk factors [14].

1.2. Prevention of devastating effects of stent thrombosis

Aspirin and thienopyridines are anti-platelet agents and have different mechanism of action. They acquire extensive impact, and combination of both is essential to prevent stent thrombosis. Thienopyridine derivates cause platelet inhibition through the P2Y12 ADP receptor whose role is to activate the glycoprotein IIb/IIIa complex. Aspirin cause an irreversible cyclooxygenase inhibiting effect and restrains synthesis of thromboxane A2.

In thrombus formation, platelets play critical role, and thus, an optimal dual antiplatelet therapy is essential preventing stent thrombosis [15]. Coating stents with cytotoxic material and polymers inhibit endothelialization, inflammation in vessel wall, and preliminary tissue factor activity. Nowadays, a pro-healing modality has been developed to achieve a natural cover of endothelium on stent surface by endothelial progenitor cells. A new approach is coating stents label with controlled releasing nitric oxide (NO) for the suppression or prevention of restenosis and thrombosis caused by implantation. NO containing liposomes control the releasing rate and prolong up to 5 days. In vitro cell studies, point NO enhances endothelial cell proliferation, while it significantly inhibits smooth muscle cell proliferation. NO-releasing stents with highly optimized release rate demonstrate improvement in arterial healing, inflammation, and neointimal thickening except thrombo-resistant effect [16].

CD133 and CD34 antibodies may be able to prevent thrombosis by promoting endothelial progenitor cells and accelerating endothelialization. The studies on novel coating strategy found that the stainless steel stents coated with vascular endothelial growth factor (VEGF) and anti-CD34 antibody less toxic on endothelial progenitor cells than single VEGF coating or bare metals [17]. Anti-CD133 antibody-coated stents have superiority in capturing endothelial progenitor cells and accelerate re-endothelialization when compared with anti-CD34 [18]. Furthermore, usage of novel biodegradable stents might also contribute the effort given against the stent thrombosis [15].

In a multicenter retrospective observational study, among 2047 STEMI patients, 1123 (54.9%) of them were received post-procedural bivalirudin full dose infusion, while the other 924 (45.1%) received low does (0.25 mg/kg/h) or null post-procedural infusion. Three acute stent thrombosis (0.3%) occurred in the group of none or low dose bivalirudin, while there was not any in the full-dose receiving group (0.3 vs 0.0%, P = 0.092). Full-dose bivalirudin infusion after PTCA procedure is safe and has protective effect against acute stent thrombosis [19].

1.3. Cardiogenic shock caused by stent thrombosis: definition, symptoms, predictors, and therapy

Cardiogenic shock is characterized by decreased end-organ perfusion due to cardiac dysfunction, and it is often caused by acute MI which may cause extensive damage of left ventricular myocardium or other mechanical complications such as free wall rupture, ventricular septal rupture, and papillary muscle rupture. It is a serious disorder with high mortality, aggressive and accurate approach increases the likelihood of treatment. The pathophysiological mechanism involves a vicious circle: ischemia causes myocardial dysfunction, which in turn aggravates myocardial ischemia (**Figure 1**). Cardiogenic shock contains three parameters: persistent hypotension (systolic blood pressure <80–90 mm Hg or mean arterial pressure <30 mm Hg) with severe reduction in cardiac index (<1.8 L min^{-1} m^{-2} without support or <2.0–2.2 L min^{-1} m^{-2} with support) and sufficient or elevated filling pressure (egg, left ventricular end-diastolic pressure > 18 mm Hg, or right ventricular end-diastolic pressure >10–15 mm Hg) [20].

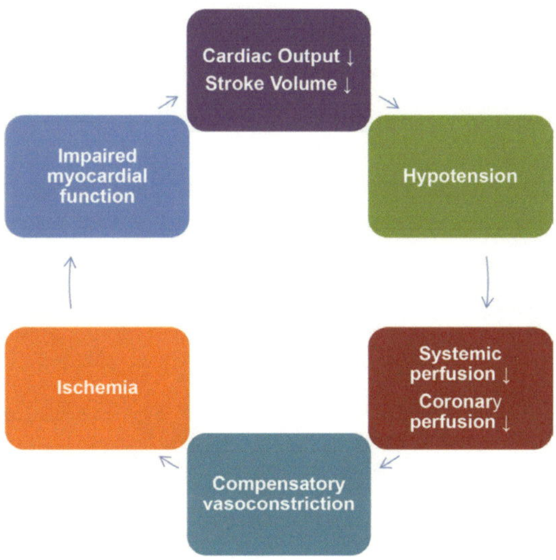

Figure 1. Vicious circle in cardiogenic shock.

Acute MI due to stent thrombosis may lead cardiogenic shock with severe ventricular dysfunction (**Figure 2**). Early revascularization such as thrombus aspiration with thrombectomy catheter and PTCA plays key role to improve the survival (**Figure 3** and **4A–F**).

1.4. Patophysiology of cardiogenic shock due to stent thrombosis

Stent thrombosis occurs as a result of variety of factors inducing thrombogenesis, clinical, and anatomical variability. BMS complete endothelization nearly 3–4 months, this returns with risk reduction of stent thrombosis. Antineoplastic stent material, hypersensitivity reaction, inflammatory response, and delayed endothelialization facilitate the risk of stent thrombosis in DES. Endothelial cells in the vessel lumen maintain vascular flow with providing a barrier to avoid aggregation and coagulation. The most frequent reason is early discontinuation of antiplatelet therapy. Mechanical factors, factors effecting coagulation cascade and response to medication, influence the risk of stent thrombosis. Evolution of intracoronary thrombus especially in acute coronary syndrome cases is related to high risk of stent thrombosis. Stent placement at injury sides increases the platelet deposition. At initial phase, the stent side covered with a thin highly platelet rich thrombus label. The neo-intimal structure mainly contains smooth muscle cells, and this occurs nearly in 6 weeks and may continue up to 12 weeks. In thrombus lesions, the elastic lamina layer is significantly thicker especially in plaque and stent area. Also, eosinophil density is apparently higher when compared to other lesions without stent [15]. Stent thrombus often ends off with ST elevation MI that can easily ruin the contraction of extensive myocardial tissue. This sudden power dissipation may break the hemodynamic stability and cause deep hypotension. As a vicious circle, hypotension reduces the coronary perfusion and enhances ischemia that result with hemodynamic collapse. Also, mechanical complications aggravate and facilitate clinical deterioration. Myocardial stunning and hibernating augment myocardial dysfunction. Increased ischemia leads the release of inflammatory mediators like interleukine-6 and cytokines thus brings barrier injuries and disrupts microcirculation. Low pressures of blood in vessels initiate multiple organ failure [20].

1.5. Cardiogenic shock caused by stent thrombosis: treatment and literature review

Thrombus aspiration has been associated with retrieving dense thrombus load away from coronary arterials to preserve myocardial performance by enhancing epicardial and microvascular

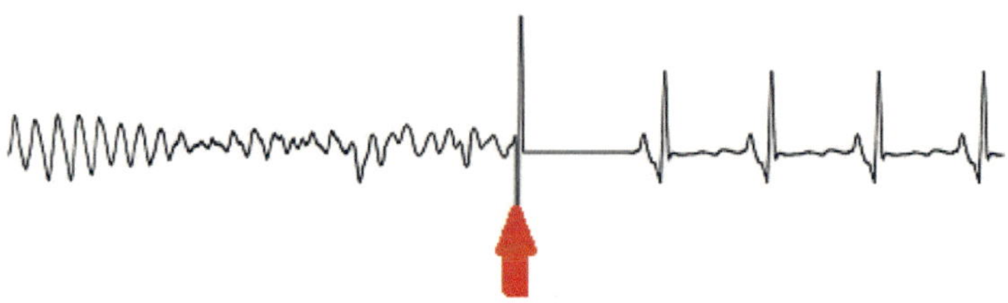

Figure 2. Ventricular fibrillation due to acute stent thrombosis. Successful defibrillation made in this patient (arrow).

http://dx.doi.org/10.5772/intechopen.68362

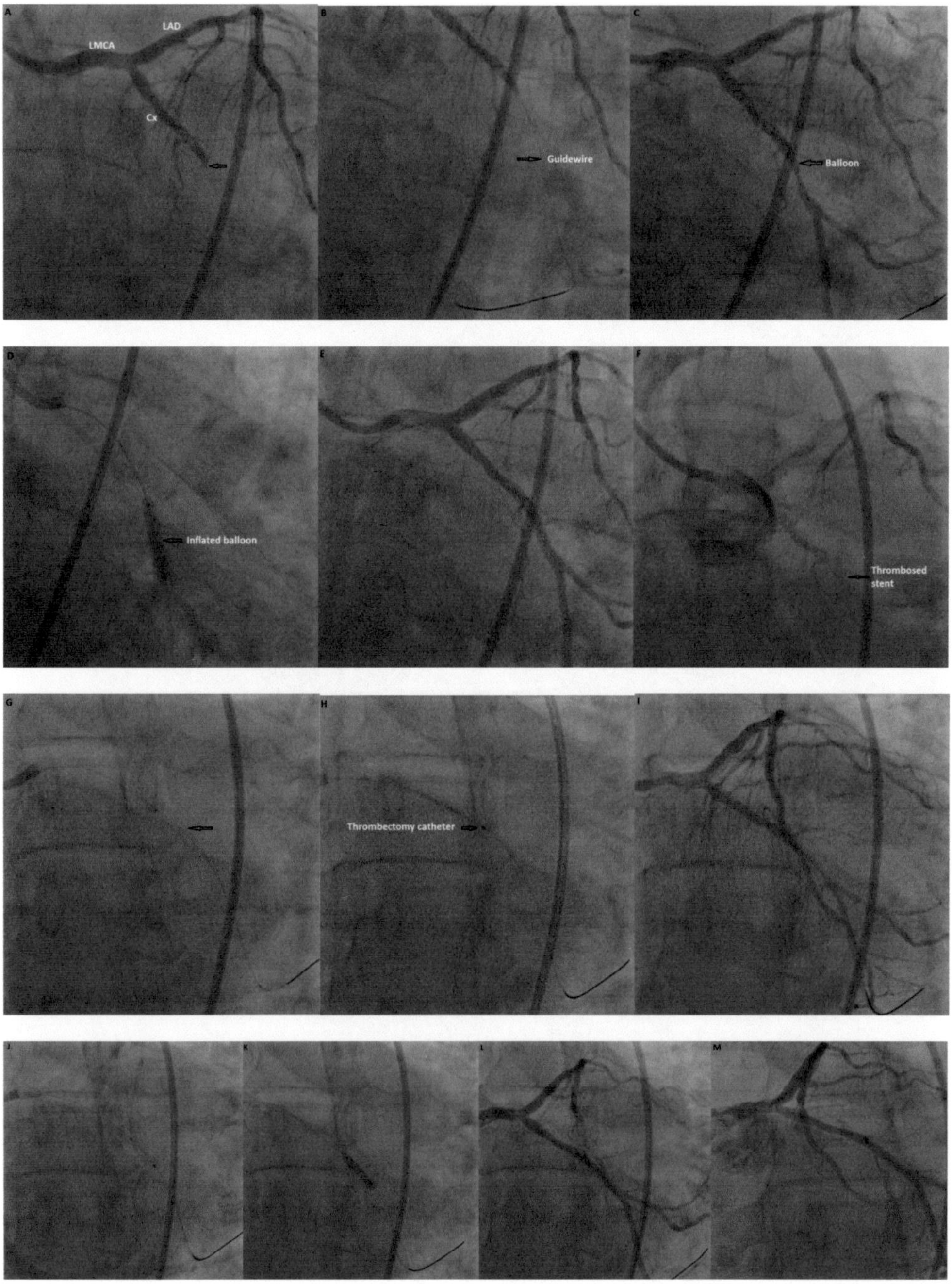

Figure 3. A. Total occlusion in Cx (arrow). B. Occlusion was passed with a guidewire (arrow). C. A coronary balloon was inflated in the occluded segment (arrow). D. The stent was implanted (arrow). E. The occluded segment was opened. F. Acute stent thrombosis of Cx stent (arrow). G. Occlusion was passed with a guidewire (arrow). H. Thrombus aspiration with thrombectomy catheter (arrow). I. Flow was reenabled. J, K. A coronary balloon was inflated in the stent. L, M. The stent was reopened. LMCA: left main coronary artery, LAD: left anterior descending coronary artery, Cx: circumflex artery.

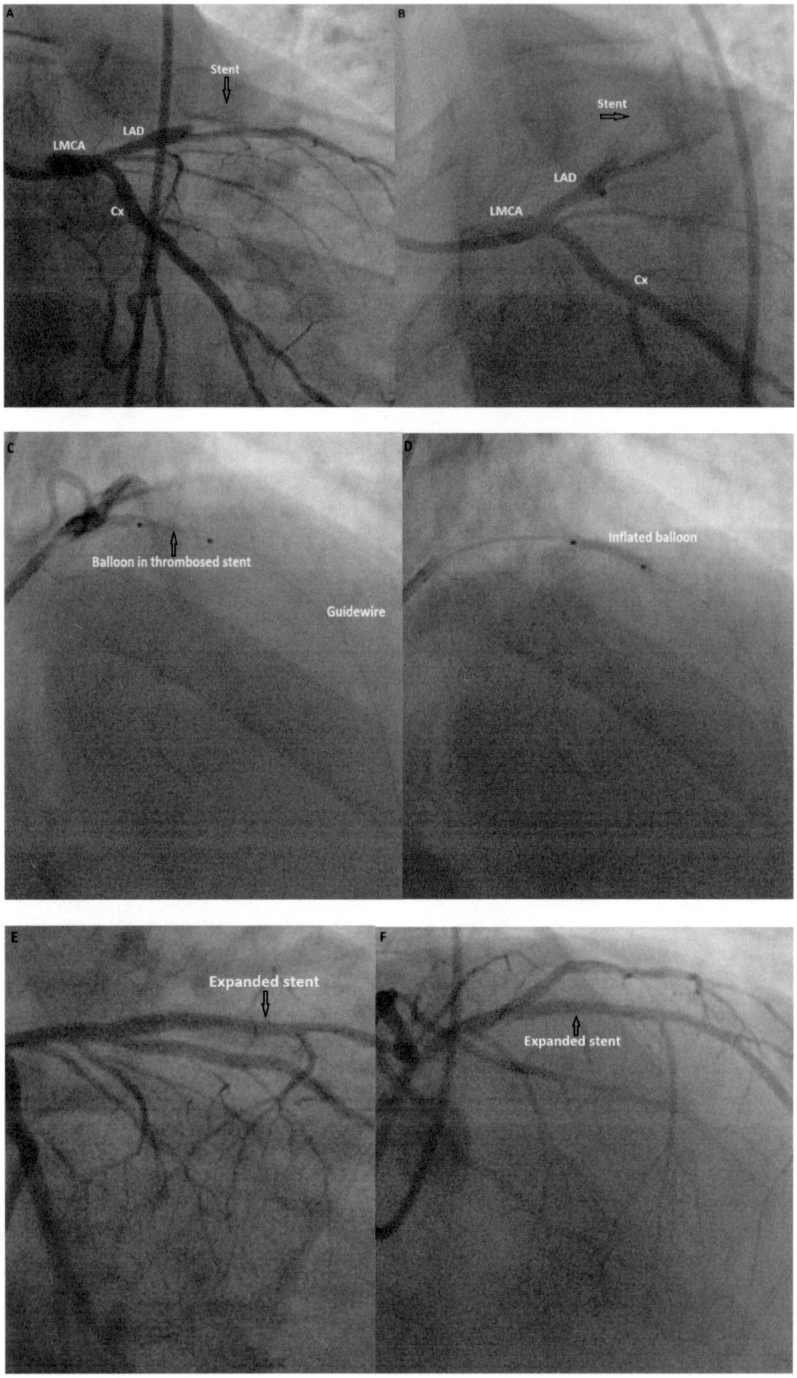

Figure 4. A, B. Total occlusion in stent (acute stent thrombosis) of mid-portion of left anterior descending coronary artery (arrow). LMCA: left main coronary artery, LAD: left anterior descending coronary artery, Cx: circumflex artery. C. Thrombosis was passed with a guidewire (arrow). D. A coronary balloon was inflated in the thrombosed stent (arrow). E, F. The stent was opened (arrows).

perfusion. A retrospective study systematically reviewed 13 stent thrombosis cases underwent angiography between January 2002 and May 2010. Thrombus aspiration performed 51 patients and 62 of them received conventional angiography. Distal embolization was significantly lower in thrombus aspiration group when compared with conventional PTCA. Mostly aspirated thrombus material included platelet and erythrocyte components at histopathologic analysis. Mortality rates in thrombus aspiration group lower but not statistically significant when compared with conventional angiography group (9.8 vs. 16% p: 0.351 at 30 days; 12 vs. 21% p: 0.220 at 1 year) [21].

Neurohormonal and cytokine systems contribute in the pathogenesis and clinical progress. As a result of hemodynamic abnormalities, hypoperfusion symptoms such as mental abnormalities, oliguria, anuria, and cool extremites can be seen. Mortality rates are between 10 and 80%, changes with demographic, initial clinical status, and hemodynamic factors. Early revascularization has a significant effect on survey [20, 22]. In the Arbeitsgemeinschaft Leitende Kardiologische Krankenhausarzte (ALKK) registry, in-hospital mortality of patients with acute myocardial infarction complicated by cardiogenic shock remained high, especially younger patient early invasive approach was the best strategy; however, in elderly patients are still a matter of debate [23].

National Cardiovascular Data Registry (NCDR) trial published data from 1,208,137 patients PCI procedures performed. In-hospital mortality was 1.4%, ranging from 0.2% within elective cases (45.1% of total PCI) to 65.9% among patients with shock and recent cardiac arrest (0.2% of total cases). Cardiogenic shock and emergent cases constitute the most predictive inpatient mortality. Intervention to chronic total occlusions, stent thrombosis, and left main lesions were the angiographic predictors of mortality [24].

Left ventricular ejection fraction (LVEF) is a prognostic indicator in cardiogenic shock. Picard et al. [25] performed echocardiography to 175 cardiogenic shock patients, 169 of them were suitable for analysis. Patients randomized into two arms: early revascularization or initial medical stabilization. In terms of echocardiography, two groups were similar. Mean LVEF was 31%, and moderate or greater mitral regurgitation was noted in 39.1%. Both short- and long-term mortality estimation according to echocardiographic indicators associated with initial left ventricular systolic function and mitral regurgitation.

Pulmonary arterial catheterization (PAC) is occasionally performed to confirm the diagnosis of cardiogenic shock. In hypotensive cases, clinical assessment of catheterization more reliable than echocardiography [26]. Performing pulmonary arterial catheterization was associated with lower short-term mortality [hazard ratio (HR) = 0.55, 95% confidence interval (CI), 0.35–0.86, p = 0.008] as well as lower mortality rates in the long-term follow-up (HR = 0.63, 95% CI 0.41–0.97, p = 0.035). However, according to subgroup analysis, the use of PAC has benefits in patients without acute coronary syndrome [26].

The main treatment to deal with cardiogenic shock is early revascularization. Patient's risk factors should be evaluated and closely followed up in case of any impending situation especially high heart rate and low blood pressure. Hypoperfusion induces catecholaminergic release but catecholamines increase myocardial oxygen demand so ischemia that causes vicious circle. Using inotropic agents temporarily increase the cardiac output therewith peripheral perfusion but unfortunately cannot interrupt the vicious circle. Intra-aortic balloon pump is a temporary solution, improves circulation, peripheral perfusion, and relieve ischemia; however, this is not long-term complete solution. Calcium-sensitizing agents such as levosimendan have some beneficial effects including positive inotropy, increases in tissue perfusion, and anti-stunning and anti-inflammatory effects. In clinical trials, levosimendan improves symptoms, cardiac function, hemodynamics, and end-organ function [27].

The Should We Emergently Revascularize Occluded Coronaries for Cardiogenic Shock (SHOCK) trial enrolled 302 patients presented with cardiogenic shock due to left ventricular failure complicating MI. Patients were randomized in emergency revascularization (152 patients) or initial medical stabilization (150 patients) groups. Intra-aortic balloon counterpulsation was performed 86% patients. At 30 days, there was not any significant difference between revascularization and medical therapy groups (46.7 and 56%, respectively; $p = 0.11$). In revascularization group, the mortality rates were significantly lower than medication group at 6-month follow-ups (50.3 vs. 63.1%, respectively; $p = 0{,}027$). Interventional cardiologist should strongly considered early revascularization for the patients with MI complicated by cardiogenic shock [28].

Stent thrombosis is a rare disorder while depending on the extensity of ischemic surface, cardiogenic shock can be occur with ventricular dysfunction and become life-threatening. Cardiogenic shock mainly associated with the infarct-related territories. A study observed 92 ST segment elevated patients from January 2004 to March 2007 [29]. Of the total, 15.2% ($n = 14$) presented with cardiogenic shock and 85.7% ($n = 12$) were DES thrombosis. Coronary collateral growth is injured with DES which inhibits formation of cytokines, chemotactic proteins, and proliferation of vascular smooth muscle cells. Mean time passed from stent implantation procedure to stent thrombosis was 4.5 ± 7.6 months. 57% of the stent thrombosis occurred less than 30 days (early stent thrombosis). In 35.7% cases, MI related to left main or multivessel stent thrombosis. Before coronary angiography, all patients underwent intra-aortic balloon pump implantation [enlarges during diastole, prior to systole, and the balloon is deflated. Therefore, device augments diastolic pressure, reduces afterload, enhances coronary perfusion, and improves cardiac output [30]. In 80% of cases, revascularization was achieved, and 21% of cases, Impella LP 2.5 pump was used because of the low cardiac output persistence. In-hospital survival was 28.6%, and in the majority of cases, death occurred within the first 48 h. All the patients who survived in the acute phase were alive at 6 months visit and had significantly lower thrombus grade after wire passage ($p = 0.03$). However, they showed a higher rate of very late stent thrombosis, longer times from symptoms onset to revascularization, and higher TIMI flow grade both before and after percutaneous coronary intervention [29].

The IMPRESS trial compares the 30-day mortality rates of Impella CP and intra-aortic balloon pump devices in patients with severe shock complicating acute MI. Forty eight patients randomized to Impella CP ($n = 24$) or intra-aortic balloon pump ($n = 24$). At 30 days, mortality in patients treated with either intra-aortic balloon pump or Impella CP was similar (50 and 46%, respectively, $p = 0.92$). At 6 months, mortality rates for both Impella CP and intra-aortic balloon pump were 50% ($p = 0.923$) [31].

Mechanical circulatory support device implantation when in early cardiogenic shock manifestation, before inotropic and vasopressor agents or coronary intervention, is independently associated with decreased mortality rates. An immediate and adequate device assists cardiac support especially Impella or intra-aortic balloon pump and supplies reperfusion without any delay are the key points of improving survival of these patients under high risk [29].

Therapeutic hypothermia is beneficial of care after cardiac arrest. ISAR-SHOCK registry included 145 patients with acute MI, cardiogenic shock, and primary percutaneous coronary intervention, 64 (44%) patients received therapeutic hypothermia treatment. After 30-day follow-up, no significant differences were observed between both groups for mortality (42 vs. 44%, HR: 0.93, 95% CI [0.56–1.53], $p = 0.77$) and MI (6 vs. 6%, HR: 0.99 95% CI [0.27–3.7], $p = 0.99$). Three definite stent thrombosis were observed, and all of them belonged to therapeutic hypothermia group ($p = 0.09$). Therapeutic hypothermia does not have a negative effect in patients who receives clopidogrel or prasugrel [32].

2. Conclusion

Stent thrombosis is the nightmare of interventional cardiologists with fatal complications such as cardiogenic shock. It occurs rarely but has significantly high incidence of in-hospital mortality. Primary strategy should avoid all the predisposing factors. The main reason of cardiogenic shock due to stent thrombosis is extensiveness of infarct-related myocardial tissue. Early revascularization and intensive life support to supply cardiac output with inotropic agents and/or mechanical circulatory devices are the beneficial strategies.

3. In the future

Developments in stent technology and novel drugs inhibits platelet aggregation are decreasing the complications of stent implantation. By completely absorption of stent material in novel stents, dual anti-platelet therapy shortens and overall late stent thrombosis and revascularization rates decreases. Recently, endothelial progenitor cell-capturing stent technology contributes re-endothelialization. With the improvement in therapeutic modulations, incidences of cardiogenic shock due to stent thrombosis and mortality rates are in decreasing tendency.

4. Take home messages

- Choice of stent type depends on clinical properties, patient and angiographic features, and carries significant weight.
- Appropriate use of dual anti-platelet therapy is essential and should be explained to patient carefully.

- In case of any cardiogenic shock presentation, patient should promptly transport to catheterization laboratory for urgent revascularization.
- Revascularization is the keystone of cardiogenic shock management due to stent thrombosis.
- To maintain end organ perfusion, inotropic agents and mechanical circulatory support devices are the only bullets for surviving from cardiogenic shock.

Author details

Mustafa Yildiz[1]*, Dogac Oksen[1] and Ibrahim Akin[2]

*Address all correspondence to: mustafayilldiz@yahoo.com

1 Department of Cardiology, Istanbul University Cardiology Institute, Istanbul, Turkey

2 First Department of Medicine, University Medical Center Mannheim, University of Heidelberg, Germany

References

[1] Kastrati A, Mehilli J, Dirschinger J, Dotzer F, Schühlen H, Neumann FJ, Fleckenstein M, Pfafferott C, Seyfarth M, Schömig A. Intracoronary stenting and angiographic results: strut thickness effect on restenosis outcome (ISAR-STEREO) trial. Circulation. 2001;**103**(23):2816-2821

[2] Stolker JM, Cohen DJ, Kennedy KF, Pencina MJ, Arnold SV, Kleiman NS, Spertus JA; EVENT Investigators. Combining clinical and angiographic variables for estimating risk of target lesion revascularization after drug eluting stent placement. Cardiovascular Revascularization Medicine. 2016 Dec 18. pii: S1553-8389(16)30350-5

[3] Iakovou I, Schmidt T, Bonizzoni E, Ge L, Sangiorgi GM, Stankovic G, Airoldi F, Chieffo A, Montorfano M, Carlino M, Michev I, Corvaja N, Briguori C, Gerckens U, Grube E, Colombo A. Incidence, predictors, and outcome of thrombosis after successful implantation of drug-eluting stents. JAMA. 2005;**293**(17):2126-2130

[4] Nakazawa G, Finn AV, Joner M, Ladich E, Kutys R, Mont EK, Gold HK, Burke AP, Kolodgie FD, Virmani R. Delayed arterial healing and increased late stent thrombosis at culprit sites after drug-eluting stent placement for acute myocardial infarction patients: An autopsy study. Circulation. 2008;**118**(11):1138-1145

[5] Croce K, Libby P. Intertwining of thrombosis and inflammation in atherosclerosis. Current Opinion in Hematology. 2007;**14**(1):55-61

[6] Lagerqvist B, Carlsson J, Fröbert O, Lindbäck J, Schersten F, Stenestrand U, James SK; Swedish Coronary Angiography and Angioplasty Registry Study Group. Stent thrombosis in Sweden: A report from the Swedish Coronary Angiography and Angioplasty Registry. Circulation: Cardiovascular Interventions. 2009;**2**(5):401-408

[7] Wenaweser P, Daemen J, Zwahlen M, van Domburg R, Jüni P, Vaina S, Hellige G, Tsuchida K, Morger C, Boersma E, Kukreja N, Meier B, Serruys PW, Windecker S. Incidence and correlates of drug-eluting stent thrombosis in routine clinical practice. 4-year results from a large 2-institutional cohort study. Journal of the American College of Cardiology. 2008;**52**(14):1134-1140

[8] Sarno G, Lagerqvist B, Fröbert O, Nilsson J, Olivecrona G, Omerovic E, Saleh N, Venetzanos D, James S. Lower risk of stent thrombosis and restenosis with unrestricted use of 'new-generation' drug-eluting stents: A report from the nationwide Swedish Coronary Angiography and Angioplasty Registry (SCAAR). European Heart Journal. 2012;**33**(5):606-613

[9] Palmerini T, Biondi-Zoccai G, Della Riva D, Mariani A, Sabaté M, Smits PC, Kaiser C, D'Ascenzo F, Frati G, Mancone M, Genereux P, Stone GW. Clinical outcomes with bioabsorbable polymer- versus durable polymer-based drug-eluting and bare-metal stents: Evidence from a comprehensive network meta-analysis. Journal of the American College of Cardiology. 2014;**63**(4):299-307

[10] Eisenstein EL, Anstrom KJ, Kong DF, Shaw LK, Tuttle RH, Mark DB, Kramer JM, Harrington RA, Matchar DB, Kandzari DE, Peterson ED, Schulman KA, Califf RM. Clopidogrel use and long-term clinical outcomes after drug-eluting stent implantation. JAMA. 2007;**297**(2):159-168

[11] Verheye S, Ormiston JA, Stewart J, Webster M, Sanidas E, Costa R, Costa JR Jr, Chamie D, Abizaid AS, Pinto I, Morrison L, Toyloy S, Bhat V, Yan J, Abizaid A. A next-generation bioresorbable coronary scaffold system: From bench to first clinical evaluation: 6- and 12-month clinical and multimodality imaging results. JACC: Cardiovascular Interventions. 2014;**7**(1):89-99

[12] Cassese S, Byrne RA, Ndrepepa G, Kufner S, Wiebe J, Repp J, Schunkert H, Fusaro M, Kimura T, Kastrati. Everolimus-eluting bioresorbable vascular scaffolds versus everolimus-eluting metallic stents: A meta-analysis of randomised controlled trials. Lancet. 2016;**387**(10018):537-544

[13] Schouten O, van Domburg RT, Bax JJ, de Jaegere PJ, Dunkelgrun M, Feringa HH, Hoeks SE, Poldermans D. Non cardiac surgery after coronary stenting: early surgery and interruption of antiplatelet therapy are associated with an increase in major adverse cardiac events. Journal of the American College of Cardiology. 2007;**49**:122-124

[14] Cheneau E, Leborgne L, Mintz GS, Kotani J, Pichard AD, Satler LF, Canos D, Castagna M, Weissman NJ, Waksman R. Predictors of subacute stent thrombosis: Results of a systematic intravascular ultrasound study. Circulation. 2003;**108**:43-47

[15] Yildiz M, Yildiz BS, Aydin E, Akin I. Stent thrombosis--mythy and facts. Cardiovascular & Hematological Disorders-Drug Targets. 2014;**14**(3):231-234

[16] Elnaggar MA, Seo SH, Gobaa S, Lim KS, Bae IH, Jeong MH, Han DK, Joung YK. Nitric oxide releasing coronary stent: A new approach using layer-by-layer coating and liposomal encapsulation. Small. 2016;**12**(43):6012-6023

[17] Song C, Li Q, Zhang JC, Wang JP, Xue X, Wang G, Shi YF, Diao HY, Liu B. Study of a novel coating strategy for coronary stents: Evaluation of stainless metallic steel coated with VEGF and anti-CD34 antibody in vitro. European Review for Medical and Pharmacological Sciences.. 2016;**20**(2):311-316

[18] Wu X, Yin T, Tian J, Tang C, Huang J, Zhao Y, Zhang X, Deng X, Fan Y, Yu D, Wang G. Distinctive effects of CD34- and CD133-specific antibody-coated stents on re-endothelialization and in-stent restenosis at the early phase of vascular injury. Regenerative Biomaterials. 2015;**2**(2):87-96

[19] Wang H, Liang Z, Li Y, Li B, Liu J, Hong X, Lu X, Wu J, Zhao W, Liu Q, An J, Li L, Pu F, Ming Q, Han Y. Effect of post-procedural full does infusion of bivalirudin on acute stent thrombosis in patients with ST-elevation myocardial infarction undergoing primary percutaneous coronary intervention: Outcomes in a large real-world population. Cardiovascular Therapeutics. 2017 Jan 13. doi:10.1111/1755-5922.12251

[20] Reynolds HR, Hochman JS. Cardiogenic shock: Current concepts and improving outcomes. Circulation. 2008;**117**:686-697

[21] Mahmoud KD, Vlaar PJ, van den Heuvel AF, Hillege HL, Zijlstra F, de Smet BJ. Usefulness of thrombus aspiration for the treatment of coronary stent thrombosis. American Journal of Cardiology. 2011;**108**(12):1721-1727

[22] Sleeper LA, Jacobs AK, LeJemtel TH, Webb JG, Hochman JS. A mortality model and severity scoring system for cardiogenic shock complicating acute myocardial infarction. Circulation. 2000;**102**(suppl II):II-795

[23] Zeymer U, Vogt A, Zahn R, Weber MA, Tebbe U, Gottwik M, Bonzel T, Senges J, Neuhaus KL; Arbeitsgemeinschaft Leitende Kardiologische Krankenhausärzte (ALKK). Predictors of in-hospital mortality in 1333 patients with acute myocardial infarction complicated by cardiogenic shock treated with primary percutaneous coronary intervention (PCI); Results of the primary PCI registry of the Arbeitsgemeinschaft Leitende Kardiologische Krankenhausärzte (ALKK). European Heart Journal. 2004;**25**(4):322-328

[24] Brennan JM, Curtis JP, Dai D, Fitzgerald S, Khandelwal AK, Spertus JA, Rao SV, Singh M, Shaw RE, Ho KK, Krone RJ, Weintraub WS, Weaver WD, Peterson ED; National Cardiovascular Data Registry. Enhanced mortality risk prediction with a focus on high-risk percutaneous coronary intervention: Results from 1,208,137 procedures in the NCDR (National Cardiovascular Data Registry). JACC: Cardiovascular Interventions. 2013;**6**(8):790-799

[25] Picard MH, Davidoff R, Sleeper LA, Mendes LA, Thompson CR, Dzavik V, Steingart R, Gin K, White HD, Hochman JS; SHOCK Trial. Should we emergently revascularize Occluded Coronaries for cardiogenic shock. Echocardiographic predictors of survival and response to early revascularization in cardiogenic shock. Circulation. 2003;**107**(2): 279-284

[26] Rossello X, Vila M, Rivas-Lasarte M, Ferrero-Gregori A, Sans-Roselló J, Duran-Cambra A, Sionis A. Impact of pulmonary artery catheter use on short- and long-term mortality in patients with cardiogenicshock. Cardiology. 2017;**136**(1):61-69

[27] Nieminen MS, Buerke M, Cohen-Solál A, Costa S, Édes I, Erlikh A, Franco F, Gibson C, Gorjup V, Guarracino F, Gustafsson F, Harjola VP, Husebye T, Karason K, Katsytadze I, Kaul S, Kivikko M, Marenzi G, Masip J, Matskeplishvili S, Mebazaa A, Møller JE, Nessler J, Nessler B, Ntalianis A, Oliva F, Pichler-Cetin E, Põder P, Recio-Mayoral A, Rex S, Rokyta R, Strasser RH, Zima E, Pollesello P. The role of levosimendan in acute heart failure complicating acute coronary syndrome: A review and expert consensus opinion. International Journal of Cardiology. 2016;**218**:150-157

[28] Hochman JS, Sleeper LA, Webb JG, Sanborn TA, White HD, Talley JD, Buller CE, Jacobs AK, Slater JN, Col J, McKinlay SM, LeJemtel TH. Early revascularization in acute myocardial infarction complicated by cardiogenic shock. SHOCK Investigators. Should We Emergently Revascularize Occluded Coronaries for Cardiogenic Shock. The New England Journal of Medicine. 1999;**341**(9):625-634

[29] Lilli A, Vecchio S, Chechi T, Vittori G, Giuliani G, Spaziani G, Consoli L, Giannotti F, Baldereschi G, Margheri M. Left ventricular support device for cardiogenic shock during myocardial infarction due to stent thrombosis: A single centre experience. International Journal of Cardiology. 2011;**148**(3):337-340

[30] Cove ME, MacLaren G. Clinical review: Mechanical circulatory support for cardiogenic shock complicating acute myocardial infarction. Critical Care. 2010;**14**(5):235

[31] Ouweneel DM, Eriksen E, Sjauw KD, van Dongen IM, Hirsch A, Packer EJ, Vis MM, Wykrzykowska JJ, Koch KT1, Baan J, de Winter RJ, Piek JJ, Lagrand WK, de Mol BA, Tijssen JG, Henriques JP. Impella CP versus ıntra-aortic balloon pump in acute myocardial ınfarction complicated by cardiogenic shock: The IMPRESS trial. Journal of the American College of Cardiology. 2016 Oct 27. pii: S0735-1097(16)36767-5

[32] Orban M, Mayer K, Morath T, Bernlochner I, Hadamitzky M, Braun S, Schulz S, Hoppmann P, Hausleiter J, Tiroch K, Mehilli J, Schunkert H, Massberg S, Laugwitz KL, Sibbing D, Kastrati A. The impact of therapeutic hypothermia on on-treatment platelet reactivity and clinical outcome in cardiogenic shock patients undergoing primary PCI for acute myocardial infarction: Results from the ISAR-SHOCK registry. Thrombosis Research. 2015;**136**(1):87-93

Chapter 9

Peripheral Ventricular Assist Devices in Interventional Cardiology: The Impella® Micro-Axial Pump

Tobias Becher, Stefan Baumann, Frederik Eder,
Christian Fastner, Michael Behnes, Dirk Loßnitzer,
Christina Dösch and Martin Borggrefe

Additional information is available at the end of the chapter

http://dx.doi.org/10.5772/67883

Abstract

Coronary artery disease (CAD) presents an ever-growing burden on health systems especially in the Western world. While percutaneous coronary intervention (PCI) is feasible in increasingly complex CAD, certain patient groups possess a high risk for major cardiac adverse events (MACE) during PCI. Poor outcome is associated with significantly depressed left ventricular function, complexity of relevant lesions, and increasing incidence of pre-existing cerebrovascular comorbidities and poor pre-interventional status. However, these risk factors also translate into a high peri-operative risk for coronary artery bypass graft (CABG) rendering some of these patients inoperable. Peripheral ventricular assist devices (pVADs) are temporarily inserted axial or centrifugal pumps that support ventricular output during PCI. The Impella® micro-axial device (Abiomed, Danvers, Massachusetts, USA) is an easily implantable pVAD that may improve patient outcome during PCI in high-risk patients (termed "protected PCI") and in patients with cardiogenic shock (CS). pVADs in general and the Impella® system in particular play important roles in interventional cardiology and its indications and use will likely expand in the future. This chapter outlines in detail the indications, applications, and future trends concerning the Impella® system. Practical advice is given on the correct implantation of the device.

Keywords: peripheral ventricular assist device, protected PCI, Impella®, interventional cardiology

1. Introduction

The Impella® system consists of a miniaturized micro-axial pump of varying size reaching from 11 French (F) to 21 F in diameter mounted on a 9 F catheter (**Figure 1**). The propeller contained in the pump revolves at up to 50,000 rounds per minute (rpm) and draws blood into the inlet area to expel it through the outlet area of the device. The micro-axial pump itself is connected through the catheter to an automated Impella® controller (AIC) that steers the pumps output as well as the required purge fluid flow and integrates information on the pumps position (**Figure 2**). The Impella® catheter is inserted either through the femoral or axillary artery by surgical cut down or percutaneously using a modified Seldinger technique. Being forwarded into the left ventricle under fluoroscopic guidance, the Impella® is positioned to expel blood bypassing the aortic valve.

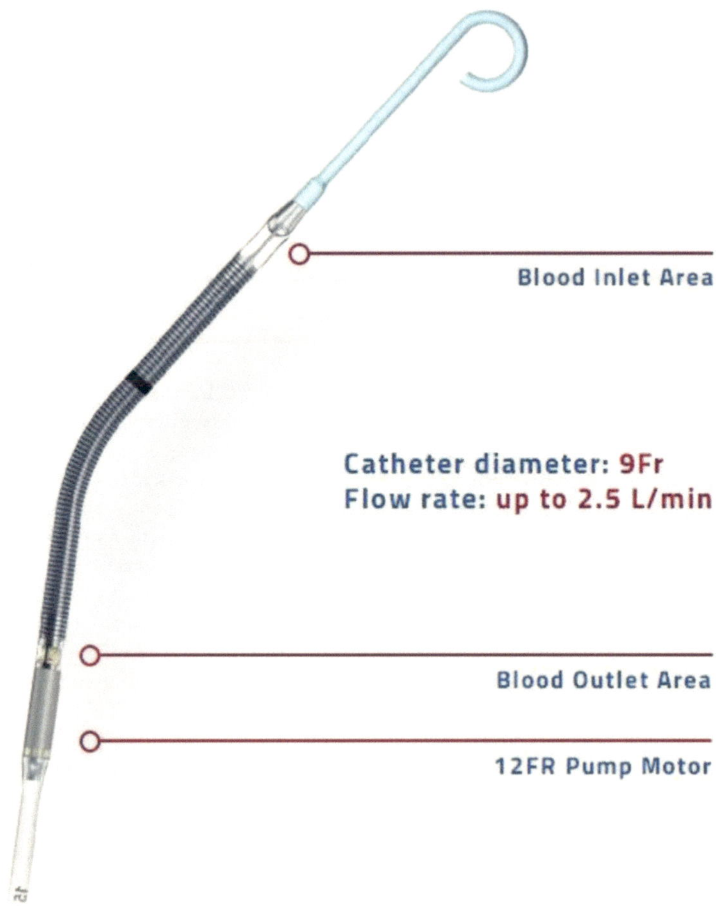

Figure 1. An Impella® 2.5 micro-axial peripheral ventricular assist device consisting of a blood inlet and an outlet area as well as the 12 Fr pump motor mounted on a 9 Fr catheter (Image courtesy of Abiomed, Danvers, Massachusetts, USA).

http://dx.doi.org/10.5772/67883

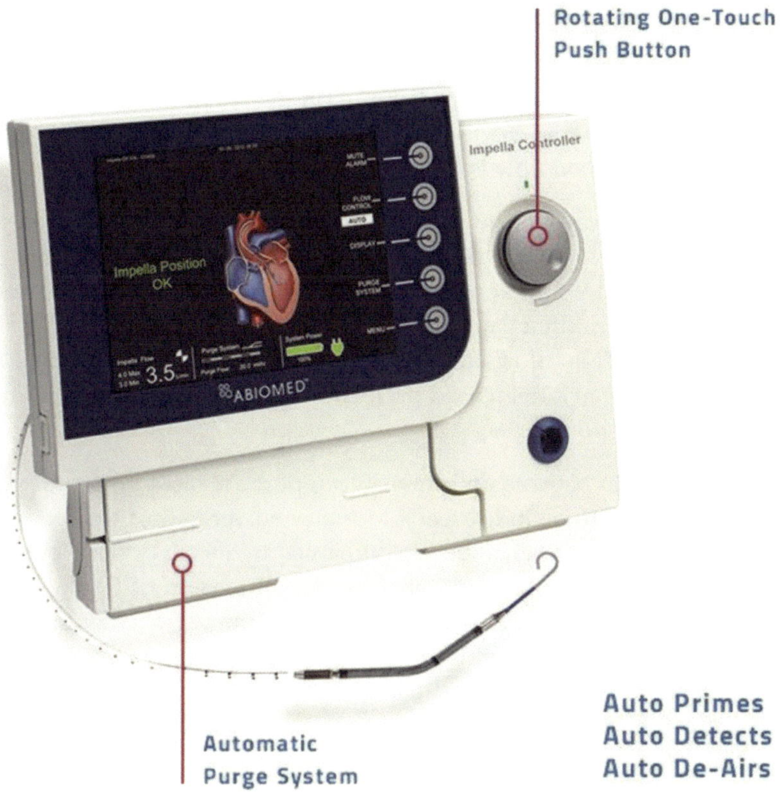

Figure 2. The Automated Impella Controller® steers the pumps output as well as the required purge fluid flow and integrates information on the pumps positions (Image courtesy of Abiomed, Danvers, Massachusetts, USA).

The Impella® platform consists of multiple devices featuring maximal output of up to 5.0 l/min and may be selected according to the required hemodynamic support. While the Impella® 2.5 (2.5 l/min of transvalvular flow) is designed to deliver support in patients mainly undergoing protected percutaneous coronary intervention (PCI), the 3.5 CP (cardiac power, 3.5 l/min of transvalvular blood flow) and 5.0 LP/LD (LP: left peripheral and LD: left direct, 5.0 l/min of transvalvular blood flow) are designed for patients in cardiogenic shock (CS). The Impella® 5.0 LD is the only device that is inserted through an open cardiac procedure into the aorta while the Impella® 5.0 LP is inserted by surgical cut down of the femoral or axillary artery.

A 3.5 l/min Impella® RP (right percutaneous) is implanted through a transvenous femoral approach into the right ventricle to support patients with right ventricular failure (RVF). The Impella® RP transports blood from an inlet in the inferior vena cava (IVC) to an outlet in the pulmonary artery bypassing the right atrium and ventricle and is currently the only device available for percutaneous hemodynamic support of the right heart. Both left and right ventricular pumps may be implanted simultaneously for support during biventricular cardiac failure [1].

2. Hemodynamic effects of Impella® support

Impella® hemodynamic support exhibits effects on intracardiac volumes and pressures as well as on systemic circulation, leading to augmentation of blood flow independent from heart rhythm. However, blood flow is dependent on after and preload.

During systole, the pressure gradient between aorta and LV is at its lowest, accounting for the highest pump flow and motor current. Vice versa, the increased pressure gradient during diastole between LV and aorta leads to diminished motor current and transvalvular blood flow. These periodic changes result in a sinus-like curve of motor current and blood flow on the AIC. This information is integrated and used by the AIC to control the pumps position. Accordingly, decreased preload may therefore result in reduced Impella® output.

Hemodynamic changes in patients on Impella® support are most profound in patients with CS. In CS, a decreased cardiac index leads to volume overload of the left ventricle resulting in a dilating left ventricular chamber accompanied by increased left ventricular end-diastolic pressure (LVEDP). Concomitantly, increased wall tension of the LV causes increased myocardial oxygen consumption. The increased LVEDP may also result in heart failure with lung edema, further decreasing overall oxygen supply. The positive effects of LV unloading by Impella® support are best explained using pressure-volume (PV) loops. Impella® support leads to a left shift of the PV loop resulting in a reduction of LVEDP and a reduction of area under the PV loop curve. This resembles reduced cardiac work, overall consistent with decreased cardiac oxygen consumption.

In a study by Schiller et al., cardiac index improved from 2.1 l/min/m2 to 3.8 l/min/m^2 [2]. Additionally, mixed venous saturation increased from 56 to 68% and diuresis increased from 69 ml/h at device insertion to 105 ml/h on support indicating improved systemic perfusion. Central venous pressure, lactate levels, and inotropic support, all consequently decreased.

Apart from patients in CS, a case study by Arain and O'Meallie demonstrated an increase in coronary artery circulation on Impella® support in a patient undergoing protected PCI. Fractional-flow reserve (FFR) and coronary flow reserve (CFR) were measured in a hemodynamically significant stenotic left anterior descending (LAD) coronary artery using a pressure wire. While FFR remained the same comparing on- and off Impella® support time points, CFR significantly increased. This demonstrates beneficial effects of Impella® support on coronary perfusion during protected PCI.

3. Implantation of an Impella® device

In general, the implantation of an Impella® device is comparatively easy procedure that is performed in a cath lab. However, pitfalls and limitations should be well known and implantation should be performed by an experienced team, including an interventional cardiologist, cath lab assistance, and a nurse.

http://dx.doi.org/10.5772/67883

Several contraindications that include vascular pathologies reaching from the femoral artery up to the aortic valve as well as aortic valve pathologies must be observed prior to implantation. These include, but are not limited to, severe peripheral artery vessel disease (pAVD) that may increase the likelihood of vascular access complications or may render the implantation of a large sheet and thereof the Impella® impossible, as well as aortic aneurism both abdominal and thoracic. Aortic insufficiency (moderate to severe degree), severe aortic stenosis, pathologies that increase the likelihood of thromboembolic events (valve endocarditis, LV thrombus) or a mechanical aortic valve may present further contraindications. Due to the administration of aPTT-relevant doses of unfractionated heparins in the purge fluid, bleeding risk may be increased. In patients with contraindications to unfractionated heparins, such as heparin-induced thrombocytopenia (HIT), using an alternative anticoagulant through a systemic line is at the discretion of the treating physician. Furthermore, pathologies that decrease right ventricular function may concomitantly decrease left ventricular preload, leading to insufficient Impella® output.

Prior to implantation of the Impella device, we therefore recommend duplex-angiography of the respective arterial vessel considered for vascular access to: (I) measure vessel diameter and (II) exclude relevant pAVD and heavy calcifications. If bedside duplex-angiography is not available, and in case of a femoral approach, vascular access at the contralateral femoral artery and placement of a 6 F sheet may be performed. The status of the ipsilateral femoral artery may be determined via angiography through a 5 F pigtail catheter placed just above the origin of the two iliac arteries. This technique may also help to determine the location of the common femoral artery (CFA) and the best spot for needle introduction. The contralateral sheath may be left in place and later be used for introducing guide catheters and wires for coronary interventions. To exclude relevant pathologies of the aortic valve and to exclude the presence of intraventricular thrombi, echocardiography is recommended to determine whether Impella® support is feasible.

The respective Impella® device is assembled according to the manufacturers' instructions and following the steps laid out on the AIC by the cath lab assistance. For the Impella® 2.5 and CP, the CFA is punctured and a sheath is inserted after dilatation using the provided set. Before insertion of the sheath, we recommend using a pre-close technique to facilitate sheath removal. This technique requires the insertion of two Perclose Proglide® devices prior to placing the sheaths. A needle is used to puncture the CFA and a wire is introduced into the vessel. Two 6 F Perclose Proglide® devices are then introduced. The first device is placed at a 30–45° angle and before complete removal of the first carrier device, the 0.035-inch guide wire is reinserted into the CFA. A second Perclose Proglide® device is then introduced at a 90° angle in relation to the first device and introduced. Following the end of the procedure, the sutures are cinched down after catheter removal to close the arteriotomy. This technique is only feasible in patients undergoing protected PCI, as long indwelling times render the vascular closure set unsterile.

A pigtail catheter is now advanced into the LV, followed by a 0.018-inch wire and the pigtail catheter is removed again over the wire. Under fluoroscopic guidance, the Impella® is now advanced over the wire so that the outlet area rests above the aortic valve (**Figure 3**). After removal of the guide wire, correct position should once again be confirmed using the AIC and fluoroscopy before starting the procedure. During each transfer of the patient, care should be taken to avoid Impella® movement and correct position of the Impella® should be confirmed after the transfer using bedside echocardiography.

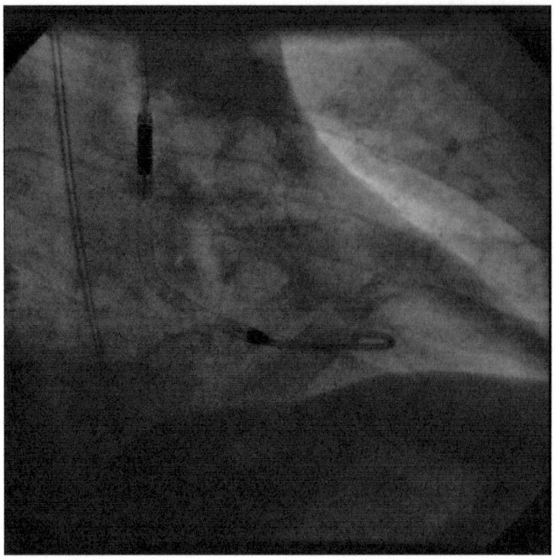

Figure 3. Correct position of the Impella 2.5 in the left ventricle with the outlet portion above the aortic valve demonstrated by fluoroscopy from an RAO (right anterior oblique) angle.

4. Adverse events

Potential adverse events following Impella® implantation or hemodynamic support with Impella® include hemolysis, functional mitral stenosis, pump displacement, malfunction and vascular site complications including bleeding and limb ischemia. Furthermore, thromboembolic events including stroke and myocardial infarction as well as acute kidney dysfunction or failure might occur. Overall incidence rate is low, seems to differ according to the indication for hemodynamic support, and is also most likely related to the duration of Impella® support. Highest rates for adverse events may accordingly be found in patients undergoing Impella® support for CS.

In 120 patients with AMI complicated by CS, The EUROSHOCK trial found major bleeding at the vascular access site in 28.6%, hemolysis in 7.5%, and pericardial tamponade in 1.7% [3]. In another study including 40 patients with end-stage heart failure and implantation of an Impella® 5.0 as bridge to transplant or bridge to left ventricular assist device (LVAD), bleeding requiring transfusion occurred in 28.0%, hemolysis in 8.0%, device malfunction in 10.0%, and limb ischemia in 3.0% [4]. Highest rates of adverse events were generally found for major bleeding at the access site and hemolysis, two complications that may usually be managed successfully while patients may remain on Impella® support.

In patients undergoing protected PCI, the frequency of adverse events is usually lower. The PROTECT trial, designed to examine the efficacy and safety of Impella® 2.5 in protected PCI, found mild, transient hemolysis in 10.0% of patients with no other major adverse events [5]. In a further study including 19 patients undergoing protected PCI, no complications occurred [6].

Recent case reports have reported mitral valve damage possibly caused by Impella support [7]. Whether this finding warrants specific precautions needs to be further evaluated. We recommend screening for signs and symptoms of acute mitral insufficiency under Impella® support and further echocardiographic examinations on a regular basis.

Davis et al. reported a case in which a patient in CS developed acquired von-Willebrand syndrome (AVWS) under Impella 5.0 support [8]. AVWS develops in situations in which high shear stress leads to excessive proteolysis of von Willebrand factor (VWF) and loss of high molecular weight multimers, in this situation attributed to high-level Impella support. The patient suffered major bleeding under surgery for long-term LVAD and required massive substitution of blood and coagulation products. Larger trials are warranted to further evaluate alterations of VWF and the incidence of AVWS under Impella support.

5. Indications

5.1. Protected PCI

Poor outcome in patients undergoing PCI is associated with depressed left ventricular function, higher complexity of lesions, multi-vessels disease, and poor pre-interventional status [9]. In these patients, even limited episodes of myocardial ischemia caused by intracoronary application of contrast medium, inflation of balloons, implantation of stents, or more sophisticated maneuvers like rotablation may provoke hypotension resulting in a vicious cycle of impaired coronary perfusion, malignant cardiac arrhythmias, and cardiac arrest. The pre-interventional implantation of an Impella® device, referred to as protected PCI, may provide hemodynamic support in case of hemodynamic compromise and augment intracoronary blood flow.

The PROTECT I trial (A Prospective Feasibility trial Investigating the Use of the IMPELLA RECOVER LP 2.5 System in Patients Undergoing High Risk PCI) was the first trial designed to evaluate the safety and feasibility of the Impella® 2.5 system in patients undergoing protected PCI [5]. Including 20 patients in a prospective, multi-center fashion, this study demonstrated that the Impella® 2.5 is safe and easy to implant with only two patients showing signs of mild hemolysis. All patients included had a poor left ventricular function and underwent PCI of an unprotected left main coronary artery or last patent coronary conduit. None of the patients developed hemodynamic compromise during PCI.

The PROTECT II trial represents the second landmark study for protected PCI via Impella® 2.5, comparing the Impella® device with intra-aortic balloon pump (IABP) in a randomized, controlled design [10]. Although the study was terminated early on grounds of futility (the study was underpowered for the primary endpoint of superiority of Impella® 2.5 compared to IABP in terms of MACCE), trends for improved outcomes were observed for Impella® 2.5-supported patients at 90 days.

Besides the mentioned trials, multiple individual experiences with the device and protected PCI, case studies, and case reports have been published [6, 11–16]. In general, the concept has been described as safe and feasible, resulting in hemodynamic improvement. Data from the USpella registry have further demonstrated the feasibility of protected PCI through Impella® 2.5 in a real-world setting [17].

5.2. Cardiogenic shock

Mortality of patients suffering from acute myocardial infarction (AMI) complicated by CS remains high. Given the potential benefits of pVADs in this specific scenario, short-term circulatory support seems to be a promising therapeutic option. Hypoperfusion caused by cardiogenic shock triggers the so called "shock spiral" by systemic hypoxemia leading to dismal systemic regulatory efforts. The implantation of a pVAD may halt this downward spiral by increasing cardiac output, decreasing LVEDP by unloading of the left ventricle, and therefore reducing oxygen consumption of the myocardium. As appealing as this approach may sound, there is currently no randomized, controlled trial available that may prove the benefit of pVADs in this scenario. The IMPRESS (IMPella versus IABP REduces mortality in STEMI patients treated with primary PCI IN SEVERE and deep cardiogenic SHOCK) trial, a recent controlled, randomized, multi-center study by Ouweneel et al. has found no difference in short-term and 6-month mortality in patients undergoing pVAD support through the Impella® CP in cardiogenic shock compared to Intra-aortic balloon pump (IABP) [18]. Furthermore, a recent meta-analysis from the same authors evaluating the three available randomized trials of Impella® usage in CS patients and comparing it to IABP also revealed no survival benefit at 30 days and 6 months [19].

Interestingly, there seems to be differences in survival in-between men and women. Data from the cVAD registry (catheter-based ventricular assist device registry), a database retrospectively enrolling patients that underwent pVAD support with Impella®, showed that early initiation of hemodynamic support in patients with AMI complicated by CS was associated with a greater survival benefit in women compared to men [20]. These data are encouraging, as women usually suffer higher unadjusted mortality rates and experience the use of guideline-recommended therapies to a lesser extent.

Although the concept of pVADs in CS seems convincing and there is ample data showing improved hemodynamic parameters, there is still no evidence from RCTs that pVADs improve survival in these patients. One issue is certainly identifying patients that might profit from pVAD implantation and selecting the appropriate pVAD. Future trials should therefore focus on identifying the "right" patient and the "right" time for Impella® implantation in CS.

5.3. Right ventricular failure

The Impella® RP received FDA approval in 2015 upon completion of the RECOVER RIGHT (The Use of Impella RP Support System in Patients with Right Heart Failure: A Clinical and Probable Benefit Study) trial, resembling the first percutaneous right ventricular assist device [21]. This prospective, multi-center, single-arm study included 32 patients from 15 institutions in the USA. Of these patients, 18 were included with right ventricular failure (RVF) after left ventricular assist device (LVAD) implantation and 12 patients presented with RVF after cardiotomy or myocardial infarction. All patients included exhibited life-threatening RVF with three vasopressors/inotrops installed and a mean cardiac index of 1.8 $l/min/m^2$.

Cardiac index increased to 3.3 $l/min/m^2$ and central venous pressure decreased from 19.2 to 12.6 mmHg under Impella® RP support. In total, 73.3% of patients survived more than 30 days after an average hemodynamic support of only 3.0 days. RECOVER RIGHT was not designed to compare Impella® RP to standard medical treatment; however, the safety and hemodynamic efficacy of the device were shown. The device is approved for a period of 14 days, warranting more durable solutions in patients that do not recover.

Besides above-mentioned causes of RVF included in the RECOVER RIGHT study, further indications for temporary right ventricular support seem appealing. Hansen et al. presented a case of a patient with sepsis induced RVF on grounds of pulmonary hypertension that initially recovered after Impella® RP implantation [22]. Again, markedly improved hemodynamic parameters were reported after initiation of hemodynamic support.

The Impella® RP therefore may serve as a valuable therapeutic option in patients presenting with life-threatening RVF of a variety of causes and under already applied standard of care. Again, patient selection plays a crucial role for the success of the treatment.

5.4. Impella® as a bridge to decision or bridge to next therapy

A growing number of patients with a severely reduced LV require temporary mechanical support to bridge time to multidisciplinary assessment of best therapeutic strategy or bridge to next therapy. Lima et al. reported their single-center experience with Impella® 5.0 for either bridge to heart transplant or bridge to durable left ventricular assist device in 40 patients [4]. The primary endpoint survival to next therapy was reached in 75.0% of patients. Compared to the predominant bridging strategy employing Extracorporeal membrane oxygenation (ECMO), this reveals a significantly higher likelihood of survival. Furthermore, critical complications are significantly lower in patients undergoing Impella® support compared to ECMO. In summary, Impella® may serve as a valuable therapeutic alternative in patients being bridged to next therapy overcoming some of ECMOs limitations.

6. Future trends

A multitude of case reports has reported potential indications for Impella. For example, Deshpande et al. reported a case of acute embolic myocardial infarction and heart failure in a Fontan patient resolved by Impella support followed by successful transplantation [23]. These descriptions on a case-by-case basis highlight promising future indications for the Impella system. However, clinical data in terms of randomized and controlled trials are missing for all of the mentioned indications. **Table 1** further reported the indications for Impella® support.

Authors	Indication for Impella® implantation	Year
Cena et al. [26]	Non-ischemic cardiomyopathy and cardiogenic shock	2016
Deshpande et al. [23]	Acute myocardial infarction and cardiogenic shock in a Fontan patient	2016
Stottrup et al. [27]	Cardiac arrest	2016
Ancona et al. [28]	Post-infarct ventricular septal rupture	2016
Burzotta et al. [29]	Bail-out use as bridge to TAVI in cardiogenic shock	2016
Desai et al. [30]	Cardiac arrest after neuraxial anesthesia	2015
Rashed et al. [31]	Cardiogenic shock secondary to takotsubo cardiomyopathy	2015
Burns and Quantz [32]	Viral myocarditis	2015
Khaliel et al. [33]	Toxic cardiomyopathy	2014
Miller et al. [34]	Hemodynamic support during VT ablation	2013

Table 1. Emerging indications for Impella® support.

6.1. Combination of ECMO and Impella

Multiple authors have introduced the concept of multi-device approaches in patients with cardiogenic shock [24, 25]. By using different pVADs either simultaneously or in a sequential order, negative effects of one individual device may be balanced by the use of another system.

This concept seems especially efficient for the simultaneous implantation of VA-ECMO and Impella. Pappalardo et al. compared in a recent study 21 patients undergoing VA-ECMO and Impella with 42 propensity-matched patients undergoing VA-ECMO alone for cardiogenic shock [24]. Hospital mortality was significantly lower in patients implanted with both devices (47.0 vs. 80.0%, $P < 0.001$).

The implantation of an Impella® device may address one of the important pitfalls of VA-ECMO, hence explaining the reported improved outcomes. VA-ECMO leads to an increased afterload due to retrograde blood flow impairing unloading of the left ventricle and increasing LVEDP. Overcoming these dismal effects and supporting unloading of the left ventricle by Impella® may therefore prove a valuable concept in the future.

7. Summary

The Impella® platform resembles a pVAD system that augments the repertoire of modern interventional cardiology. The landmark PROTECT II study presented evidence that in patients undergoing protected PCI, hemodynamic support with Impella 2.5 leads to improved outcomes at 3 months when compared to IABP. With the Impella® being easy and safe to implant and its overall low rate of adverse events, the system provides interventional cardiologists with a tool for patients at high risk for adverse events during complex PCI procedures.

Adding more powerful (up to 5.0 l/min) and right cardiac support devices to the platform, the range of indications have expanded to cardiogenic shock, right ventricular failure, and a multitude of conditions that result in impaired left ventricular output. Although the principal physiological benefits of left ventricular support of unloading of the left ventricle with Impella® have been examined extensively, there are currently no randomized, controlled trials demonstrating improved survival of patients supported with Impella® in cardiogenic shock. A promising new strategy is combining ECMO with Impella. Further studies should answer the questions of (I) what cohort of patients at (II) what time and stage of cardiogenic shock (III) profit from what respective pVAD.

Author details

Tobias Becher*, Stefan Baumann, Frederik Eder, Christian Fastner, Michael Behnes, Dirk Loßnitzer, Christina Dösch and Martin Borggrefe

*Address all correspondence to: tobias.becher@umm.de

First Medical Department, University Medical Center Mannheim (UMM), Faculty of Medicine Mannheim, University of Heidelberg, Germany

References

[1] Aghili N, Bader Y, Vest AR, et al. Biventricular circulatory support using 2 axial flow catheters for cardiogenic shock without the need for surgical vascular access. *Circulation. Cardiovascular Interventions*. 2016;9(6):e003636.

[2] Schiller P, Vikholm P, Hellgren L. The Impella(R) recover mechanical assist device in acute cardiogenic shock: a single-centre experience of 66 patients. *Interactive Cardiovascular and Thoracic Surgery*. 2016;22(4):452-458.

[3] Lauten A, Engstrom AE, Jung C, et al. Percutaneous left-ventricular support with the Impella-2.5-assist device in acute cardiogenic shock: results of the Impella-EUROSHOCK-registry. *Circulation. Heart Failure*. 2013;6(1):23-30.

[4] Lima B, Kale P, Gonzalez-Stawinski GV, Kuiper JJ, Carey S, Hall SA. Effectiveness and safety of the Impella 5.0 as a bridge to cardiac transplantation or durable left ventricular assist device. *The American Journal of Cardiology*. 2016;117(10):1622-1628.

[5] Dixon SR, Henriques JP, Mauri L, et al. A prospective feasibility trial investigating the use of the Impella 2.5 system in patients undergoing high-risk percutaneous coronary

intervention (The PROTECT I Trial): initial U.S. experience. JACC. Cardiovascular interventions. Feb 2009;2(2):91-96

[6] Henriques JP, Remmelink M, Baan J, Jr., et al. Safety and feasibility of elective high-risk percutaneous coronary intervention procedures with left ventricular support of the Impella Recover LP 2.5. *The American Journal of Cardiology*. 2006;97(7):990-992.

[7] Elhussein TA, Hutchison SJ. Acute mitral regurgitation: unforeseen new complication of the Impella LP 5.0 ventricular assist device and review of literature. *Heart, Lung & Circulation*. 2014;23(3):e100-e104.

[8] Davis ME, Haglund NA, Tricarico NM, Keebler ME, Maltais S. Development of acquired von Willebrand syndrome during short-term micro axial pump support: implications for bleeding in a patient bridged to a long-term continuous-flow left ventricular assist device. *ASAIO Journal*. 2014;60(3):355-357.

[9] Peterson ED, Dai D, DeLong ER, et al. Contemporary mortality risk prediction for percutaneous coronary intervention: results from 588,398 procedures in the National Cardiovascular Data Registry. Journal of the American College of Cardiology. May 04 2010;55(18):1923-1932.

[10] O'Neill WW, Kleiman NS, Moses J, et al. A prospective, randomized clinical trial of hemodynamic support with Impella 2.5 versus intra-aortic balloon pump in patients undergoing high-risk percutaneous coronary intervention: the PROTECT II study. Circulation. Oct 02 2012;126(14):1717-1727.

[11] Valgimigli M, Steendijk P, Serruys PW, et al. Use of Impella Recover(R) LP 2.5 left ventricular assist device during high-risk percutaneous coronary interventions; clinical, haemodynamic and biochemical findings. *EuroIntervention: Journal of EuroPCR in Collaboration with the Working Group on Interventional Cardiology of the European Society of Cardiology*. 2006;2(1):91-100.

[12] Dens J, Meyns B, Hilgers RD, et al. First experience with the Impella Recover(R) LP 2.5 micro axial pump in patients with cardiogenic shock or undergoing high-risk revascularisation. *EuroIntervention: Journal of EuroPCR in Collaboration with the Working Group on Interventional Cardiology of the European Society of Cardiology*. 2006;2(1):84-90.

[13] Minden HH, Lehmann H, Meyhofer J, Butter C. Transradial unprotected left main coronary stenting supported by percutaneous Impella Recover LP 2.5 assist device. *Clinical Research in Cardiology: Official Journal of the German Cardiac Society*. 2006;95(5):301-306.

[14] Cohen R, Domniez T, Elhadad S. High-risk left main coronary stenting supported by percutaneous Impella Recover LP 2.5 assist device. *The Journal of Invasive Cardiology*. 2007;19(10):E294-E296.

[15] Hatch J, Baklanov D. Percutaneous hemodynamic support in PCI. *Current Treatment Options in Cardiovascular Medicine*. 2014;16(4):293.

[16] Spiro J, Venugopal V, Raja Y, Ludman PF, Townend JN, Doshi SN. Feasibility and efficacy of the 2.5 L and 3.8 L Impella percutaneous left ventricular support device during high-risk, percutaneous coronary intervention in patients with severe aortic stenosis. *Catheterization and Cardiovascular Interventions: Official Journal of the Society for Cardiac Angiography & Interventions*. 2015;85(6):981-989.

[17] Maini B, Naidu SS, Mulukutla S, et al. Real-world use of the Impella 2.5 circulatory support system in complex high-risk percutaneous coronary intervention: the USpella Registry. *Catheterization and Cardiovascular Interventions: Official Journal of the Society for Cardiac Angiography & Interventions*. 2012;80(5):717-725.

[18] Ouweneel DM, Eriksen E, Sjauw KD, et al. Impella CP versus intra-aortic balloon pump in acute myocardial infarction complicated by cardiogenic shock: the IMPRESS trial. *Journal of the American College of Cardiology*. 2017 Jan 24;69(3):278-287.

[19] Ouweneel DM, Eriksen E, Seyfarth M, Henriques JP. Impella versus intra-aortic balloon pump for treatment of cardiogenic shock: a meta-analysis of randomized controlled trials. *Journal of the American College of Cardiology*. 2017 Jan 24;69(3):358-360.

[20] Joseph SM, Brisco MA, Colvin M, et al. Women with cardiogenic shock derive greater benefit from early mechanical circulatory support: an update from the cVAD registry. *Journal of Interventional Cardiology*. 2016;29(3):248-256.

[21] Anderson MB, Goldstein J, Milano C, et al. Benefits of a novel percutaneous ventricular assist device for right heart failure: the prospective RECOVER RIGHT study of the Impella RP device. *The Journal of Heart and Lung Transplantation: The Official Publication of the International Society for Heart Transplantation*. 2015;34(12):1549-1560.

[22] Hansen LN, Berg H, Schmidt H, et al. Percutaneous right ventricular assist device in sepsis due to right ventricular failure and pulmonary hypertension. *Acta Anaesthesiologica Scandinavica*. 2016;60(10):1470-1472.

[23] Deshpande SR, Dalal A, Kim DW, Babaliaros V, Jokhadar M. Acute embolic myocardial infarction and heart failure in a fontan patient: recovery with Impella device and successful transplantation. *ASAIO Journal*. 2016;62(6):e52-e54.

[24] Pappalardo F, Schulte C, Pieri M, et al. Concomitant implantation of Impella(R) on top of veno-arterial extracorporeal membrane oxygenation may improve survival of patients with cardiogenic shock. *European Journal of Heart Failure*. 2017 Mar;19(3):404-412.

[25] Pieri M, Contri R, Winterton D, et al. The contemporary role of Impella in a comprehensive mechanical circulatory support program: a single institutional experience. *BMC Cardiovascular Disorders*. 2015;15:126.

[26] Cena M, Karam F, Ramineni R, Khalife W, Barbagelata A. New Impella cardiac power device used in patient with cardiogenic shock due to nonischemic cardiomyopathy. *The International Journal of Angiology: Official Publication of the International College of Angiology, Inc*. 2016;25(4):258-262.

[27] Stottrup NB, Jakobsen L, Krusell LR, Terkelsen CJ. Utility of Impella(R) left ventricular assist device during cardiac arrest: a case report. *International Journal of Cardiology*. 2016;225:111-112.

[28] Ancona MB, Regazzoli D, Mangieri A, Monaco F, De Bonis M, Latib A. Post-infarct ventricular septal rupture: early Impella implantation to delay surgery and reduce surgical risk. *Cardiovascular Intervention and Therapeutics*. 2016 Sep 7. [Epub ahead of print].

[29] Burzotta F, Nerla R, Trani C. Bail-out use of Impella CP as a bridge to TAVI in a cardiogenic shock patient: the "pump-rewiring" technique. *The Journal of Invasive Cardiology*. 2016;28(1):E1-E5.

[30] Desai N, Chaudhry K, Aji J. Impella left ventricular assist device in cardiac arrest after spinal anaesthesia for caesarean section. *BMJ Case Reports*. Oct 28;2015.

[31] Rashed A, Won S, Saad M, Schreiber T. Use of the Impella 2.5 left ventricular assist device in a patient with cardiogenic shock secondary to takotsubo cardiomyopathy. *BMJ Case Reports*. May 7;2015.

[32] Burns DJ, Quantz MA. Use of the Impella 5.0 device as a bridge to recovery in adult fulminant viral myocarditis. *Innovations*. 2015;10(4):279-281.

[33] Khaliel F, Moss E, Demers P, Bouchard D. A bailout approach: transaxillary Impella implantation in toxic cardiomyopathy. *Asian Cardiovascular & Thoracic Annals*. 2014;22(6): 722-724.

[34] Miller MA, Dukkipati SR, Chinitz JS, et al. Percutaneous hemodynamic support with Impella 2.5 during scar-related ventricular tachycardia ablation (PERMIT 1). *Circulation. Arrhythmia and Electrophysiology*. Feb 2013;6(1):151-159.

Section 5

Coronary Imaging

Chapter 10

Coronary Computed Tomography Angiography

Stefan Baumann, Philipp Kryeziu,
Marlon Rutsch and Dirk Lossnitzer

Additional information is available at the end of the chapter

http://dx.doi.org/10.5772/67800

Abstract

Coronary computed tomographic angiography (cCTA) as a noninvasive approach underlies a rapid technological development with an impressive improvement of spatial and temporal resolution of the images. Therefore, it has become an accurate and cost-effective method to detect or exclude obstructive coronary artery disease (CAD) in patients with low to medium cardiovascular risk profile, as recommended by the ESC/AHA/ACC guidelines. The results show an excellent sensitivity, but still with a lack of specificity compared with invasive measurement. Several novel techniques like myocardial perfusion, plaque characterization or CT-based measurement of the fractional flow reserve have been developed to improve the positive predictive value and create more accurate results in detecting hemodynamically relevant stenoses. Moreover, during the last decade, the need to reduce radiation dose has become a central issue in clinical use, while the current generation of CT scanners has drastically lowered radiation dose. In conclusion, cCTA has become a promising alternative to invasive cardiac catheterization with still existing limitations. Thus, an appropriate patient selection is mandatory to utilize the advantages of this technique.

Keywords: coronary artery disease, coronary computed tomography angiography, coronary plaque, CT perfusion, CT-fractional flow reserve

1. Introduction

In the beginning of computed tomography (CT) era, the beating heart could not be examined suitably by this technique due to its motion artefacts. While scan times and consecutively temporal resolution, enhanced rapidly it has become a more accurate noninvasive imaging method for cardiac morphology. The first attempts in using CT to visualize coronary arteries have been made in the early 1980s and were followed by the back then newly emerging electron beam computed tomography (EBCT), which already had scan times lower than 100 ms [1]. Clinical relevance of the coronary CT angiography (cCTA) increased distinctly with the introduction of multi detector CT (MDCT) in the late 1990s—initially with four parallel detectors, the launch of the 64-slice MDCT generation enabled cCTA to become established in routine clinical practice [2, 3]. Nowadays, there are systems with up to 320-slices in clinical use, providing even lower scan times and a very high spatial resolution. Another landmark development was the introduction of the dual-source CT (DSCT) technology. DSCT contains of two tubes and detectors arranged in a 90° angle, also resulting in a higher temporal resolution due to the halved rotation time. The dual-energy CT (DECT) scans allow two different tube voltages, resulting in a significant lower radiation exposure for the patient [4]. As spatial and temporal resolution achieved remarkable dimensions, recent technologic improvement emphasized particularly the reduction of radiation dose on the one hand (see Section 3.1) [5], and the expansion of cCTA on additionally functional and morphological aspects, e.g., plaque characterization, myocardial perfusion imaging, or even CT-based fractional flow reserve (CT-FFR).

2. Coronary CT-angiography

2.1. Indication

Despite its many advantages, cCTA is only one out of many clinically approved methods to examine coronary arteries. Although there are notable technical developments in evaluating functional parameters as well [6–8], the current indication is predominantly the investigation of anatomical and morphological vessel characteristics. Especially in the exclusion of coronary artery disease (CAD), cCTA plays a decisive role [9–11]. Patients presenting with symptoms of CAD and low-to-intermediate risk patients undergo rapid evaluation of their coronary arteries. To estimate the suitable method for the individual patient, pre-test risk-stratification calculation plays a key role. For this purpose, Diamond-Forrester (**Table 1**) [12] and Genders (**Table 2**) [13] are well-established charts to obtain a pre-test probability of CAD based on age, sex, and chest pain constellation. However, further established cardiovascular

	Non-anginal chest pain		**Atypical angina**		**Typical angina**	
Age	**Men**	**Women**	**Men**	**Women**	**Men**	**Women**
30–39	5.2 ± 0.8	0.8 ± 0.3	21.8 ± 2.4	4.2 ± 1.3	69.7 ± 3.2	25.8 ± 6.6
40–49	14.1 ± 1.3	2.8 ± 0.7	46.1 ± 1.8	13.3 ± 2.9	87.3 ± 1.0	55.2 ± 6.5
50–59	21.5 ± 1.7	8.4 ± 1.2	58.9 ± 1.5	32.4 ± 3.0	92.0 ± 0.6	79.4 ± 2.4
60–69	28.1 ± 1.9	18.6 ± 1.9	67.1 ± 1.3	54.4 ± 2.4	94.3 ± 0.4	90.6 ± 1.0

Each value represents the percentage ± 1 standard deviation. Adapted from Diamond et al. [12].

Table 1. Pre-test likelihood of CAD in symptomatic patients according to age and sex.

http://dx.doi.org/10.5772/67800

	Non-anginal chest pain		Atypical angina		Typical angina	
Age	**Men**	**Women**	**Men**	**Women**	**Men**	**Women**
30–39	17.7	5.3	28.9	9.6	59.1	27.5
40–49	24.8	8.0	38.4	14.0	68.9	36.7
50–59	33.6	11.7	48.9	20.0	77.3	47.1
60–69	43.7	16.9	59.4	27.7	83.9	57.7
70–79	54.4	23.8	69.2	37.0	88.9	67.7
>80	64.6	32.3	77.5	47.4	92.5	76.3

Adapted from Genders et al. [13].

Table 2. Updated pre-test likelihood of CAD in symptomatic patients according to age and sex.

risk factors such as smoking, dyslipidemia, hypertension, diabetes, and family history of cardiac diseases should be considered in the risk stratification as well. Depending on the individual risk constellation, cCTA may be the suitable modality in low-to-intermediate risk patients, as for high-risk patients, invasive coronary angiography remains still the gold standard, as recommended by the ESC/AHA/ACC guidelines [9, 10]. Due to the three-dimensional visualization that can be constructed by cCTA, it can also be even used in planning and evaluating coronary artery bypass grafts (CABG) and detecting in-stent restenosis (ISR).

2.1.1. Suspected coronary artery disease

cCTA is excellent in visualizing coronary morphology and has emerged to an appropriate method of ruling out obstructive CAD. But by cCTA alone, the pathophysiological relevance of a detected CAD remains often unclear. Despite the remarkable advancements regarding functional parameters as for example perfusion imaging achieved by new DECT approaches, many conventional cCTAs show a rather moderate specificity regarding the functional assessment of cCTA measured stenosis. The methodical approach, as proposed by the SCCT guidelines for the interpretation and reporting of cCTA, consists of a systematic inspection of each coronary segment in multiple planes, the contemplation of image quality and artifacts and finally the evaluation of the respective lesions in regard of morphology, composition, and stenosis severity. A modified version of the well-established 1975 American Heart Association (AHA) model is used to refer to the certain segments [14]. Coronary abnormalities, plaque description or insufficient interpretability due to artifacts should be mentioned. Following this, a qualitative assessment for each segment is obtained and should be reported according to **Table 3**. Subsequently, a quantitative assessment of the stenosis severity is performed; the findings should be reported according to **Table 4**.

It has to be mentioned that these classifications are founded on morphological features only and, based on these findings, conclusions about functional or ischemic insufficiencies are not to be inferred.

0	Normal	Absence of plaque and no luminal stenosis
1	Minimal	Plaque with negligible impact on lumen
2	Mild	Plaque with mild narrowing of the lumen
3	Moderate	Plaque with moderate stenosis that may be of hemodynamic significance
4	Severe	Plaque with probable flow limiting disease
5	Occluded	

According to SCCT guidelines.

Table 3. Descriptors of qualitative stenosis severity.

2.1.2. Coronary artery stent

Due to the limited spatial resolution of the first electronic beam CT, it was initially not possible to visualize of the stented lumen and an indirect approach was applied to assess the stent patency. For this reason, contrast density was measured distally to the stent and compared with the density pattern proximal to the stented segment, in the aorta or the left ventricle, while stent patency was assumed when the contrast enhancement matched [15].

With the introduction of 64-slice scanners, a high negative predictive value could be reached for the evaluation of in-stent restenosis, while the positive predictive value is still rather worse as demonstrated by meta-analysis [16, 17]. However, there are specific technical limitations such as blooming caused by metal artifacts resulting in an underestimation of the stent lumen.

2.1.3. Coronary artery bypass graft

The value of cCTA in the assessment of coronary artery bypass graft (CABG) and native coronary arteries after bypass graft surgery continues to grow with advances in CT technology [18, 19]. The improvement of spatial resolution allows the cardiovascular radiologist and cardiac surgeon to evaluate the patency of CAGB in a rapid and noninvasive manner [20]. The major advantage of cCTA over invasive angiography is the ability to simultaneously evaluate for alternate postoperative complications like malposition, kinking, or pericardial effusion.

0	Normal	Absence of plaque and no luminal stenosis
1	Minimal	Plaque with <25% stenosis
2	Mild	25–49% stenosis
3	Moderate	50–69% stenosis
4	Severe	70–99% stenosis
5	Occluded	100% stenosis

According to SCCT guidelines.

Table 4. Descriptors of quantitative stenosis severity.

http://dx.doi.org/10.5772/67800

2.2. Benefits and limitation

The main benefit of cCTA is its noninvasive character. Although invasive coronary angiography (ICA) is an approved and secure procedure, it still involves the possibility of serious complications such as bleeding, stroke, or coronary dissection [6]. In comparison, the risks of cCTA, such as extravasation or allergic reaction to the contrast agent are less severe and common. As previously mentioned, cCTA is able to rule out CAD with excellent sensitivity and negative predictive value, both up to 99% in several studies [9, 21, 22]. Therefore, a preceding cCTA can reduce the share of unnecessarily performed ICA [11]. On the other hand, currently, the moderate specificity of cCTA causes a following ICA to validate the findings [9]. Recent developments seek to solve this issue. Further limitations result from technical conditions of computed tomography:

Although the temporal resolution has achieved levels below 80 ms, it is still necessary for the patient to maintain a heart frequency under 70 beats per minute to obtain a sufficient image quality. This might be accomplished using beta-blockers, but not all patients are suitable for auxiliary agents. Regarding patients who are unable to follow breathing orders, but especially patients with cardiac arrhythmias, prospectively electrocardiogram (ECG)-triggered images are prone to artifacts. New approaches in ECG triggering seek to react flexibly to arrhythmia but have to be implemented in the clinical routine. Retrospectively ECG-gated image acquisition is less interference-prone, but is along going with higher radiation doses. ECG-dependent dose reduction is required. Furthermore, a high coronary calcification or iatrogenic metallic material may lead to so-called blooming or streak artifacts, which tend to over-estimate the severity of stenoses [23, 24]. A better temporal resolution, acquired e.g., by using DSCT allows reduction of blooming artifacts. Radiation dose represents another important disbenefit of cCTA, which is explained later in detail.

3. Technical development

3.1. Radiation dose

Since its introduction into clinical use, a constantly mentioned point of criticism of cCTA is the radiation the patient is exposed to. While referring to this topic, one should distinguish the terms "radiation exposure," which describes the radiation emitted by the X-ray source, and "radiation dose," which indicates the amount of radiation absorbed by the patient [25]. The early concerns were not unjustified, as the novel scanners with 16 or 64 slices showed radiation doses above 10 mSv, even up to 21 mSv [26, 27], and radiation resulting of CT examinations make up a large share of the populations radiation exposure [28]. But subsequently, a substantial reduction of the applied radiation doses was achieved by different approaches: cCTA images are usually acquired using retrospective ECG gating, which requires a lower pitch and a longer duration, resulting in higher doses than prospective ECG triggering. Dose reduction is acceived using ECG gating or implementation of suitable ECG-triggering protocols. The first option is realized through ECG-dependent tube current modulation. The best image quality is obtained in the late-diastolic phase of the heart cycle; therefore, the tube current can be decreased in the remaining phase, resulting in a radiation dose lowered up to 50% [29, 30]. Under certain circumstances, it is possible to perform cCTA by prospective ECG triggering and sequential scanning. Patients with a low and stable heart rhythm and without an indication for functional testing are qualified for this technique in line with SCCT guidelines [31]. This attempt could reduce the radiation dose to 70–80% [29, 32]. Both options are optimal if either a scanner with 256 or more slices or a DSCT is used. Furthermore, use of DSCT enables further decrease due to its higher pitch rates at higher heart rates, since multisegment reconstruction is not necessary [33, 34]. Additional reduction is accomplished by a tube voltage of 100 kV or even 80 kV instead of the usual 120 kV, which can be performed depending on the patient's body mass [30, 31]. The image postprocessing technique of iterative reconstruction (chapter 3.2) also contributes to reduction of radiation dose. With all these measures taken into consideration, cCTA reached radiation doses lower than 4 mSv, therefore being in the range of the average yearly background radiation dose, in certain conditions even in submillisievert range [35, 36].

3.2. Image reconstruction

Nowadays, two methods of image reconstruction are in use, analytical filtered back projection (FBP) and iterative reconstruction (IR). The initially used technique was indeed the more complex IR [37], but soon its use was limited by the computational power of erstwhile processors. The method was displaced by FBP, which still is the most widely used technique nowadays.

In FBP, the measured intensity is described as an integral function, and the reconstruction data is obtained through solution of the resulting equations, which is called back projection. Additionally, a filter component compensates low-pass signals. If a higher spatial resolution is required, the filter can be adjusted accordingly. However, this adaptation of the filter causes a higher image noise, since image sharpness and image noise are proportional [38].

IR seeks to solve this problem, and since nowadays, not only CT hardware but also software underwent enormous advances, complex computational operations are more and more available. Iterative reconstruction accomplishes the back projection through the comparison of two components; a simulated first image estimation on the one hand and the actual measured projection on the other hand. Both images are automatically compared and, in case of discrepancy, the estimation is altered and another comparison is made until a default condition is achieved [38]. The underlying complex mathematical algorithms are propriety of the respective companies. Not only was IR able to break the correlation between image noise and spatial resolution, but it does so while simultaneously reducing the applied radiation dose up to 40–70%, while maintaining or even increasing subjective image quality and diagnostic accuracy [39–42].

4. Plaque characterization

The first attempts in evaluating atherosclerotic plaques via CT have already been made 1985 [43], but this approach did not gain acceptance due to insufficient resolution and image quality. Nowadays, with a spatial resolution up to 400 μm, noninvasive detection and characterization of atherosclerotic lesion and plaque characteristics can be performed by current CT scanners. Although intravascular ultrasound (IVUS) and optical coherence tomography (OCT) provide even higher spatial resolutions up to 80 and 20 μm, respectively [44], and therefore are the reference standard, cCTA yields the advantage of its noninvasive character. This technique enables an evaluation and characterization of the individual plaque extent and composition in patients without the clear indication for invasive measures. Recent studies have shown the ability of cCTA to perform on a high level in comparison with earlier mentioned reference standards, thus making cCTA a promising noninvasive method in identifying high-risk atherosclerotic coronary plaques [45–47]. Plaque characterization is essential in risk stratification in patients with suspected or diagnosed CAD or ACS, hereby it is important to distinguish the terms "stable" and "vulnerable" plaque (**Figure 2**). The hazard in stable plaques, consisting mainly of calcifications, lies in their subsequent obstruction of vessel lumen, associated with hemodynamic insufficiency, whereas vulnerable plaques tend to rupture and can lead to occlusion of the affected vessel through the thrombogenic lesion [48]. The finding that major adverse cardiac events (MACEs) are a consequence of the hemodynamically insignificant vulnerable plaques in more of two-thirds has been already made in the end of the last century [49, 50], but only now it is possible to detect morphological correlates *in vivo* via noninvasive methods [51]. Certain morphological plaque features correlate with the presence of rupture-prone plaques, and it is yet to be examined, which of these are reliable markers of plaque vulnerability [47, 52]. Although cCTA can distinguish distinctly between calcified, noncalcified (lipid rich/fibrotic) and mixed plaques, direct visualization of thin-cap fibroatheroma (TCFA) is currently only possible via OCT. To make plaque characterization via cCTA less dependent on the examiner's experience, scoring systems [53] and semiautomated software are ready to be implemented in clinical use, increasing operator convenience of this promising method.

5. CT myocardial perfusion

Due to high sensitivity and negative predictive value [54, 55], cCTA is at present an accepted diagnostic tool in detecting CAD in patients with low pretest probability [9]. However, the major limitation of cCTA remains in its low specificity and positive predictive value and the missing correlation of detected lesions and their physiological significance [56–58].

Challenge for novel diagnostic methods is to provide data about the anatomical and functional assessment of coronary stenosis. Myocardial perfusion derived from computed tomography (CTMP) is a recent instrument in diagnosis of ischemia. Compared to other functional tests, CTMP offers the substantial advantage that it is performed during ordinary cCTA. CTMP is a "one-stop shop" approach to close the gap between anatomical and functional assessment within a single imaging and could additionally limit false-positive results of cCTA [6].

Underlying principles of CTMP is the distribution and enhancement of iodinated contrast agent within the myocardium. The iodinated contrast agent is used as an indicator for myocardial blood flow and myocardial blood volume, based on the principles of the indicator-dilution theory. Myocardial areas with reduced amounts of contrast agent are indicating perfusion defects [59].

5.1. Image acquisition and protocols

Like other functional imaging methods, ordinary acquisition of CTMP consists of three sequences: a rest acquisition, an acquisition under pharmacological stress, and an acquisition of late enhancement. This approach is used to evaluate the reversibility of the ischemia [6].

Adenosine is used during the pharmacological stress acquisition for dilation of the coronary arteries with a dose ratio of 140 μg kg^{-1} min^{-1}. This leads to a decrease of the perfusion pressure. However, compensatory dilatation of obstructed arteries is limited. Reversible ischemia is the result of decreased perfusion reserves within these vessels. This pathophysiological phenomenon is called the "steal-effect." After 2–3 min of continuous administration of adenosine with monitoring of ECG, pulse oximetry, and blood pressure, iodinated contrast agent is injected and image acquisition starts [6]. Beyond the application of iodinated contrast agent during rest and stress acquisition and adenosine during stress acquisition, beta blockers, and nitrates were administered immediately before the examination to avoid motion artifacts and to improve image quality [59]. Contraindication (e.g., contrast agent allergy, severe COPD, severe aortic valve stenosis) should be taken into consideration regarding suitability of the patient. After 5–10 min of administration of contrast agent, a delayed acquisition can provide information about nonviable myocardium [6]. Myocardial areas of ischemia or infarction are described based on the American Heart Association segmental model [14].

Regarding comparability of studies and deeper understanding, it should be noted that there is a static myocardial blood pool imaging method during first pass and apart from it a dynamic myocardial perfusion method over several time points of myocardial iodine distribution. Development in computed tomography offers with dual-energy CT a further static perfusion method. For example, differences between these techniques apply on the direct assessment of quantitative perfusion parameters or radiation exposure [6, 60].

5.2. Radiation exposure

Radiation dose of a comprehensive protocol containing rest, stress, delayed enhancement, and calcium scoring have generally been reported in the range of 12–14 mSv. This is comparable to the radiation dose during SPECT examination [6]. Modified protocols in research contain considerably lower radiation. Feuchtner et al. achieved high accuracy (sensitivity 96%, specificity 88%, PPV 93%, and NPV 94%) in a stress approach and reported radiation dose of 2.5 mSv for cCTA and perfusion imaging with pharmacological stress [61]. Radiation doses for CTMP can be expected to decrease further, as radiation doses <1 mSv on cCTA studies are still state of the art [61].

5.3. Clinical setting

As mentioned in the introduction of this chapter, CT myocardial perfusion offers additional functional data of the myocardial blood supply. In contrast, ordinary cCTA only provides anatomical evaluation of the heart. Combined cCTA plus CTMP provides incremental diagnostic value compared with cCTA alone to assess the status of the myocardial blood supply and for the detection of significant coronary stenosis [6, 57, 58].

Compared with other functional noninvasive methods such as single photon emission computed tomography (SPECT) or cardiac magnetic resonance perfusion imaging (cMRI), CTMP is a recent technology.

SPECT is a nuclear imaging technique with tracer substances, such as thallium-201 or technetium-99. Myocardial enhancement of this tracer differs in damaged myocardium. A rotating gamma camera enables three-dimensional tomographic reconstruction [6]. According to current guidelines of the American Heart Association and American College of Cardiology, SPECT is used for the diagnosis of CAD, risk stratification, myocardial viability, and left ventricular function [62]. Rest and stress SPECT acquisitions allow evaluation of ischemic reversibility.

Cardiac magnetic resonance imaging (cMRI) offers anatomical information and a variety of functional aspects, such as assessment of myocardial perfusion during rest and stress acquisition and myocardial viability. SPECT has lower temporal and spatial resolution than cMRI [6]. The large CE-MARC trial led to higher sensitivity with cMRI than with SPECT and postulated cost-effectiveness and more use of this method [63, 64]. Patients with devices such as cardiac pacemakers or internal cardiac defibrillator (ICD) are often associated with great effort, regarding cMRI requirements. For patients with a tendency to claustrophobia, cMRI is potentially not the adequate examination due to long acquisition time [65]. On the other hand, cMRI is advantageous because of no ionizing radiation.

CT myocardial perfusion or other functional techniques are not reasonable in each clinical question compared to ordinary cCTA for ruling out CAD. In a situation of acute chest pain in a patient with low pretest probability of CAD, an extensive stress examination (irrespective of the imaging technique) is potentially not indicated due to prolonged examination. The availability in case of short-term request of such a comprehensive examination represents a further doubtful aspect in the clinical setting. However, CT myocardial perfusion has the potential to overcome these obstacles.

6. Conclusion and further perspective

Myocardial perfusion derived from computed tomography is a growing diagnostic method that provides a comprehensive evaluation of coronary artery disease along with functional assessment of the myocardium with promising findings in current clinical studies. Combining cCTA with CTMP significantly improves specificity and positive predictive value [57, 58].

The multicentre DECIDE-Gold trial [66] might contribute in establishment myocardial perfusion within the clinical setting. Focus of current research is, e.g., the order and general need of all three sequences in times of modern dual energy computed tomography scanners. Meinel et al. postulates a dual energy rest-stress approach as protocol of choice. Furthermore, he achieves excellent sensitivity and specificity in a rest-only approach [67]. This would represent substantial advantage for the patient. Functional situation of myocardial blood supply could be derived simultaneously from ordinary coronary computed tomography angiography within the same examination, without additional radiation, drugs or prolonged examination.

CT myocardial perfusion imaging offers great potential to reclassify findings in cCTA and to evaluate the myocardial blood supply [68]. Regarding risk of invasive coronary angiography [69], an initial noninvasive diagnostic selection would be desirable to reduce invasive angiograms, showing no obstructive CAD. Addition of CTMP to cCTA holds highly promising potential to adopt this role and to establish CT as a single imaging examination for comprehensive evaluation of CAD and direct assessment of myocardial ischemia in one examination (**Figure 1**).

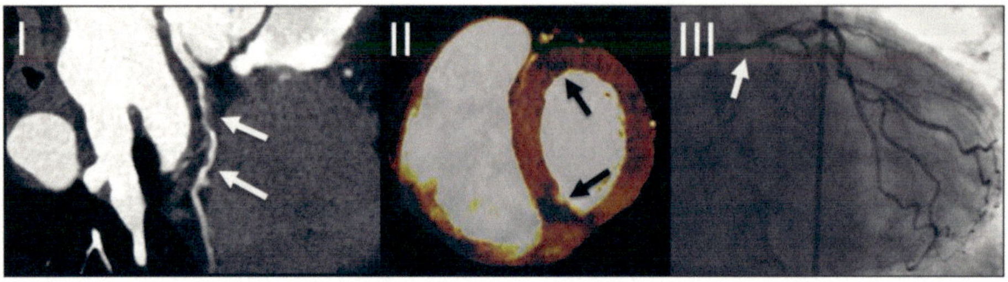

Figure 1. 59-year-old female with known hypertension presenting with chest pain. (I) cCTA show several moderate stenoses of the LAD (arrows). **(II)** DECT show minor iodine distribution within basal LAD and RCA territory as a sign of hemodynamic significance (arrows). **(III)** Invasive catheter angiography show severe artery disease of all three vessels. Subtotal stenosis of RCA, significant stenosis of the left main trunk (arrow) and 75% stenosis of mid RCX and Ramus marginalis. cCTA, coronary computed tomography; DECT, dual-energy computed tomography; LAD, left anterior descending; RCA, right coronary artery; RCX, ramus circumflexus.

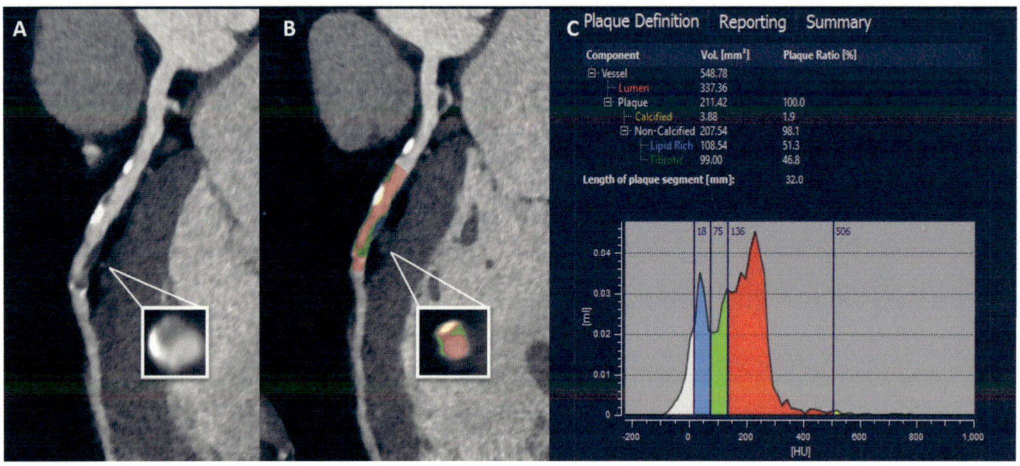

Figure 2.(A) cCTA shows stenotic noncalcified plaque of the LAD. **(B + C)** Color-coded automated plaque quantification by the analysis software showed the plaque composition as predominantly noncalcified. cCTA, coronary computed tomography angiography; LAD, left anterior descending.

7. CT-FFR

The invasive measurement of the fractional flow reserve is currently the accepted reference standard to determine, whether a coronary stenosis is hemodynamically relevant and is

http://dx.doi.org/10.5772/67800

therefore implemented in the guidelines [70]. The FAME study has proved that FFR guided coronary revascularization is associated with reduced rates of death, myocardial infarction or target vessel revascularization [71]. In clinical routine, the use of invasive FFR is associated with risks and complications such a severe bleeding, arrhythmia, stroke, and coronary dissections depending on the experience of the interventional cardiologist [72].

Novel technologies have been developed to calculate noninvasive FFR from routine cCTA datasets using computational fluid dynamics. The main advantage of this technology is the markly improvement of specificity and positive predictive value compared to standard cCTA, without additional stress medication, image protocols, and radiation exposure (**Table 5**). While the first studies concentrated on the general feasibility and diagnostic performance, further clinical studies validated the cost-effectiveness. The PLATFORM-study showed that the numbers of patients without anatomically obstructive CAD ($p < 0.0001$) could be significantly improved with the CT-FFR arm, while the secondary endpoint radiation exposure showed no difference (9.9 vs. 9.4 mSv, $p = 0.20$) [73].

There are the first head-to-head comparisons of CT-FFR compared stress CT myocardial perfusion (CTP) in patients with CAD with a per-vessel specificity of was 66% for cCTA, 77% for CT-FFR, and 91% for CTP, respectively, while the diagnostic performance of cCTA alone

	Koo et al. (DISCOVER-FLOW) [77]	**Min et al. (DeFACTO) [78]**	**Nørgaard et al. (NXT-Trial) [79]**	**Renker et al. [80]**	**Coenen et al. [81]**
Vessels	159	407	484	67	189
Vessels with intermediate stenosis (30–70%)	66/159 [25] (41.5%)	150/407 [26] (36.9%)	235/484 (48.6%)	39/67 (58.2%)	144/189 (76.2%)
Sensitivity (%)	87.9 (76.7–95.0) [91.4 (81.0–97.1)]	80 (73–86) [N.A.]	84 (75–89) [83 (74–89)]	85 (62–97) [90 (68–98)]	87.5 (78.2–93.8) [81.3 (71.0–89.1)]
Specificity (%)	82.2 (73.3–89.1) [39.6 (30.0–49.8)]	61 (54–67) [N.A.]	86 (82–89) [60 (56–65)]	85 (72–94) [34 (21–49)]	65.1 (55.4–74.0] [37.6 (28.5–47.4)]
PPV (%)	73.9 (61.9–83.7) [46.5 (37.1–56.1)]	56 (49–62) [N.A.]	61 (53–69) [33 (27–39)]	71 (49–87) [37 (23–52)]	64.8 (55.0–73.8)] [48.9 (40.1–57.7)]
NPV (%)	92.2 (84.6–96.8] [88.9 (75.9–96.3)]	84 (78–89) [N.A.]	95 (93–97) [92 (88–95)]	93 (81–98) [89 (65–98)]	87.7 (78.5–93.9) [73.2 (59.7–84.2)]
Accuracy (%)	84.3 (77.7–90.0) [58.5 (50.4–66.2)]	N.A. [N.A.]	86 (83–89) [65 (61–69)]	N.A. [N.A.]	74.6 (68.4–80.8) [56.1 (49.0–63.2)]
AUC	0.90 (N.A.) [0.75 (N.A.)] (p = 0.001)	N.A. [N.A.]	0.93 (0.91–0.95) [0.79 (0.74–0.84)] (p <0.001)	0.92 (N.A.) [0.72(N.A.)] (p <0.005)	0.83 (N.A.) [0.64 (N.A.)] (p <0.001)

CT-FFR <0.80 (95% CI) und cCTA stenosis ≥50% (95% CI) [in brackets] were defined as cut-off values. AUC, area under the curve; cCTA, coronary CT-angiography; CT-FFR, CT-based FFR; FFR, Fractional flow reserve; N.A., not available; NPV, negative predictive value; PPV, positive predictive value.

Table 5. Diagnostic accuracy of CT-FFR and cCTA compared to invasive FFR as the reference standard on a per vessel (n = 1306) basis.

was significantly improved by combination with CT-FFR or CTP [74]. Meta-analysis shows that CT-FFR can act in the context of other myocardial perfusion modalities as a potential gatekeeper for invasive revascularization (**Table 6**) in patients with suspected or known CAD using invasive FFR as the reference standard [75]. Due to time-consuming off-site calculation and transfer of the datasets to external core laboratory the clinical impact is limited. Thus, a novel solution for physician-driven CT-FFR derivation using regular on-site workstations was developed. This CT-FFR algorithm applies reduced-order models for more expeditious calculation, but is currently not commercially available [76].

	CT-FFR	CT-perfusion	SPECT	PET	MRT
Number of vessels	714	1074	924	870	1830
Sensitivity (%)	0.83 (0.79–0.87)	0.78 (0.72–0.82)	0.61 (0.56–0.66)	0.83 (0.77–0.88)	0.87 (0.84–0.90)
Specificity (%)	0.77 (0.74–0.80)	0.86 (0.83–0.88)	0.84 (0.81–0.87)	0.89 (0.86–0.91)	0.91 (0.89–0.92)
PLR	3.76 (2.17–6.54)	5.74 (3.48–9.46)	3.76 (2.74–5.16)	7.43 (5.03–10.99)	8.27 (4.93–13.87)
NLR	0.23 (0.16–0.35)	0.22 (0.12–0.39)	0.47 (0.37–0.59)	0.15 (0.05–0.44)	0.16 (0.13–0.21)
AUC	N.A.	0.91 (0.86–0.96)	0.83 (0.67–0.98)	0.95 (0.91–0.99)	0.95 (0.93–0.97)

Adapted from von Gonzalez et al. [82] and Takx et al. [75]. AUC, area under the curve; cCTA, coronary CT-angiography; CT-FFR, CT based fractional flow reserve; FFR, fractional flow reserve; N.A., not available; NLR, negative likelihood ratio; PLR, positive likelihood ratio.

Table 6. Diagnostic accuracy of CT-FFR and other non-invasive modalities compared to invasive FFR.

Currently, CT-FFR is an interesting and sophisticated approach to identify functionally significant CAD in a noninvasive way. However, this promising technique is still in development and searching for its clinical application, and further evidence studies are necessary before CT-FFR is implemented for clinical use.

Author details

Stefan Baumann*, Philipp Kryeziu, Marlon Rutsch and Dirk Lossnitzer

*Address all correspondence to: stefanbaumann@gmx.at

First Department of Medicine-Cardiology, University Medical Centre Mannheim, Mannheim, Germany

References

[1] Boyd, D.P. and M.J. Lipton, *Cardiac Computed Tomography*. Proceedings of the IEEE, 1983. **71**(3): pp. 298-307.

[2] Rubin, G.D., et al., *CT angiography after 20 years: a transformation in cardiovascular disease characterization continues to advance*. Radiology, 2014. **271**(3): pp. 633-52.

[3] Apfaltrer, P., et al., *Coronary computed tomography—present status and future directions*. Int J Clin Pract Suppl, 2011(173): pp. 3-13.

[4] Halliburton, S., et al., *State-of-the-art in CT hardware and scan modes for cardiovascular CT*. J Cardiovasc Comput Tomogr, 2012. **6**(3): pp. 154-63.

[5] Heydari, B., et al., *Diagnostic performance of high-definition coronary computed tomography angiography performed with multiple radiation dose reduction strategies*. Can J Cardiol, 2011. **27**(5): pp. 606-12.

[6] Bucher, A.M., et al., *Cardiac CT for myocardial ischaemia detection and characterization--comparative analysis*. Br J Radiol, 2014. **87**(1043): p. 20140159.

[7] Douglas, P.S., et al., *Outcomes of anatomical versus functional testing for coronary artery disease*. N Engl J Med, 2015. **372**(14): pp. 1291-300.

[8] Norgaard, B.L., et al., *Coronary computed tomography angiography derived fractional flow reserve and plaque stress*. Curr Cardiovasc Imaging Rep, 2016. **9**: p. 2.

[9] Montalescot, G., et al., *2013 ESC guidelines on the management of stable coronary artery disease: the task force on the management of stable coronary artery disease of the European Society of Cardiology*. Eur Heart J, 2013. **34**(38): pp. 2949-3003.

[10] Wolk, M.J., et al., *ACCF/AHA/ASE/ASNC/HFSA/HRS/SCAI/SCCT/SCMR/STS 2013 multimodality appropriate use criteria for the detection and risk assessment of stable ischemic heart disease: a report of the American College of Cardiology Foundation Appropriate Use Criteria Task Force, American Heart Association, American Society of Echocardiography, American Society of Nuclear Cardiology, Heart Failure Society of America, Heart Rhythm Society, Society for Cardiovascular Angiography and Interventions, Society of Cardiovascular Computed Tomography, Society for Cardiovascular Magnetic Resonance, and Society of Thoracic Surgeons*. J Am Coll Cardiol, 2014. **63**(4): pp. 380-406.

[11] Shaw, L.J., et al., *Coronary computed tomographic angiography as a gatekeeper to invasive diagnostic and surgical procedures: results from the multicenter CONFIRM (Coronary CT angiography evaluation for clinical outcomes: an International multicenter) registry*. J Am Coll Cardiol, 2012. **60**(20): pp. 2103-14.

[12] Diamond, G.A. and J.S. Forrester, *Analysis of probability as an aid in the clinical diagnosis of coronary-artery disease*. N Engl J Med, 1979. **300**(24): pp. 1350-8.

[13] Genders, T.S., et al., *A clinical prediction rule for the diagnosis of coronary artery disease: validation, updating, and extension*. Eur Heart J, 2011. **32**(11): pp. 1316-30.

[14] Cerqueira, M.D., et al., *Standardized myocardial segmentation and nomenclature for tomographic imaging of the heart. A statement for healthcare professionals from the Cardiac Imaging Committee of the Council on Clinical Cardiology of the American Heart Association*. Circulation, 2002. **105**(4): pp. 539-42.

[15] Schmermund, A., et al., *Non-invasive assessment of coronary Palmaz-Schatz stents by contrast enhanced electron beam computed tomography.* Eur Heart J, 1996. **17**(10): pp. 1546-53.

[16] Sun, Z. and A.M. Almutairi, *Diagnostic accuracy of 64 multislice CT angiography in the assessment of coronary in-stent restenosis: a meta-analysis.* Eur J Radiol, 2010. **73**(2): pp. 266-73.

[17] Kumbhani, D.J., et al., *Meta-analysis of diagnostic efficacy of 64-slice computed tomography in the evaluation of coronary in-stent restenosis.* Am J Cardiol, 2009. **103**(12): pp. 1675-81.

[18] Malagutti, P., et al., *Use of 64-slice CT in symptomatic patients after coronary bypass surgery: evaluation of grafts and coronary arteries.* Eur Heart J, 2007. **28**(15): pp. 1879-85.

[19] Engelmann, M.G., et al., *Non-invasive coronary bypass graft imaging after multivessel revascularisation.* Int J Cardiol, 2000. **76**(1): pp. 65-74.

[20] Frazier, A.A., et al., *Coronary artery bypass grafts: assessment with multidetector CT in the early and late postoperative settings.* Radiographics, 2005. **25**(4): pp. 881-96.

[21] Budoff, M.J., et al., *Diagnostic performance of 64-multidetector row coronary computed tomographic angiography for evaluation of coronary artery stenosis in individuals without known coronary artery disease: results from the prospective multicenter ACCURACY (Assessment by Coronary Computed Tomographic Angiography of Individuals Undergoing Invasive Coronary Angiography) trial.* J Am Coll Cardiol, 2008. **52**(21): pp. 1724-32.

[22] Min, J.K., L.J. Shaw, and D.S. Berman, *The present state of coronary computed tomography angiography a process in evolution.* J Am Coll Cardiol, 2010. **55**(10): pp. 957-65.

[23] Sarwar, A., et al., *Calcified plaque: measurement of area at thin-section flat-panel CT and 64-section multidetector CT and comparison with histopathologic findings.* Radiology, 2008. **249**(1): pp. 301-6.

[24] Hoffmann, U., et al., *Predictive value of 16-slice multidetector spiral computed tomography to detect significant obstructive coronary artery disease in patients at high risk for coronary artery disease: patient-versus segment-based analysis.* Circulation, 2004. **110**(17): pp. 2638-43.

[25] Morin, R.L., T.C. Gerber, and C.H. McCollough, *Radiation dose in computed tomography of the heart.* Circulation, 2003. **107**(6): pp. 917-22.

[26] Sun, Z. and K.H. Ng, *Multislice CT angiography in cardiac imaging. Part III: radiation risk and dose reduction.* Singapore Med J, 2010. **51**(5): pp. 374-80.

[27] Peebles, C., *Computed tomographic coronary angiography: how many slices do you need?* Heart, 2006. **92**(5): pp. 582-4.

[28] Brenner, D.J. and E.J. Hall, *Computed tomography—an increasing source of radiation exposure.* N Engl J Med, 2007. **357**(22): pp. 2277-84.

[29] Earls, J.P., et al., *Prospectively gated transverse coronary CT angiography versus retrospectively gated helical technique: improved image quality and reduced radiation dose.* Radiology, 2008. **246**(3): pp. 742-53.

[30] Hausleiter, J. and T. Meyer, *Tips to minimize radiation exposure*. J Cardiovasc Comput Tomogr, 2008. **2**(5): pp. 325-7.

[31] Halliburton, S.S., et al., *SCCT guidelines on radiation dose and dose-optimization strategies in cardiovascular CT*. J Cardiovasc Comput Tomogr, 2011. **5**(4): pp. 198-224.

[32] Menke, J., et al., *Head-to-head comparison of prospectively triggered vs retrospectively gated coronary computed tomography angiography: Meta-analysis of diagnostic accuracy, image quality, and radiation dose*. Am Heart J, 2013. **165**(2): pp. 154-63 e3.

[33] Linsen, P.V., et al., *Computed tomography angiography with a 192-slice dual-source computed tomography system: improvements in image quality and radiation dose*. J Clin Imaging Sci, 2016. **6**: p. 44.

[34] Sun, K., et al., *Prospectively electrocardiogram-gated high-pitch spiral acquisition mode dual-source CT coronary angiography in patients with high heart rates: comparison with retrospective electrocardiogram-gated spiral acquisition mode*. Korean J Radiol, 2012. **13**(6): pp. 684-93.

[35] Achenbach, S., et al., *Coronary computed tomography angiography with a consistent dose below 1 mSv using prospectively electrocardiogram-triggered high-pitch spiral acquisition*. Eur Heart J, 2010. **31**(3): pp. 340-6.

[36] Chen, M.Y., S.M. Shanbhag, and A.E. Arai, *Submillisievert median radiation dose for coronary angiography with a second-generation 320-detector row CT scanner in 107 consecutive patients*. Radiology, 2013. **267**(1): pp. 76-85.

[37] Hounsfield, G.N., *Computerized transverse axial scanning (tomography). 1. Description of system*. Br J Radiol, 1973. **46**(552): pp. 1016-22.

[38] Geyer, L.L., et al., *State of the art: iterative CT reconstruction techniques*. Radiology, 2015. **276**(2): pp. 339-57.

[39] Renker, M., et al., *Iterative image reconstruction techniques: applications for cardiac CT*. J Cardiovasc Comput Tomogr, 2011. **5**(4): pp. 225-30.

[40] Hou, Y., et al., *The optimal dose reduction level using iterative reconstruction with prospective ECG-triggered coronary CTA using 256-slice MDCT*. Eur J Radiol, 2012. **81**(12): pp. 3905-11.

[41] Pontone, G., et al., *Feasibility and diagnostic accuracy of a low radiation exposure protocol for prospective ECG-triggering coronary MDCT angiography*. Clin Radiol, 2012. **67**(3): pp. 207-15.

[42] Takx, R.A., et al., *Coronary CT angiography: comparison of a novel iterative reconstruction with filtered back projection for reconstruction of low-dose CT-Initial experience*. Eur J Radiol, 2013. **82**(2): pp. 275-80.

[43] Leeson, M.D., et al., *Atheromatous extracranial carotid arteries: CT evaluation correlated with arteriography and pathologic examination*. Radiology, 1985. **156**(2): pp. 397-402.

[44] Baumann, S., et al., *Computed tomography imaging of coronary artery plaque: characterization and prognosis*. Radiol Clin North Am, 2015. **53**(2): pp. 307-15.

[45] Fischer, C., et al., *Coronary CT angiography versus intravascular ultrasound for estimation of coronary stenosis and atherosclerotic plaque burden: a meta-analysis.* J Cardiovasc Comput Tomogr, 2013. **7**(4): pp. 256-66.

[46] Achenbach, S., et al., *Detection of calcified and noncalcified coronary atherosclerotic plaque by contrast-enhanced, submillimeter multidetector spiral computed tomography: a segment-based comparison with intravascular ultrasound.* Circulation, 2004. **109**(1): pp. 14-7.

[47] Nakazato, R., et al., *Quantification and characterisation of coronary artery plaque volume and adverse plaque features by coronary computed tomographic angiography: a direct comparison to intravascular ultrasound.* Eur Radiol, 2013. **23**(8): pp. 2109-17.

[48] Finn, A.V., et al., *Concept of vulnerable/unstable plaque.* Arterioscler Thromb Vasc Biol, 2010. **30**(7): pp. 1282-92.

[49] Muller, J.E., G.H. Tofler, and P.H. Stone, *Circadian variation and triggers of onset of acute cardiovascular disease.* Circulation, 1989. **79**(4): pp. 733-43.

[50] Virmani, R., et al., *Lessons from sudden coronary death: a comprehensive morphological classification scheme for atherosclerotic lesions.* Arterioscler Thromb Vasc Biol, 2000. **20**(5): pp. 1262-75.

[51] Stone, G.W., et al., *A prospective natural-history study of coronary atherosclerosis.* N Engl J Med, 2011. **364**(3): pp. 226-35.

[52] Tesche, C., et al., *Prognostic implications of coronary CT angiography-derived quantitative markers for the prediction of major adverse cardiac events.* J Cardiovasc Comput Tomogr, 2016. 10(6): pp. 458-465.

[53] Cavalcante, R., et al., *Validation of coronary computed tomography angiography scores for non-invasive assessment of atherosclerotic burden through a comparison with multivessel intravascular ultrasound.* Atherosclerosis, 2016. **247**: pp. 21-7.

[54] Gorenoi, V., M.P. Schonermark, and A. Hagen, *CT coronary angiography vs. invasive coronary angiography in CHD.* GMS Health Technol Assess, 2012. **8**: p. Doc02.

[55] Jacobs, J.E., et al., *ACR practice guideline for the performance and interpretation of cardiac computed tomography (CT).* J Am Coll Radiol, 2006. **3**(9): pp. 677-85.

[56] Kristensen, T.S., et al., *Correlation between coronary computed tomographic angiography and fractional flow reserve.* Int J Cardiol, 2010. **144**(2): pp. 200-5.

[57] Sorgaard, M.H., et al., *Diagnostic accuracy of static CT perfusion for the detection of myocardial ischemia. A systematic review and meta-analysis.* J Cardiovasc Comput Tomogr, 2016.

[58] Caruso, D., et al., *Dynamic CT myocardial perfusion imaging.* Eur J Radiol, 2016. **85**(10): pp. 1893-9.

[59] Ambrose, M.S., et al., *CT perfusion: ready for prime time.* Curr Cardiol Rep, 2011. **13**(1): pp. 57-66.

[60] Pelgrim, G.J., et al., *The dream of a one-stop-shop: meta-analysis on myocardial perfusion CT.* Eur J Radiol, 2015. **84**(12): pp. 2411-20.

[61] Feuchtner, G., et al., *Adenosine stress high-pitch 128-slice dual-source myocardial computed tomography perfusion for imaging of reversible myocardial ischemia: comparison with magnetic resonance imaging*. Circ Cardiovasc Imaging, 2011. **4**(5): pp. 540-9.

[62] Klocke, F.J., et al., *ACC/AHA/ASNC guidelines for the clinical use of cardiac radionuclide imaging—executive summary*. J Am Coll Cardiol, 2003. **42**(7): pp. 1318-1333.

[63] Greenwood, J.P., et al., *Comparison of cardiovascular magnetic resonance and single-photon emission computed tomography in women with suspected coronary artery disease from the Clinical Evaluation of Magnetic Resonance Imaging in Coronary Heart Disease (CE-MARC) Trial*. Circulation, 2014. **129**(10): pp. 1129-38.

[64] Walker, S., et al., *Cost-effectiveness of cardiovascular magnetic resonance in the diagnosis of coronary heart disease: an economic evaluation using data from the CE-MARC study*. Heart, 2013. **99**(12): pp. 873-81.

[65] Bluemke, D.A., et al., *Noninvasive coronary artery imaging: magnetic resonance angiography and multidetector computed tomography angiography: a scientific statement from the american heart association committee on cardiovascular imaging and intervention of the council on cardiovascular radiology and intervention, and the councils on clinical cardiology and cardiovascular disease in the young*. Circulation, 2008. **118**(5): pp. 586-606.

[66] Truong, Q.A., et al., *Rationale and design of the dual-energy computed tomography for ischemia determination compared to "gold standard" non-invasive and invasive techniques (DECIDE-Gold):a multicenter international efficacy diagnostic study of rest-stress dual-energy computed tomography angiography with perfusion*. J Nucl Cardiol, 2015. **22**(5): pp. 1031-40.

[67] Meinel, F.G., et al., *First-arterial-pass dual-energy CT for assessment of myocardial blood supply: do we need rest, stress, and delayed acquisition? Comparison with SPECT*. Radiology, 2014. **270**(3): pp. 708-16.

[68] Osawa, K., et al., *Diagnostic performance of first-pass myocardial perfusion imaging without stress with computed tomography (CT) compared with coronary CT angiography alone, with fractional flow reserve as the reference standard*. PLoS One, 2016. **11**(2): p. e0149170.

[69] Noto, T.J., Jr., et al., *Cardiac catheterization 1990: a report of the registry of the Society for Cardiac Angiography and Interventions (SCA&I)*. Cathet Cardiovasc Diagn, 1991. **24**(2): pp. 75-83.

[70] Authors/Task Force, m., et al., *2014 ESC/EACTS Guidelines on myocardial revascularization: the task force on myocardial revascularization of the European Society of Cardiology (ESC) and the European Association for Cardio-Thoracic Surgery (EACTS)developed with the special contribution of the European Association of Percutaneous Cardiovascular Interventions (EAPCI)*. Eur Heart J, 2014. **35**(37): pp. 2541-619.

[71] Tonino, P.A., et al., *Fractional flow reserve versus angiography for guiding percutaneous coronary intervention*. N Engl J Med, 2009. **360**(3): pp. 213-24.

[72] Park, S.J., et al., *Trends in the outcomes of percutaneous coronary intervention with the routine incorporation of fractional flow reserve in real practice*. Eur Heart J, 2013. **34**(43): pp. 3353-61.

[73] Douglas, P.S., et al., *Clinical outcomes of fractional flow reserve by computed tomographic angiography-guided diagnostic strategies vs. usual care in patients with suspected coronary artery disease: the prospective longitudinal trial of FFR(CT): outcome and resource impacts study*. Eur Heart J, 2015. **36**(47): pp. 3359-67.

[74] Yang, D.H., et al., *Diagnostic performance of on-site CT-derived fractional flow reserve versus CT perfusion*. Eur Heart J Cardiovasc Imaging, 2016. 35: pp. 1120-30.

[75] Takx, R.A., et al., *Diagnostic accuracy of stress myocardial perfusion imaging compared to invasive coronary angiography with fractional flow reserve meta-analysis*. Circ Cardiovasc Imaging, 2015. **8**(1).

[76] Baumann, S., et al., *Different approaches for coronary computed tomography angiography-derived versus invasive fractional flow reserve assessment*. Am J Cardiol, 2016. **117**(3): p. 486.

[77] Koo, B.K., et al., *Diagnosis of ischemia-causing coronary stenoses by noninvasive fractional flow reserve computed from coronary computed tomographic angiograms. Results from the prospective multicenter DISCOVER-FLOW (Diagnosis of Ischemia-Causing Stenoses Obtained Via Noninvasive Fractional Flow Reserve) study*. J Am Coll Cardiol, 2011. **58**(19): pp. 1989-97.

[78] Min, J.K., et al., *Diagnostic accuracy of fractional flow reserve from anatomic CT angiography*. Jama, 2012. **308**(12): pp. 1237-45.

[79] Norgaard, B.L., et al., *Diagnostic performance of noninvasive fractional flow reserve derived from coronary computed tomography angiography in suspected coronary artery disease: the NXT trial (Analysis of Coronary Blood Flow Using CT Angiography: Next Steps)*. J Am Coll Cardiol, 2014. **63**(12): pp. 1145-55.

[80] Renker, M., et al., *Comparison of diagnostic value of a novel noninvasive coronary computed tomography angiography method versus standard coronary angiography for assessing fractional flow reserve*. Am J Cardiol, 2014. **114**(9): pp. 1303-8.

[81] Coenen, A., et al., *Fractional flow reserve computed from noninvasive CT angiography data: diagnostic performance of an on-site clinician-operated computational fluid dynamics algorithm*. Radiology, 2015. **274**(3): pp. 674-83.

[82] Gonzalez, J.A., et al., *Meta-Analysis of diagnostic performance of coronary computed tomography angiography, computed tomography perfusion, and computed tomography-fractional flow reserve in functional myocardial ischemia assessment versus invasive fractional flow reserve*. Am J Cardiol, 2015. **116**(9): pp. 1469-78.

Section 6

Acute Myocardial Infarction Mimicking Syndrome

Chapter 11

The Clinical Manifestations, Diagnosis and Management of Takotsubo Syndrome

Uzair Ansari and Ibrahim El-Battrawy

Additional information is available at the end of the chapter

http://dx.doi.org/10.5772/68037

Abstract

The Takotsubo syndrome (TTS) is a transient cardiac dysfunction characterised by a variety of ventricular wall-motion abnormalities. Alternative nomenclatures for this disorder include stress-induced cardiomyopathy, apical ballooning syndrome and 'broken heart syndrome'. TTS bears stark resemblance to an acute coronary syndrome, wherein patients present with acute chest pain and initial diagnostic workup correlates to abnormalities suggesting significant coronary stenosis. Interestingly, the distinguishing factor in TTS is the absence of an occlusive coronary vascular disease, which could correlate with these changes. The underlying pathophysiology explaining the evolution of TTS is still debatable; however, results from various recent studies and registers have shed more light on this obscure clinical entity. The detailed description of a criterion which demonstrably includes most patients with probable TTS has helped tune management strategies in ensuring necessary supportive care and early therapeutic interventions of complications, which could arise in course of the disease.

Keywords: Takotsubo cardiomyopathy, pathophysiology, catecholamines, complication, diagnosis, treatment

1. Introduction

The *Takotsubo* syndrome (TTS), first described in 1990 by Sato et al., is a transient cardiac dysfunction characterised by a variety of ventricular wall-motion abnormalities [1, 2]. Its name is derived from the resemblance of the left ventricle at end-systole to the octopus-pots of Japanese fishermen in the Hiroshima fish markets [3]; however, alternative nomenclatures such as stress or stress-induced cardiomyopathy, apical ballooning syndrome and 'broken heart syndrome' have also been used to label this usually reversible form of acute heart failure [4–7]. This clinical entity essentially mimics an acute coronary syndrome, wherein patients present with acute chest pain, and demonstrates the typical biomarker profile (release of cardiac troponin and creatine kinase) and/or electrocardiographic abnormalities suggesting significant coronary stenosis. Interestingly, the distinguishing factor in Takotsubo syndrome is the absence of an occlusive coronary vascular disease, which correlates with these changes [8]. Although, the pathophysiology of this disorder remains unclear, recent hypotheses have suggested a form of acute catecholaminergic myocardial stunning to explain the pattern of temporary LV dysfunction and regional wall-motion abnormality commonly seen at the time of presentation [9].

2. Definition

The Takotsubo syndrome is an acute and usually reversible form of heart failure, precipitated by physical and/or emotional stresses or in some cases without any evident preceding trigger. In recent years, various institutions and working groups such as the Mayo Clinic, the Gothenburg group, the Japanese Circulation Society and the Takotsubo Italian Network have proposed their diagnostic criteria to better define this disease; however, in 2015, the Heart Failure Association for the European Society of Cardiology (HFA) outlined its conclusive version. This has been outlined in **Table 1** [8, 10]. A significant feature of this criterion is the inclusion of pheochromocytoma as a trigger for this syndrome. Patients diagnosed with this disorder could suffer from an acute Takotsubo syndrome in the event of a catecholamine storm, analogous to the response incited by other emotional or physical stresses.

- Transient regional wall-motion abnormalities of LV or RV myocardium which are frequently, but not always, preceded by a stressful trigger (emotional or physical).
- The regional wall-motion abnormalities usually[a] extend beyond a single epicardial vascular distribution, and often result in circumferential dysfunction of the ventricular segments involved.
- The absence of culprit atherosclerotic coronary artery disease including acute plaque rupture, thrombus formation, and coronary dissection or other pathological conditions to explain the pattern of temporary LV dysfunction observed (e.g. hypertrophic cardiomyopathy, viral myocarditis).
- New and reversible electrocardiography (ECG) abnormalities (ST-segment elevation, ST depression, LBBB,[b] T-wave inversion, and/or QTc prolongation) during the acute phase (3 months).
- Significantly elevated serum natriuretic peptide (BNP or NT-proBNP) during the acute phase.
- Positive but relatively small elevation in cardiac troponin measured with a conventional assay (i.e. disparity between the troponin level and the amount of dysfunctional myocardium present).[c]
- Recovery of ventricular systolic function on cardiac imaging at follow-up (3–6 months).[d]

[a]Acute, reversible dysfunction of a single coronary territory has been reported.

[b]Left bundle branch block may be permanent after Takotsubo syndrome, but should also alert clinicians to exclude other cardiomyopathies. T-wave changes and QTc prolongation may take many weeks to months to normalise after recovery of LV function.

[c]Troponin-negative cases have been reported, but are atypical.

dSmall apical infarcts have been reported. Bystander sub-endocardial infarcts have been reported, involving a small proportion of the acutely dysfunctional myocardium. These infarcts are insufficient to explain the acute regional wall-motion abnormality observed.

Table 1. Heart Failure Association diagnostic criteria for Takotsubo syndrome [10].

http://dx.doi.org/10.5772/68037

3. Clinical subtypes: the primary and secondary Takotsubo syndrome

An attempt to classify Takotsubo patients based on the evolving clinical scenario has helped outline two elemental subtypes. The primary form of the syndrome includes patients developing acute cardiac symptoms, possibly in the wake of a stressful trigger, as also those whose co-morbid conditions act as predisposing factors indirectly contributing to rising levels of catecholamines. The secondary form comprises patients, wherein the result is essentially a response to either a primary medical condition or treatment, and the pathophysiological process is probably mediated by a sudden activation of the sympathetic nervous system or at times by an increased catecholamine activity [11]. Some examples of triggers for the secondary Takotsubo syndrome include acute neuromuscular crises, especially if involving acute respiratory failure (acute myasthenia gravis, acute Guillain-Barre syndrome), attempted suicide, severe sepsis, infection, babesiosis, pacemaker implantation, electrical DC conversion for atrial fibrillation, acute pulmonary embolism, acute pneumothorax, pheochromocytoma, Addisonian crisis, hyperglycaemic hyperosmolar state, blood transfusions, thrombotic thrombocytopenic purpura, acute exacerbation of asthma or COPD, induction of general anaesthesia, cocaine abuse, acute cholecystitis, acute pancreatitis, surgery, dobutamine stress echocardiography, etc.

4. Anatomical variants

A study describing the varying morphological presentations of the left ventricle in patients diagnosed with the Takotsubo syndrome has led to the identification of at least four major anatomical variants [12, 13]. The classical pattern defined by an apical ballooning of the left ventricle at end-systole is present in at least 50–80% of the cases. The inverted Takotsubo (basal) variant with a predominantly hypokinetic circumferential base; the mid left ventricular variant with a hypokinetic circumferential mid ventricle; and the focal variant constitute other forms of presentation. Rarer variations include cases with a pronounced dysfunction of the biventricular apex and those with an isolated right ventricular involvement [14–16].

5. Epidemiology

A retrospective review of studies reporting cases of the Takotsubo syndrome has estimated that these patients account for approximately 2% of all suspected cases of an acute coronary syndrome [17]. The average age of the TTS patient at presentation was around 68 years and the gender bias skewed to a female preponderance for disease, with 90% of the diagnosed population constituting postmenopausal women. The Nationwide Inpatient Sample Database (NIS-USA) reported that 24,701 patients were diagnosed with the Takotsubo syndrome between 2008 and 2009 in the United States, and an extrapolation of this data suggests that there could be as many as 50,000–100,000 cases per annum in the United States alone [11].

6. Pathophysiology

There have been several hypotheses postulated in contemporary literature, insinuating the complex pathophysiological evolution of the Takotsubo syndrome from either possible coronary microvascular dysfunction, coronary artery spasm, catecholamine-induced myocardial stunning, acute left ventricular outflow obstruction, acute increased ventricular afterload, myocardial microinfarction or abnormalities in cardiac fatty acid metabolism [10]. The potential for excessive hypothalamic-pituitary-adrenal axis (HPA) gain and epinephrine release in the event of a stressful trigger, and the corresponding response of the cardiovascular system and the sympathetic nervous system to the following surge in levels of catecholamines is the driving theory currently attributed to the pathophysiological evolution of TTS [10, 18].

The consistent presence of microvascular dysfunction in TTS patients has been effectively elucidated in the studies by Uchida et al. (report of extensive endothelial cell apoptosis on myocardial biopsy) and Afonso et al. (demonstrated circulatory disturbance on myocardial contrast echocardiography). A detailed study describing coronary microvascular dysfunction in patients diagnosed with the Takotsubo syndrome suggested abnormalities consistent with endothelium-dependent vasodilation, excessive vasoconstriction and impairment of myocardial perfusion [19]. Additionally, myocardial biopsy of these patients showed regions with contraction band necrosis, inflammatory cell infiltration and localised fibrosis [20]. These changes have been attributed to direct catecholamine toxicity on cardiac muscle cells [21]. Kurisu et al. demonstrated using the TIMI frame count method, which impaired coronary blood flow corresponding to LV wall-motion abnormalities immediately after onset of TTS and improved on the resolution of the LV dysfunction, giving credence to the theory of coronary microvascular impairment.

In another study, Morel et al. suggested that an increase in C-reactive protein levels and white blood cell counts corresponded to increased levels of catecholamines in TTS patients [22]. The possible role of systemic inflammation mediated by catecholamine-induced proinflammatory cytokines like TNF-alpha and interleukin-6 has been used to explain the myocardial oedema observed in cardiac MRI [23].

Recent studies conducted by Wittstein et al. (proving catecholamine levels are two to three times greater in patients with TTS as compared to those with myocardial infarction) and Lyon et al. (proposing '*stimulus trafficking*' as the cause of decline of myocyte contractile function in TTS patients) give support to the theory that catecholamine-induced cardiotoxicity plays a significant role in the development of the Takotsubo syndrome [17]. It is currently hypothesised that the pathophysiology of TTS could be dictated by changes in beta-adrenergic receptor (AR) signalling [24–26]. A switch in intracellular signal trafficking from Gs protein to Gi protein (signalling through the β2AR) mediates a negative inotropic effect, greatest at the apical myocardium where the density of β-adrenoceptors is the highest. This mechanism of stimulus trafficking is triggered by excessively high levels of catecholamines and has been used to explain the acute apical cardio-depression in TTS [26].

7. Risk factors

Lack of oestrogen has often been cited as a risk factor contributing to the development of TTS. The preponderance of postmenopausal women affected by this syndrome has led to studies investigating the use of hormone replacement theory among these patients. One such study by Kuo et al., although constituting a small sample size, showed that none of their TTS patients received any form of oestrogen replacement [27]. Recent work by Ueyema et al. in ovariectomised rats subjected to stress showed that decrease in LV function was more pronounced in those receiving estradiol supplements [28].

Patients with mood disorders and those using antidepressants tend to have an increased risk of developing TTS [29]. There is also an attempt to identify genetic factors that could suggest susceptibility to this syndrome. Although adrenoceptor polymorphisms are yet to be identified, patients with TTS have been shown to have a L41Q polymorphism of G protein coupled receptor kinase (GRK5) more frequently as compared to the normal population [30].

8. Clinical features of the Takotsubo syndrome

The definitive patient with a primary Takotsubo syndrome would be represented by a postmenopausal woman with experience of an acute, unexpected emotional or physical stress [31]. This bias, however, does not preclude men, younger women and patients with no identifiable trigger from a possible TTS. Consequently, gender, menopausal status and stressful triggers are not mandatory features included in the HFA criteria.

Patients typically present with acute chest pain are consistent with symptoms of angina pectoris, dyspnoea and palpitations. Pre-syncope and syncope due to ventricular tachyarrhythmia, severe left ventricular outflow tract obstruction and cardiogenic shock are more serious manifestations of this syndrome. Non-specific symptoms such as weakness, cough and fever have also been reported [32–34].

9. Diagnosis

9.1. Laboratory investigations

The measurement of cardiac enzymes such as serum troponin and creatinine kinase is essential to the diagnosis of the Takotsubo syndrome. Although, cardiac troponin levels are elevated in most patients with TTS, the rise in its levels is disproportionately low relative to the extent of regional wall-motion abnormality and cardiac dysfunction [24, 35]. In contrast, elevated values of cardiac natriuretic peptides, such as pro-BNP and NT-proBNP, serve as a better correlate for degree of ventricular wall dysfunction in the acute phase of TTS [36–38]. Normal values of NT-proBNP are extremely rare in Takotsubo syndrome, thus helping it serve as a valuable marker of myocardial deterioration and recovery.

Recent studies have suggested the potential of circulating microRNAs to differentiate between TTS and STEMI patients; however, conclusive research is needed to establish this as a routine diagnostic biomarker [39].

9.2. Electrocardiography

The acute phase of TTS is characterised by ECG abnormalities such as ST-segment elevation, ST-segment depression, new left bundle branch block, Q-waves, T-wave inversions and significant QT-interval prolongation developing 24–48 hours after onset. These changes are reflected in almost 95% of all patients diagnosed with the Takotsubo syndrome [40]. It is not uncommon for the QTc-interval to be prolonged more than 500 ms, predisposing the patient to torsades de pointes and ventricular fibrillation, see **Figure 1**.

9.3. Echocardiography

The initial assessment of LV morphology and function with the use of thoracic echocardiography is inherent to the diagnostic cascade of Takotsubo syndrome. Standard, colour and tissue Doppler techniques assist in the identification of anatomical variants, monitor recovery and help detect potential complications such as left ventricular outflow tract obstructions, RV involvement, mitral regurgitation and cardiac rupture [41–43].

The echocardiographic examination of patient in the acute phase of TTS shows a large area of poorly functioning myocardium extending beyond the territory of a single coronary artery.

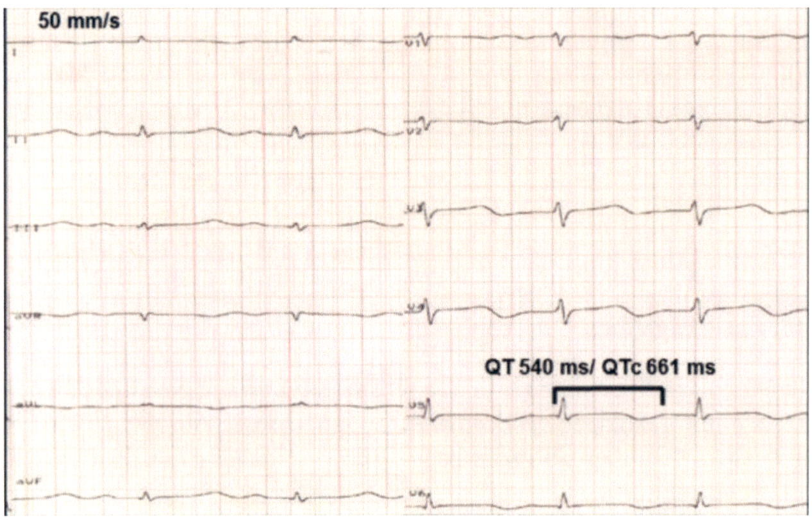

Figure 1. Electrocardiogram of TTS patient with acquired long QT syndrome at admission.

The typical regional wall-motion abnormality is found in the apical to mid segments of the left ventricle, extending equally into the anterior, inferior and lateral walls. This 'circumferential pattern' is considered the hallmark of TTS. In certain cases, the use of a contrast agent for LV opacification eases assessment of the RWMA, while, myocardial deformation imaging with the speckle tracking method has been used to demonstrate a transient circular impairment of not only longitudinal LV function, but also circumferential and radial LV function [44–46].

9.4. Cardiac magnetic resonance

The use of cardiac magnetic resonance imaging (CMR) has been advocated in the first 7 days (acute phase) to accurately assess both LV and RV regional function and demonstrate the typical patterns of RWMA, permitted by the full visualisation of the ventricles in the main long axes. Cardiac magnetic resonance imaging has a distinct advantage over standard transthoracic echocardiography in offering better views of the right ventricle and in detection of apical LV thrombi [47].

In CMR, tissue characterisation of acute myocardial changes occurring in the TTS patient shows a high signal intensity with a diffuse or transmural distribution, indicative of oedema of the hypokinetic LV myocardium. This oedema corresponds to the region of the wall-motion abnormality and is not restricted by the boundaries of a single coronary artery territory, unlike an acute myocardial infraction in which oedema is always coherent with a vascular distribution [42].

Late Gadolinium Enhancement (LGE) is typically absent in both the acute phase as well as follow-up, serving as an important criterion to distinguish between AMI and TTS. Recently, there has been some debate concerning the presence of minor LGE in the acute phase; however, this is dependent on the threshold of signal intensity used to define LGE presence [48, 49], see **Figure 2**.

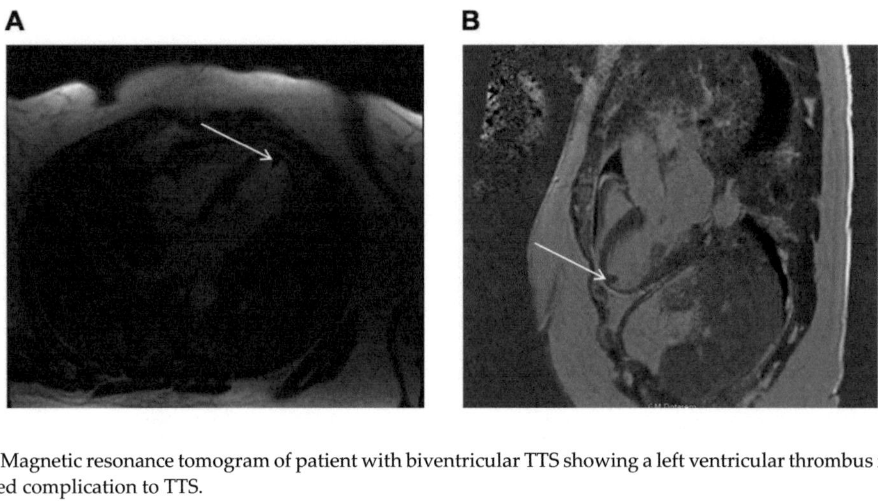

Figure 2. Magnetic resonance tomogram of patient with biventricular TTS showing a left ventricular thrombus formation as a related complication to TTS.

9.5. Coronary angiography and left ventriculography

The necessity to exclude an acute myocardial infarction in patients presenting with angina-like symptoms and typical ECG-changes predicates the use of coronary angiography. In TTS, the epicardial coronary arteries typically do not have any significant stenoses; however, there is possibility of bystander CAD considering the older age group of the presenting patients. A co-existing CAD has been reported in almost 10% of all TTS cases [50, 51]. The coronary stenosis in this scenario may or may not be hemodynamically significant; however, it is generally insufficient to explain the acute LV dysfunction and regional wall-motion abnormalities transpiring in the Takotsubo syndrome.

The exclusion of occlusive coronary artery disease, acute plaque rupture, thrombus formation and coronary dissection should be followed by a left ventriculography (if not contraindicated). This is necessary to confirm the pattern of LV wall-motion abnormality and diagnose, if any, mitral regurgitation. It also allows direct measurement of the pressure gradient across the LVOT [42], see **Figure 3**.

9.6. Coronary computed tomography angiography

The role of coronary computed tomography angiography (CCTA) is limited to cases where a delay in access to urgent invasive coronary angiography is expected. Information acquired throughout the cardiac cycle (spiral or helical acquisition mode) during the acute phase could demonstrate the typical pattern of systolic dysfunction [52]; however, this would come at the cost of greater radiation exposure. Retrospective evaluation of patients with typical history of TTS could also theoretically include CCTA to exclude significant coronary stenosis.

9.7. Radionuclide imaging

Single-photon emission tomography (SPECT) with ^{201}Thallium or ^{99m}Technetium-labelled radiopharmaceuticals and ^{123}I-metaIodobenzyl-guanidine (mIBG) has been used to demonstrate

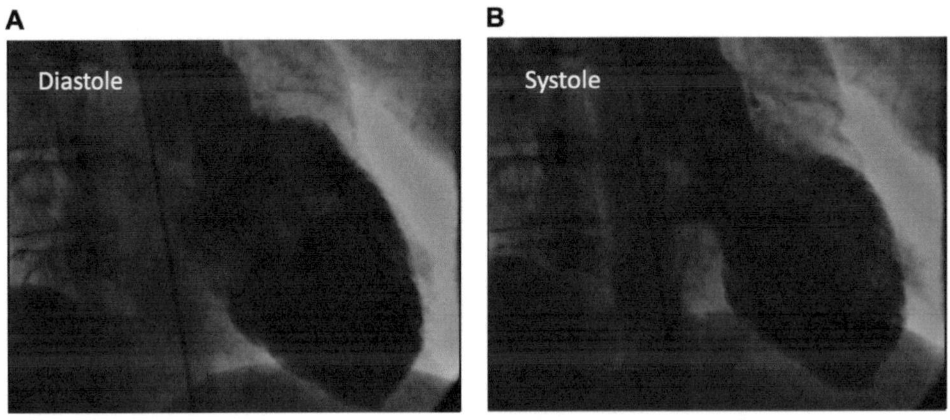

Figure 3. Laevocardiography of TTS patient with typical apical ballooning triggered by emotional stress.

myocardial perfusion and sympathetic innervation. A reduced mIBG in the dysfunctional myocardial segments during the acute phase is consistent with disturbances in regional sympathetic neuronal activity [53, 54], and its use in diagnosing TTS has been suggested in combination with myocardial perfusion scintigraphy to exclude infarction.

^{18}F-fluorodeoxyglucose (FDG) has been used to study myocardial glucose metabolism by positron emission tomography (PET); however, its current use has been relegated to scientific research [55].

10. Clinical management and therapeutic strategies

The clinical management protocol for Takotsubo syndrome is poorly defined as the debate explaining its pathophysiological evolution is yet to be resolved. As most patients present initially with symptoms of angina pectoris, it has been recommended that the first line of management be directed towards the treatment of possible myocardial ischemia. This essentially entails treatment with anticoagulants such as aspirin and heparin. Once occlusive coronary artery disease has been excluded, the objective of treatment is to minimise complications and ensure optimal supportive care. Patients are usually admitted to the coronary care unit to enable seamless continuous ECG-monitoring, serial lab tests and repeated echocardiographic examinations.

Takotsubo patients constituting a low-risk profile, with insignificant compromise to cardiac function (LVEF > 45%) could be discharged from the hospital early, however, only after a thorough review of the cardiovascular risk factors and heart failure medication. Recent pre-clinical trials have advocated therapy with beta-blockers such as metoprolol and carvedilol in patients with low-risk [26, 56], unless contraindications to use pre-exist.

Interesting observations in this regard are the results published from a study by Templin et al., where the use of angiotensin-converting enzyme-inhibitors or angiotensin-receptor-blockers, and not beta-blockers, were associated with improved survival [9].

In patients presenting with severely depressed cardiac output and complications associated with the Takotsubo syndrome, it is advised to stop drugs with sympathomimetic properties (e.g. catecholamines and beta-2-agonists). A therapy with beta-blockers has been recommended in hemodynamically stable patients with atrial and ventricular tachyarrhythmias [10], as also in patients with a hemodynamically significant LVOT obstruction (in combination with an alpha-1-recpetor agonist). In severe manifestations like acute cardiogenic shock, options like use of temporary left ventricular assist devices and extracorporeal membrane oxygenation could be considered. The potential of IABP in this scenario has taken a backseat considering the neutral data presented in the recently concluded IABP-SHOCK II Trial.

The use of inotropes, like norepinephrine or dobutamine, is mostly contraindicated in the Takotsubo syndrome; however, experts have recommended treatment with Levosimendan in patients with advancing cardiogenic shock and multi-organ failure [57–61]. The role of prophylactic anticoagulation with unfractionated or low-molecular weight heparin is also debatable, but experts have suggested that TTS patients with extensive segmental akinesia could be started on a regimen with therapeutic doses of LMWH.

11. Complications

Takotsubo syndrome has been associated with a growing list of complications of varied severity, contributing to its mortality rate. Almost 52% of all patients have been reported to develop some form of complication in course of this disease [62, 63]. These include acute heart failure, left ventricular outflow tract obstruction, cardiogenic shock, arrhythmias, thrombus formation, pericardial effusion, right ventricular involvement and ventricular wall rupture.

Acute heart failure develops in almost 12–45% of all patients with TTS and, in some patients, it is exacerbated by mitral regurgitation and/or left ventricular tract obstruction. Patients could have significantly elevated LVOT gradients (20–140 mmHg), and those with values greater than 40 mmHg are predisposed to develop hypotension and cardiogenic shock. It has been demonstrated that the use of inotropic drugs exacerbates this LVOT obstruction, while beta-blockers decrease it. Around 4–20% of all TTS patients show symptoms of cardiogenic shock, while almost 9% of them document ventricular arrhythmias during the acute phase. Thrombi develop generally 2–5 days after the index event and are known to resolve after 2 weeks of therapeutic anticoagulation (treatment regimen of at least 3 months). There are also instances of patients presenting with a biventricular involvement, which has been associated with a poorer prognosis and a higher frequency of heart failure [10].

12. Prognosis and conclusion

The Takotsubo syndrome is essentially a benign disease and the prognosis is favourable in most patients. The regional wall-motion abnormalities usually resolve spontaneously within a few days to weeks; however, there have been instances where TTS has persisted due to complications associated with apical thrombus formation [64, 65]. Recent studies have demonstrated that the in-hospital death rate ranges between 0 and 8%, while recurrence rates fluctuate anywhere between 0 and 15% [66, 67].

These results have eschewed renewed interest into the study of Takotsubo syndrome and mechanisms contributing to its pathophysiology. Patients are now recommended routine follow-ups after 3–6 months to evaluate the progress of disease and help better understand its evolutionary dynamics.

Limited current knowledge and often contradictory data have fuelled the debate surrounding the Takotsubo syndrome. There is an urgent need for multiple randomised controlled trials and large registries to optimise existing clinical goals and management strategies, and the launch of InterTAK registry is a step forward in this regard.

http://dx.doi.org/10.5772/68037

Author details

Uzair Ansari* and Ibrahim El-Battrawy

*Address all correspondence to: uzair.ansari@yahoo.com

First Department of Medicine, Medical Faculty Mannheim, University Heidelberg, Mannheim, Germany

References

[1] Hurst RT, Prasad A, Askew JW III, Sengupta PP, Tajik AJ. Takotsubo cardiomyopathy: A unique cardiomyopathy with variable ventricular morphology. JACC: Cardiovascular Imaging. 2010;**3**:641-649

[2] Medeiros K, O'Connor MJ, Baicu CF, et al. Systolic and diastolic mechanics in stress cardiomyopathy. Circulation. 2014;**129**:1659-1667

[3] Sharkey SW, Lesser JR, Maron MS, Maron BJ. Why not just call it tako-tsubo cardiomyopathy: A discussion of nomenclature. Journal of the American College of Cardiology. 2011;**57**:1496-1497

[4] Maron BJ, Towbin JA, Thiene G, Antzelevitch C, Corrado D, Arnett D, Moss AJ, Seidman CE, Young JB. Contemporary definitions and classification of the cardiomyopathies: An American Heart Association Scientific Statement from the Council on Clinical Cardiology, Heart Failure and Transplantation Committee; Quality of Care and Outcomes Research and Functional Genomics and Translational Biology Interdisciplinary Working Groups; and Council on Epidemiology and Prevention. Circulation. 2006;**113**:1807-1816

[5] Kawai S, Suzuki H, Yamaguchi H, Tanaka K, Sawada H, Aizawa T, Watanabe M, Tamura T, Umawatari K, Kawata M, Nakamura T, Yamanaka O, Okada R. Ampulla cardiomyopathy ('Takotusbo' cardiomyopathy)–reversible left ventricular dysfunction: With ST segment elevation. Japanese Circulation Journal. 2000;**64**:156-159

[6] Owa M, Aizawa K, Urasawa N, Ichinose H, Yamamoto K, Karasawa K, Kagoshima M, Koyama J, Ikeda S. Emotional stress-induced 'ampulla cardiomyoopathy': Discrepancy between the metabolic and sympathetic innervation imaging performed during the recovery course. Japanese Circulation Journal. 2001;**65**:349-352

[7] Mukherjee A, Sunkel-Laing B, Dewhurst N. 'Broken Heart' syndrome in Scotland: A case of Takotsubo cardiomyopathy in a recently widowed lady. Scottish Medical Journal. 2013;**58**:e15-e19

[8] Prasad A. Apical ballooning syndrome: An important differential diagnosis of acute myocardial infarction. Circulation. 2007;**115**:e56-e59

[9] Templin C, Ghadri JR, Diekmann J, Napp LC, Bataiosu DR, Jaguszewski M, ... Lüscher TF. Clinical features and outcomes of Takotsubo (stress) cardiomyopathy. New England Journal of Medicine. 2015;**373**(10):929-938

[10] Lyon AR, Bossone E, Schneider B, Sechtem U, Citro R, Underwood SR, ... Omerovic E. Current state of knowledge on Takotsubo syndrome: A Position Statement from the Taskforce on Takotsubo Syndrome of the Heart Failure Association of the European Society of Cardiology. European Journal of Heart Failure. 2016;**18**(1):8-27

[11] Eitel I, von Knobelsdorff-Brenkenhoff F, Bernhardt P, Carbone I, Muellerleile K, Aldrovandi A, Francone M, Desch S, Gutberlet M, Strohm O, Schuler G, Schulz-Menger J, Thiele H, Friedrich MG. Clinical characteristics and cardiovascular magnetic resonance findings in stress (takotsubo) cardiomyopathy. JAMA. 2011;**306**:277-286

[12] Haghi D, Athanasiadis A, Papavassiliu T, Suselbeck T, Fluechter S, Mahrholdt H, Borggrefe M, Sechtem U. Right ventricular involvement in Takotsubo cardiomyopathy. European Heart Journal. 2006;**27**:2433-2439

[13] Kurowski V, Kaiser A, von Hof K, Killermann DP, Mayer B, Hartmann F, Schunkert H, Radke PW. Apical and midventricular transient left ventricular dysfunction syndrome (tako-tsubo cardiomyopathy): Frequency, mechanisms, and prognosis. Chest. 2007;**132**:809-816

[14] Ennezat PV, Pesenti-Rossi D, Aubert JM, Rachenne V, Bauchart JJ, Auffray JL, Logeart D, Cohen-Solal A, Asseman P. Transient left ventricular basal dysfunction without coronary stenosis in acute cerebral disorders: A novel heart syndrome (inverted Takotsubo). Echocardiography. 2005;**22**:599-602

[15] Van de Walle SO, Gevaert SA, Gheeraert PJ, De Pauw M, Gillebert TC. Transient stress-induced cardiomyopathy with an 'inverted takotsubo' contractile pattern. Mayo Clinic Proceedings. 2006;**81**:1499-1502

[16] Cacciotti L, Camastra GS, Beni S,Giannantoni P,Musaro S, Proietti I, De Angelis L, Semeraro R, Ansalone G. A new variant of Tako-tsubo cardiomyopathy: Transient midventricular ballooning. Journal of Cardiovascular Medicine. 2007;**8**:1052-1054

[17] Komamura K. Takotsubo cardiomyopathy: Pathophysiology, diagnosis and treatment. World Journal of Cardiology. 2014;**6**(7), 602-609

[18] Wittstein IS, Thiemann DR, Lima JAC, Baughman KL, Schulman SP, Gerstenblith G, Wu KC, Rade JJ, Bivalacqua TJ, Champion HC. Neurohumoral features of myocardial stunning due to sudden emotional stress. New England Journal of Medicine. 2005;**352**:539-548

[19] Galiuto L, De Caterina AR, Porfidia A, Paraggio L, Barchetta S, Locorotondo G, Rebuzzi AG, Crea F. Reversible coronary microvascular dysfunction: A common pathogenetic mechanism in Apical Ballooning or Tako-Tsubo Syndrome. European Heart Journal. 2010;**31**:1319-1327. [PMID: 20215125 DOI: 10.1093/eurheartj/ehq039]

[20] Nef HM, Möllmann H, Kostin S, Troidl C, Voss S, Weber M, Dill T, Rolf A, Brandt R, Hamm CW, Elsässer A. Takotsubo cardiomyopathy: Intra-individual structural analysis in the acute phase and after functional recovery. European Heart Journal. 2007;**28**:2456-2464 [PMID: 17395683 DOI: 10.1093/eurheartj/ehl570]

[21] Khullar M, Datta BN, Wahi PL, Chakravarti RN. Catecholamine-induced experimental cardiomyopathy—A histopathological, histochemical and ultrastructural study. Indian Heart Journal. 1989;**41**:307-313 [PMID: 2599540]

[22] Morel O, Sauer F, Imperiale A, Cimarelli S, Blondet C, Jesel L, Trinh A, De Poli F, Ohlmann P, Constantinesco A, Bareiss P. Importance of inflammation and neurohumoral activation in Takotsubo cardiomyopathy. Journal of Cardiac Failure. 2009;**15**:206-213 [PMID: 19327622 DOI: 10.1016/j.cardfail.2008.10.031]

[23] Avegliano G, Huguet M, Costabel JP, Ronderos R, Bijnens B, Kuschnir P, Thierer J, Tobón-Gomez C, Martinez GO, Frangi A. Morphologic pattern of late gadolinium enhancement in Takotsubo cardiomyopathy detected by early cardiovascular magnetic resonance. Clinical Cardiology. 2011;**34**:178-182 [PMID: 21400545 DOI: 10.1002/clc.20877

[24] Lyon AR, Rees PSC, Prasad S, Poole-Wilson PA, Harding SE. Stress (Takotsubo) cardiomyopathy—A novel pathophysiological hypothesis to explain catecholamine-induced acute myocardial stunning. Nature Clinical Practice. Cardiovascular Medicine. 2008;**5**:22-29

[25] Scantlebury D, Prasad A. Diagnosis of Takotsubo cardiomyopathy. Circulation Journal. 2014;**78**(9):2129-2139

[26] Paur H, Wright PT, Sikkel MB, Tranter MH, Mansfield C, O'Gara P, et al. High levels of circulating epinephrine trigger apical cardiodepression in a β2-adrenergic receptor/Gi-dependent manner: A new model of Takotsubo cardiomyopathy. Circulation. 2012;**126**:697-706

[27] Kuo BT, Choubey R, Novaro GM. Reduced estrogen in menopause may predispose women to takotsubo cardiomyopathy. Gender Medicine. 2010;**7**:71-77 [PMID: 20189157 DOI: 10.1016/j.genm.2010.01.006]

[28] Ueyama T, Hano T, Kasamatsu K, Yamamoto K, Tsuruo Y, Nishio I. Estrogen attenuates the emotional stress-induced cardiac responses in the animal model of Takotsubo (Ampulla) cardiomyopathy. Journal of Cardiovascular Pharmacology. 2003;**42**(Suppl 1):S117-S119 [PMID: 14871041]

[29] Abraham J, Mudd JO, Kapur NK, Klein K, Champion HC, Wittstein IS. Stress cardiomyopathy after intravenous administration of catecholamines and beta-receptor agonists. Journal of American College of Cardiology. 2009;**53**:1320-1325 [PMID: 19358948 DOI: 10.1016/j.jacc.2009.02.020]

[30] Spinelli L, Trimarco V, Di Marino S, Marino M, Iaccarino G, Trimarco B. L41Q polymorphism of the G protein coupled receptor kinase 5 is associated with left ventricular apical ballooning syndrome. European Journal of Heart Failure. 2010;**12**:13-16 [PMID: 20023040 DOI: 10.1093/eurjhf/hfp173]

[31] Bybee KA, Kara T, Prasad A, Lerman A, Barsness GW, Wright RS, Rihal CS. Systematic review: Transient left ventricular apical ballooning: A syndrome that mimics ST-segment elevation myocardial infarction. Annals of Internal Medicine. 2004;**141**:858-865

[32] Kara T, Bybee K, Prasad A, et al. Transient left ventricular apical ballooning syndrome: A mimic of ST-segment elevation myocardial infarction. Annals of Internal Medicine. 2004;**141**:858-865

[33] Yamasa T, Ikeda S, Ninomiya A, et al. Characteristic clinical findings of reversible left ventricular dysfunction. Internal Medicine 2002;**41**:789-792

[34] Elesber A, Prasad A, Bybee K, et al. Transient cardiac apical ballooning syndrome: Prevalence and clinical implications of right ventricular involvement. Journal of the American College of Cardiology. 2006;**47**:1082-1083

[35] Pilgrim TM, Wyss TR. Takotsubo cardiomyopathy or transient left ventricular apical ballooning syndrome: A systematic review. International Journal of Cardiology. 2008;**124**: 283-292

[36] Madhavan M, Borlaug BA, Lerman A, Rihal CS, Prasad A. Stress hormone and circulating biomarker profile of apical ballooning syndrome (Takotsubo cardiomyopathy): Insights into the clinical significance of B-type natriuretic peptide and troponin levels. Heart. 2009;**95**:1436-1341

[37] Ahmed KA, Madhavan M, Prasad A. Brain natriuretic peptide in apical ballooning syndrome (Takotsubo/stress cardiomyopathy): Comparison with acute myocardial infarction. Coronary Artery Disease. 2012;**23**:259-264

[38] Frohlich GM, Schoch B, Schmid F, Keller P, Sudano I, Luscher TF, Noll G, Ruschitzka F, Enseleit F. Takotsubo cardiomyopathy has a unique cardiac biomarker profile: NT-proBNP/myoglobin and NT-proBNP/troponin T ratios for the differential diagnosis of acute coronary syndromes and stress induced cardiomyopathy. International Journal of Cardiology. 2012;**154**:328-332

[39] Jaguszewski M, Osipova J, Ghadri JR, Napp LC,Widera C, Franke J, Fijalkowski M, Nowak R, Fijalkowska M, Volkmann I, Katus HA, Wollert KC, Bauersachs J, Erne P, Luscher TF, Thum T, Templin C. A signature of circulating microRNAs differentiates takotsubo cardiomyopathy from acute myocardial infarction. European Heart Journal. 2014;**35**:999-1006

[40] Kurisu S, Inoue I, Kawagoe T, Ishihara M, Shimatani Y, Nakamura S, Yoshida M, Mitsuba N, Hata T, Sato H. Time course of electrocardiographic changes in patients with takotsubo syndrome: Comparison with acute myocardial infarction with minimal enzymatic release. Circulation Journal. 2004;**68**:77-81

[41] Citro R, Rigo F, Ciampi Q, D'Andrea A, Provenza G, Mirra M, Giudice R, Silvestri F, Di Benedetto G, Bossone E. Echocardiographic assessment of regional left ventricular wall motion abnormalities in patients with tako-tsubo cardiomyopathy: Comparison with anterior myocardial infarction. European Journal of Echocardiography. 2011;**12**:542-549

[42] Bossone E, Lyon A, Citro R, Athanasiadis A, Meimoun P, Parodi G, Cimarelli S, Omerovic E, Ferrara F, Limongelli G, Cittadini A, Salerno-Uriarte JA, Perrone Filardi P, Schneider B, Sechtem U, Erbel R. Takotsubo cardiomyopathy: An integrated multi-imaging approach. European Heart Journal. Cardiovascular Imaging. 2014;**15**:366-377

[43] Meimoun P, Clerc J, Vincent C, Flahaut F, Germain AL, Elmkies F, Zemir H, Luycx-Bore A. Non-invasive detection of tako-tsubo cardiomyopathy vs. acute anterior myocardial infarction by transthoracic Doppler echocardiography. European Heart Journal. Cardiovascular Imaging. 2013;**14**:464-470

[44] Mansencal N, Abbou N, Pilliere R, El Mahmoud R, Farcot JC, Dubourg O. Usefulness of two-dimensional speckle tracking echocardiography for assessment of Tako-Tsubo cardiomyopathy. American Journal of Cardiology. 2009;**103**:1020-1024

[45] Meimoun P, Passos P, Benali T, Boulanger J, Elmkies F, Zemir H, et al. Assessment of left ventricular twist mechanics in Tako-Tsubo cardiomyopathy by two-dimensional speckle tracking echocardiography. European Journal of Echocardiography. 2011;**12**:931-939

[46] Heggemann F,Weiss C, Hamm K, Kaden J, Suselbeck T, Papavassiliu T et al. Global and regional myocardial function quantification by two-dimensional strain in Tako-Tsubo cardiomyopathy. European Journal of Echocardiography. 2009;**10**:760-764

[47] Eitel I, von Knobelsdorff-Brenkenhoff F, Bernhardt P, Carbone I, Muellerleile K, Aldrovandi A et al. Clinical characteristics and cardiovascular magnetic resonance findings in stress (Takotsubo) cardiomyopathy. JAMA. 2011;**306**:277-286

[48] Naruse Y, Sato A, Kasahara K, Makino K, Sano M, Takeuchi Y, Nagasaka S, Wakabayashi Y, Katoh H, Satoh H, Hayashi H, Aonuma K. The clinical impact of late gadolinium enhancement in Takotsubo cardiomyopathy: Serial analysis of cardiovascular magnetic resonance images. Journal of Cardiovascular Magnetic Resonance. 2011;**13**:67

[49] Alter P, Figiel JH, Rominger MB. Increased ventricular wall stress and late gadolinium enhancement in Takotsubo cardiomyopathy. International Journal of Cardiology. 2014;**172**: e184–e186

[50] Gaibazzi N, Ugo F, Vignali L, Zoni A, Reverberi C, Gherli T. Tako-Tsubo cardiomyopathy with coronary artery stenosis: A case-series challenging the original definition. International Journal of Cardiology. 2009;**133**:205-212

[51] Previtali M, Repetto A, Panigada S, Camporotondo R, Tavazzi L. Left ventricular apical ballooning syndrome: Prevalence, clinical characteristics and pathogenetic mechanisms in a European population. International Journal of Cardiology. 2009;**134**:91-96

[52] Nance JW, Schoepf UJ, Ramos-Duran L. Tako-tsubo cardiomyopathy: Findings on cardiac CT and coronary catheterisation. Heart. 2010;**96**:406-407

[53] Cimarelli S, Sauer F, Morel O, Ohlmann P, Constantinesco A, Imperiale A. Transient left ventricular dysfunction syndrome: Patho-physiological bases through nuclear medicine imaging. International Journal of Cardiology. 2010;**144**:212-218

[54] Ito K, Sugihara H, Kinoshita N, Azuma A, Matsubara H. Assessment of Takotsubo cardiomyopathy (transient left ventricular apical ballooning) using 99mTc-tetrofosmin, 123I-BMIPP, 123I-MIBG and 99mTc-PYP myocardial SPECT. Annals of Nuclear Medicine. 2005;**19**:435-445

[55] Christensen TE, Bang LE, Holmvang L, Ghotbi AA, Lassen ML, Andersen F, Ihlemann N, Andersson H, Grande P, Kjaer A, Hasbak P. Cardiac Tc sestamibi SPECT and F FDG PET as viability markers in Takotsubo cardiomyopathy. International Journal of Cardiovascular Imaging. 2014;**30**:1407-1416

[56] Izumi Y, Okatani H, Shiota M, Nakao T, Ise R, Kito G, Miura K, Iwao H. Effects of metoprolol on epinephrine-induced Takotsubo-like left ventricular dysfunction in non-human primates. Hypertension Research. 2009;**32**:339-346

[57] Santoro F, Ieva R, Ferraretti A, Ienco V, Carpagnano G, Lodispoto M, Di Biase L, Di Biase M, Brunetti ND. Safety and feasibility of levosimendan administration in takotsubo cardiomyopathy: A case series. Cardiovascular Therapeutics. 2013;**31**:e133-e137

[58] Karvouniaris M, Papanikolaou J, Makris D, Zakynthinos E. Sepsis-associated takotsubo cardiomyopathy can be reversed with levosimendan. American Journal of Emergency Medicine. 2012;**30**:832.e5-832.e7

[59] Antonini M, Stazi GV, Cirasa MT, Garotto G, Frustaci A. Efficacy of levosimendan in Takotsubo-related cardiogenic shock. Acta Anaesthesiologica Scandinavica. 2010;**54**: 119-120

[60] De Santis V, Vitale D, Tritapepe L, Greco C, Pietropaoli P. Use of levosimendan for cardiogenic shock in a patient with the apical ballooning syndrome. Annals of Internal Medicine. 2008;**149**:365-367

[61] Padayachee L. Levosimendan: The inotrope of choice in cardiogenic shock secondary to takotsubo cardiomyopathy? Heart, Lung & Circulation. 2007;**16**(Suppl 3):S65-S70

[62] Redfors B, Vedad R, Angerås O, Råmunddal T, Petursson P, Haraldsson I, Ali A, Dworeck C, Odenstedt J, Ioaness D, Libungan B, Shao Y, Albertsson P, Stone GW, Omerovic E. Mortality in takotsubo syndrome is similar to mortality in myocardial infarction—A report from the SWEDEHEART1 registry. International Journal of Cardiology. 2015;**185**:282-289

[63] Schneider B, Athanasiadis A, Schwab J, Pistner W, Gottwald U, Schoeller R, Toepel W, Winter KD, Stellbrink C, Muller-Honold T,Wegner C, Sechtem U. Complications in the clinical course of tako-tsubo cardiomyopathy. International Journal of Cardiology. 2014;**176**:199-205

[64] Lee PH, Song JK, Park IK, Sun BJ, Lee SG, Yim JH, et al. Takotsubo cardiomyopathy: A case of persistent apical ballooning complicated by an apical mural thrombus. Korean Journal of Internal Medicine. 2011;**26**:455-459

[65] Shim IK, Kim BJ, Kim H, Lee JW, Cha TJ, Heo JH. A case of persistent apical ballooning complicated by apical thrombus in takotsubo cardiomyopathy of systemic lupus erythematosus patient. Journal of Cardiovascular Ultrasound. 2013;**21**:137-139

[66] Bietry R, Reyentovich A, Katz SD. Clinical management of Takotsubo cardiomyopathy. Heart Failure Clinics. 2013;**9**(2):177-186. DOI: https://doi.org/10.1016/j.hfc.2012.12.003

[67] Eitel I, Lücke C, Grothoff M, Sareban M, Schuler G, Thiele H, Gutberlet M. Inflammation in takotsubo cardiomyopathy: Insights from cardiovascular magnetic resonance imaging. European Radiology. 2010;**20**:422-431 [PMID: 19705125 DOI: 10.1007/s00330-009-1549-5]

Section 7

Interventional Treatment for Stroke Prevention in Atrial Fibrillation

Chapter 12

Interventional Left Atrial Appendage Closure: Focus on Practical Implications

Christian Fastner, Michael Behnes, Uzair Ansari,
Ibrahim El-Battrawy and Martin Borggrefe

Additional information is available at the end of the chapter

http://dx.doi.org/10.5772/67773

Abstract

Catheter-based left atrial appendage closure is an evolving therapy for the prophylaxis of thromboembolic complications in nonvalvular atrial fibrillation patients, which are ineligible for long-term oral anticoagulation. For this indication, it is recommended by the current European guidelines. This review of the existing literature should facilitate the understanding of the therapy's practical implications. It presents a clinical approach toward a correct patient selection, gives an overview of the different devices and the procedural aspects, reflects differences and benefits between several postprocedural regimens for device surveillance as well as antithrombotic medication and rounds off with a summary of the relevant studies concerning efficacy and safety outcome measures.

Keywords: atrial fibrillation, left atrial appendage closure, thromboembolism, stroke, oral anticoagulation

1. Atrial fibrillation, thromboembolic risk, and prevention

Atrial fibrillation (AF) is the most common cardiac arrhythmia with a significant burden of disease. The prevalence is age-dependent and increases with the age [1, 2]. While it is uncommon in patients younger than 40, about 10% of the 80-year olds are affected [1, 2]. AF nowadays is prevalent in about 3% of the western population, but it is estimated that the incidence will rise over the next decades linked to the increased life expectancy [1, 2]. As in the case of other cardiovascular diseases, males are more frequently affected than females [1, 2]. Though AF rather rarely causes acute fatal complications at the time of onset, medium-term prognostic complications such as left ventricular dysfunction, cognitive decline, and utmost important cerebral ischemic stroke change AF toward a harmful cardiac disease [3]. AF accounts for 20–30% of all strokes and many patients are diagnosed with AF for the first time after they have been affected by a stroke (so-called "silent" AF) [3]. Therefore, the prognosis of AF patients is substantially determined by the risk for thromboembolic events.

1.1. Thrombogenesis during atrial fibrillation

Due to the electrical storm occurring on the atrial myocardium and the irregular ventricular excitation during AF episodes, the atrial mechanical function is impaired. Consecutively, the atrial cavities are distended, the intraatrial pressure is increased and the blood flow is reduced. These mechanisms connected to the Virchow's triad are only part of a multifactorial network leading to thrombogenesis also including the expression of prothrombotic factors [4–6]. The changes are especially prominent in the blind-ended left atrial appendage (LAA) located in front of the anterior wall of the left atrium (LA) with its ostium between the left upper pulmonary vein and the mitral valve annulus [6, 7]. The walls of the LAA are highly trabeculated which renders them thrombogenic [7]. Four general LAA shapes are described in the literature, i.e., the chicken wing, cactus, windsock, and cauliflower shaped LAA (**Figure 1A**), whereby the data of the proportional distribution substantially vary within the literature [8]. Certain LAA morphologies were identified as an independent risk factor for thromboembolic events [9, 10]. Altogether, in patients with nonrheumatic AF more than 90% of all atrial thrombi occur in the left atrial appendage (**Figure 1B**) [11].

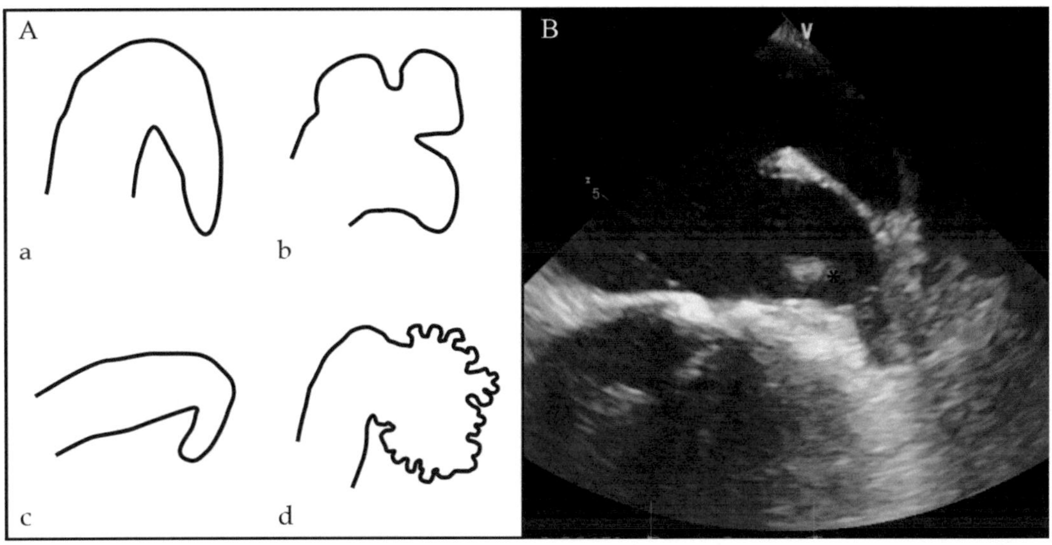

Figure 1. (A) The four different left atrial appendage morphologies with (a) the chicken wing, (b) the cactus, (c) the windsock and (d) the cauliflower type. (B) Echocardiographic visualization of a left atrial appendage thrombus (*).

1.2. Pros and cons of an oral anticoagulation therapy for thromboembolic prophylaxis

Because of these interrelationships, the risk stratification for thromboembolic events and a risk-based indication for thromboembolic prophylaxis are important pillars in the AF patient's therapy. For this purpose, the CHA_2DS_2-VASc score is recommended (IA) [3]. It incorporates all the relevant risk factors for stroke in AF patients: congestive heart failure (+1), hypertension (+1), age (65–74 +1 and ≥ 75 years +2, respectively), diabetes mellitus (+1), prior stroke, transient ischemic attack (TIA) or thromboembolism (+2), vascular disease (+1), and female gender (+1). According to the current European guideline recommendations, a thromboembolic prophylaxis by oral anticoagulants is recommended for all males with a CHA_2DS_2-VASc score ≥ 2 and for all females with a CHA_2DS_2-VASc score ≥ 3 (IA). Furthermore, this prophylaxis should be considered in males with a CHA_2DS_2-VASc score = 1 and in females with a CHA_2DS_2-VASc score = 2 according to the individual characteristics and the patient's preferences (IIaB) [3]. The evaluation of biomarkers, e.g., high-sensitive troponins and natriuretic peptides, can be helpful in this context (IIbB) [3]. For several decades, vitamin K antagonists have served as the gold standard for thromboembolic prophylaxis in AF patients [12], but their clinical use is limited by an increased and substantial bleeding risk which especially harms vulnerable patients [13, 14]. The vulnerability to bleedings can be assessed by the HAS-BLED score including arterial hypertension (+1), abnormal renal (+1) or liver (+1) function, prior stroke (+1), bleeding history or predisposition (+1), labile international normalized ratio (INR) (+1), age > 65 (+1) and drugs (+1) or alcohol (+1) concomitantly [15]. While dual antiplatelet agents failed to be an effective and safe alternative to vitamin K antagonists [16], recently, non-vitamin K antagonist oral anticoagulants (NOACs), i.e., dabigatran, rivaroxaban, apixaban, and edoxaban, were gaining ground [17–20]. In the current European guidelines, these substances are preferentially recommended for all eligible nonvalvular AF patients (IA) [3]. However, stoked by a higher incidence of gastrointestinal bleedings in comparison to vitamin K antagonists and other side effects [21], patients' adherence to NOAC therapy was also shown to be limited [22].

1.3. Alternatives to an oral anticoagulation therapy

By the implication of the LAA as a primary source of thrombi for thromboembolic events in nonvalvular AF, locoregional techniques to avoid thromboembolism out of the LAA were developed. Besides the surgical resection of the LAA during open heart surgery and the epicardial LARIAT® Suture Delivery Device (SentreHEART, Redwood City, CA, USA) with limited evidence for efficacy and safety [23, 24], six CE-marked devices for transvenous catheter-based LAA closure are currently available: the WATCHMAN™ left atrial appendage closure device (Boston Scientific, Natick, MA, USA), the AMPLATZER™ Cardiac Plug (ACP) and its next generation the AMPLATZER™ Amulet™ left atrial appendage occluder (both St. Jude Medical, Minneapolis, MN, USA), the WaveCrest™ LAA Occlusion System (Coherex Medical, Salt Lake City, UT, USA), the Occlutech® LAA occluder (Occlutech, Jena, Germany) and the LAmbre™ LAA Closure System (Lifetech Science, Shenzhen, China), respectively. However, only the WATCHMAN™ device was compared to oral anticoagulation (OAC), i.e., warfarin, in a prospective randomized controlled trial (RCT) in patients eligible for OAC

[25]. Long-term data revealed a noninferiority and superiority compared to OAC for preventing the combined outcome of stroke, systemic embolism, and cardiovascular death as well as superiority for cardiovascular and all-cause mortality [26]. Moreover, the PREVAIL trial stated adequate safety of the WATCHMAN™ procedure [27]. The efficacy and safety of other devices were exclusively evaluated by observational studies.

2. The interventional left atrial appendage closure

2.1. Indications and decision-making

Worthy of note, the patients with the strongest indication for a thromboembolic prophylaxis often also have a relevantly increased bleeding risk, represented by a major intersection of the risk factors included in the CHA_2DS_2-VASc and the HAS-BLED score. Based on the different approval procedures the necessary indications for the interventional closure of the LAA vary geographically and will subsequently be presented in the European context. The current European guidelines recommend the interventional LAA closure (LAAC) as an alternative to OAC for nonvalvular AF patients with an indication for OAC but on the other hand contraindications for a long-term treatment with this substances (IIbB) [3]. They note that, for example, patients with a prior life-threatening bleeding without a reversible cause may have a contraindication for long-term OAC [3]. However, further examples for the practical implementation are not given. Furthermore, the indication is impeded by the fact that numerous patients that formerly have been considered unsuitable for long-term OAC nowadays can take an oral prophylactic medication due to an adequate management [3, 28].

As the two currently available RCTs in the field of interventional LAAC only included, by their nature, patients which were eligible for long-term OAC [25, 27], they do not appear suitable for the identification of guideline-conform reasons for an interventional approach. The best practical help may be provided by the EHRA/EAPCI expert consensus statement [29] from which the presented decision-making algorithm is derived (**Figure 2**). If possible contraindications for a long-term anticoagulation arise and the individual CHA_2DS_2-VASc score is low, i.e., 1 in males and 2 in females, the necessity for OAC should be strictly checked in a risk-tailored approach with the aid of biomarkers (cf. 1.2 and [3]). Only patients with a persisting indication should be further evaluated.

In a *first step*, patients, which are presented for the LAAC evaluation, should be divided into those who are per se eligible for OAC and those who are not. All eligible patients should be well informed about the guideline recommendation for a prophylaxis by OAC, preferentially by a NOAC whenever possible. Some patients, however, will still refuse to take one of these substances due to various reasons, e.g., subjective anxiety, increased professional bleeding risk, OAC intolerance due to other side-effects than bleedings or noncompliance with OAC. If so, patients' refusal may be considered as an adequate contraindication for long-term OAC.

http://dx.doi.org/10.5772/67773

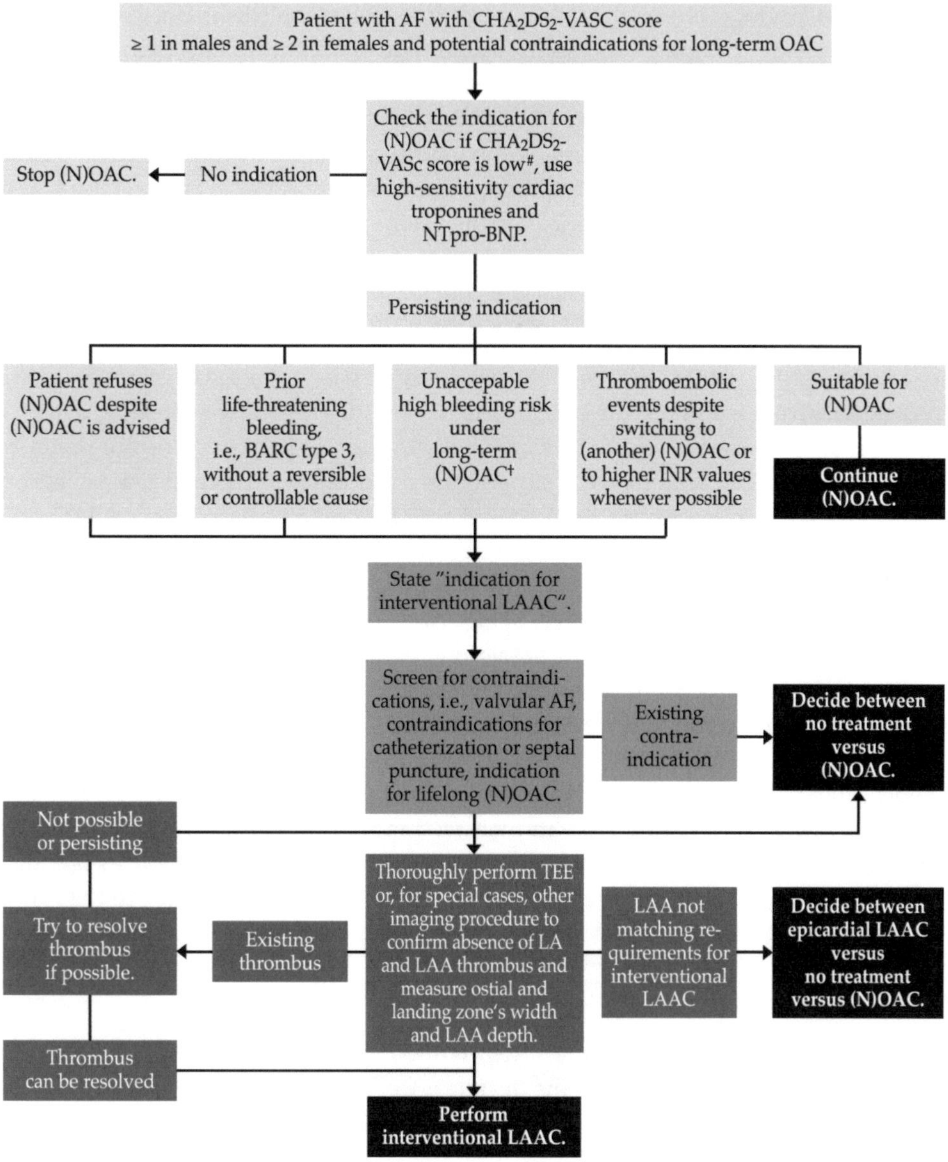

Figure 2. Decision-making algorithm derived from Ref. [29]; # = 1 in males or 2 in females; † = HAS-BLED score ≥ 3, bleeding risk not reflected by the HAS-BLED score, prolonged triple therapy or recurrent minor bleedings under (N)OAC, e.g., gastrointestinal bleedings.

Two prospective, observational studies demonstrated safety and efficacy of LAAC in patients who were ineligible for any OAC [30, 31]. This indication is depicted most clearly by the formulation in the European guidelines [3]. It covers, in particular, prior life-threatening bleedings according to Bleeding Academic Research Consortium (BARC) type 3 [32] without a reversible or controllable cause. This includes bleedings due to angiodysplasia, amyloid angiopathy, malignoma, chronic inflammatory bowel disease, thrombocytopenia, platelet dysfunctions, or other coagulation disorders as well as recurrent falling in the course of epilepsy or frailty [30, 31, 33, 34]. As well as for the patients refusing OAC, it must be stated, that a postinterventional temporary intake of at least two antiplatelet agents regularly followed by a lifelong single antiplatelet therapy is mandatory in most centers and cases of relevant postinterventional bleedings under dual antiplatelet therapy (DAPT) can be found in literature [35, 36]. There is growing evidence for the efficacy of a single antiplatelet therapy following LAAC but a strategy of discontinuation of any antiplatelet therapy is still based on single-center experience [37–40]. In this context, at least the bleeding risk under acetylsalicylic acid (ASA) should be included in the considerations [29, 41].

In other patients, the risk for a severe bleeding under long-term OAC might be estimated unacceptably high even without the existence of a prior life-threatening bleeding event. These patients with an increased HAS-BLED score (≥ 3 according to [29]) or recurrent minor bleedings (according to BARC type 1 and 2 [32]) require a thorough individual risk-benefit profile evaluation by taking into account the lowered bleeding event rates under NOAC therapy. But, thereby, especially patients with recurrent minor gastrointestinal (GI) bleedings as well as those with a risk for GI bleedings perform very poor [21]. Due to the practical necessity of a postinterventional lifelong ASA intake, again, the risk for bleedings under ASA should be determined [29, 41]. In addition to the above-mentioned causes for bleedings and the ones depicted by the HAS-BLED score, a prolonged triple therapy due to a complex coronary artery disease may be a particularly relevant indication in this group of patients. AF patients with a highly impaired renal function, i.e., glomerular filtration rate <15 ml/min, or those with chronic renal replacement therapy reflect special cases. In these patients, both a high bleeding risk and a high stroke risk are associated with an increased mortality [42, 43]. These patients cannot be treated by NOACs and the benefit of a treatment with vitamin K antagonists is controversially discussed [44–46]. The value of an interventional closure of the LAA in these patients cannot be stated at this point. However, promising data concerning safety and efficacy exist in patients with chronic kidney disease compared to the estimated TIA, stroke and bleedings rates of the collective even in patients with an end-stage renal disease [47].

Special cases where a LAAC may be indicated without a contraindication for long-term OAC are patients with thromboembolic events despite a well monitored treatment with OAC even after switching to another substance or to higher INR values. In these patients, and especially if it is likely that the thrombus originated from the LAA, LAAC can be an alternative or an additional treatment to OAC [29].

In a European multicenter observational trial consecutively including slightly more than 1000 patients with a LAAC procedure, 47% had suffered a major hemorrhage, 35% were defined as being prone to a high bleeding risk, 22% had an indication for a triple therapy, 16% suffered a stroke under OAC, and 8% had an elevated risk of falling [33]. By reflecting the above-presented indications in a real-life cohort, it was emphasized that in some patients the combination of several reasons resulted in the indication.

In a *second step*, after establishing the indication, the patients' medical documents should be screened for contraindications for catheter-based LAAC. These are valvular or rheumatic AF as, in these patients, thrombi do not originate from the LAA in up to 60% of cases [11, 48], contraindications for catheterization and transseptal puncture such as active infection, left atrial thrombus or tumor as well as the presence of a closure device on the atrial septal puncture site and indications for lifelong OAC besides AF such as mechanical heart valves, recurrent pulmonary embolism and deep vein thrombosis.

In a *third step*, if these contraindications can be excluded, anatomical feasibility should be checked by thorough two- and three-dimensional transesophageal (TEE) measurements prior to the intervention [49–51]. Not only the absence of a thrombus in the LA and LAA must be confirmed but also LAA dimensions must fulfill certain device-specific requirements. Ultrasound contrast agent use may facilitate the detection of a thrombus [52]. Therefore, the LAA is visualized and measured in multiple views (0, 45, 90 and 135°) at the end of the atrial diastole when the LAA volume is largest to avoid undersizing. First of all, the maximal ostial width is measured from a point right next to the left circumflex coronary artery or the mitral valve annulus to a point 1–2 cm from the tip of the left superior pulmonary vein limbus (**Figure 3**). While the orifice usually is oval shaped, the largest diameter is of procedural interest for the WATCHMAN™ device implantation. For the Amplatzer™ devices a so-called landing zone 10–12 mm from the orifice into the LAA is important. Furthermore, the LAA depth is measured perpendicular to the ostial plane. The WATCHMAN™ device is unsuitable if the depth-width ratio is < 1, the Amplatzer™ Amulet™ is limited to a depth of ≥ 7.5 mm. An orifice of 30 mm for the WATCHMAN™ device and a landing zone of 31 mm for the Amplatzer™

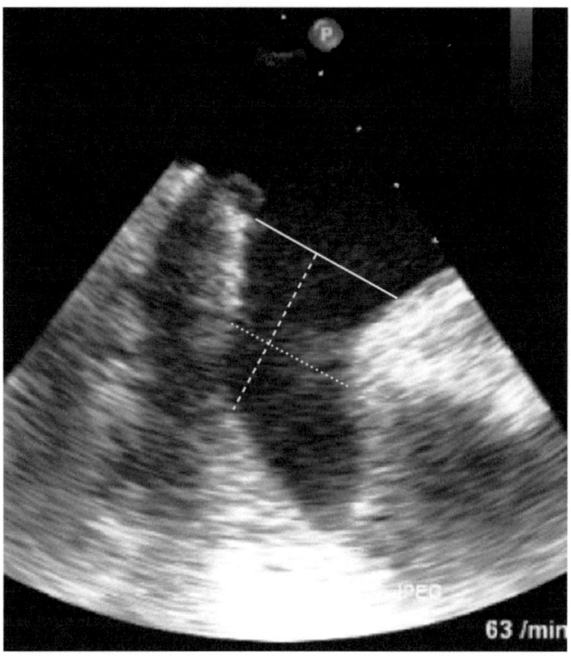

Figure 3. Echocardiographic measurements prior to the left atrial appendage closure; solid line = orifice diameter, dashed line = depth, dotted line = landing zone.

Amulet™, respectively, are the upper limitations concerning the LAA width. Large secondary lobes should be assessed accurately as they might impede the complete sealing of the LAA orifice, especially when a second large lobe branches off close to the ostium.

In cases where the LAA evaluation by TEE is difficult, especially if multiple lobes are present, further imaging methods, e.g., computed tomography (CT) angiography, may help to ensure correct measurements [53–57]. In case of an existing LAA thrombus, several attempts with different substances can become necessary to resolve it [58], but this effort will not be possible in patients with absolute contraindications to even short-term (N)OAC treatment.

2.2. Device types and procedural aspects

The five CE-marked devices for catheter-based LAAC can be divided into two groups, the ball and the disk type, respectively. The WATCHMAN™ device, the WaveCrest™ system and the Occlutech® occluder form the ball-type group while the Amplatzer™ devices and the Lambre™ system form the disk-type group. All devices consist of a self-expanding nitinol mesh with wires to anchor in the LAA walls and they are covered by different patches. The disk-type group is characterized by a so-called waist connecting a proximal disk with a distal lobe. Newer LAAC devices are optimized for intraprocedural repositioning by retractable anchors, for instance, to facilitate the procedure in complex anatomies. The WaveCrest™ system has a foam coat to minimize residual leaks after implantation. Operators evaluated the ACP's "pacifier principle" was particularly user-friendly, which might be reflected by high success rates in the early trials [29]. Furthermore, it might have advantages in anatomies with two large main lobes originating from one ostium. But these assertions are mainly based on expert opinions and ongoing studies will have to further evaluate the individual advantages of the latest developments on the device market and the value of a certain device type for different morphologies.

The catheter-based LAAC procedure (**Figure 4**) is usually performed under deep conscious sedation or general anesthesia. Antibiotic prophylaxis is recommended prior to the intervention. The procedure is guided by fluoroscopy, angiography, and TEE. Some centers use additional intracardiac echocardiography (ICE) [59]. The correct device type and size (10–30% larger than the measured diameter to allow device stabilization by compression forces) is chosen by the above mentioned preinterventional TEE or CT measurements. In Seldinger technique, vascular access is taken via the right femoral vein and the transseptal puncture is performed in a standard fashion in the posterior and inferior atrial septum. This allows to easily access the LAA ostium. If a patent foramen ovale is present, this "natural" way can also be used for transseptal crossing provided it is suitable for the LAA access [33]. Again, the freedom from thrombus is confirmed by angiography via an intraatrial pigtail catheter (right anterior oblique 30°/cranial 30°) and by TEE or ICE. Prior to the transseptal puncture, unfractionated heparin is administered to achieve an activated clotting time >250 s. Via the transseptal wire the device delivery sheath (8–14 French) is inserted. It is particularly important to avoid air embolism by flushing the sheath and the device with isotonic saline prior to the insertion. All devices are preinstalled on the catheters. The device is deployed by retracting the delivery sheath over the device which then self-expands. The deployment is conducted by fluoroscopy and echocardiography. In case of incorrect positioning, all current devices can be repositioned by retraction into the delivery

http://dx.doi.org/10.5772/67773

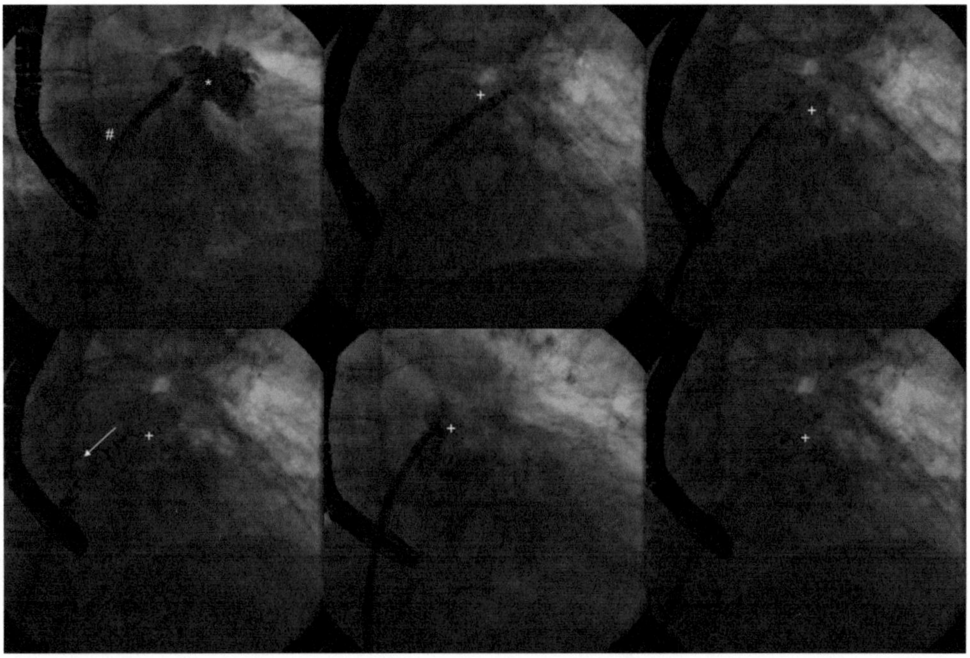

Figure 4. Fluoroscopic and angiographic images of the left atrial appendage closure procedure. (A) Angiographic illustration of the cauliflower shaped left atrial appendage (*); # = delivery sheath. (B) The WATCHMAN™ device (+) is pushed forward through the delivery sheath. (C) The device (+) is implanted in the left atrial appendage. (D) Stable anchoring is confirmed by pulling the device (+) in the direction of the white arrow ("tug test"). (E) The correct sealing of the left atrial appendage by the device (+) is illustrated by angiography. (F) The released left atrial appendage occluder (+).

sheath prior to device releasement. When the correct landing position is achieved, the stable device anchoring is confirmed by a so-called "tug test" and correct sealing of the LAA ostium is illustrated by angiography and color Doppler imaging. After complete device deployment and before TEE retraction, a pericardial effusion should be ruled out. It is naturally clear that the procedural steps might slightly vary between the different devices. In relation to procedural success, an operator-related learning curve could be demonstrated [33, 60, 61]. Procedures combined with other cardiac interventions, e.g., percutaneous coronary intervention, closure of a persistent foramen ovale or an atrial septum defect, atrial fibrillation ablation, or even transcatheter aortic valve implantation, are not untypical in clinical practice [33]. The value of combined procedures especially of those which both require a transseptal puncture is currently not completely elucidated. Moreover, despite the knowledge of the chicken wing morphology being a highly challenging LAA anatomy [62], procedural characteristics and outcomes related to different LAA morphologies still remain to be evaluated.

2.3. Postprocedural measures and antithrombotic regimens

It is a frequent practice to perform a chest X-ray as well as a transthoracic echocardiography 24 hours after the procedure to reconfirm the device position and the absence of a pericardial effusion prior to the patients' discharge from hospital. The average length of stay is around 2–5 days [63, 64]. Endocarditis prophylaxis is usually considered prior to at-risk procedures for 6 months after the implantation.

The follow-up visits as well as the imaging modalities for device surveillance are closely linked to the initiated postinterventional antithrombotic regimen. Subsequently, different regimens for the most common devices, the WATCHMAN™ and the Amplatzer™ devices, respectively, are presented. For the other devices, regimens must be adopted by having regard to the instructions for use.

If the patient is eligible for short-term OAC after the WATCHMAN™ device implantation, it is usually conducted for 45 days reflected by the two RCTs [25, 27], two observational studies with NOACs [65, 66] and the instructions for use. TEE is performed after this period to rule out device thrombus prior to switching to DAPT and again after 6 months when switching from DAPT to ASA therapy is intended. In the PROTECT-AF trial, 86% of all implanted patients could be discontinued with warfarin after 45 days and 92% after 6 months as the TEE criterion (peridevice leak <5 mm) was met. In the more recent PREVAIL trial, 92 and 98% of all implanted patients were able to discontinue warfarin after 45 days and 6 months, respectively. While there is no evidence for increased thromboembolic event rates associated to peridevice leaks <5 mm independent of OAC discontinuation based on a limited source of evidence [67], peridevice leaks ≥ 5 mm remain an indication for continuation or reinitiation of OAC whenever possible or for a second occlusion attempt [29, 68].

As many patients are ineligible to even short-term OAC, postinterventional regimens without OAC prescription had been urgently needed. Therefore, two smaller prospective observational studies evaluated a DAPT after LAAC and revealed adequate efficacy and safety for such regimen with the WATCHMAN™ device and the ACP [30, 31]. This regimen is also adopted in the instructions for use for the Amplatzer™ devices. DAPT was prescribed 1–6 months after the procedure and then switched to an indefinite single antiplatelet therapy. As above-stated, the efficacy of a single antiplatelet therapy following LAAC for specific high-risk patients appears adequate but the complete discontinuation of antithrombotic treatment at some point is based on limited experience [37–40]. While the optimal timing for postinterventional device surveillance cannot be completely justified by the existing literature, a follow-up between a minimum of 1.5 and a maximum of 6 months as a compromise between the fast switch to minimal antithrombotic therapy after ensuring adequate LAA occlusion and the secure identification of device-related thrombi appears reasonable [69]. Platelet count, CHA_2DS_2-VASc score and reduced ejection fraction were identified as risk factors for device-related thrombi under DAPT [70]. Although the thrombus-associated stroke rate appears low [61], it is recommended to resolve it by a new initiated or continued anticoagulation whenever possible [29]. Additional clinical visits or imaging procedures may not be mandatory apart from study protocols, but by bearing in mind late device embolizations [71] (cf. 2.4) and the underlying cardiovascular disease of the intervened patients, it appears reasonable to follow them up regularly.

TEE currently remains the gold standard for postimplant device surveillance. Magnetic resonance tomography imagining is hindered by artefacts from the device and especially in light of radiation exposure and the need for contrast agent use [72], the value of CT angiography compared to TEE for postimplant imaging has not been finally clarified [73, 74].

2.4. Procedure-related complications and short-term outcome

Procedure-related complications are mainly associated with bleedings such as pericardial effusion and tamponade and access site complications, i.e., hematoma, overt bleeding, AV fistula, and pseudoaneurysm. Moreover, periinterventional TIA and stroke as well as early device embolization and air embolism have also been reported. Additional late device embolizations have been observed and there are several surgical and interventional techniques to retrieve an embolized device in relation to its location [71, 75]. **Table 1** summarizes the reported complications from the most representative studies for the most common devices. The presented

Study	Patients in the treatment arm [n]	Successful implantation [%]	Relevant pericardial effusion [%]	Access site complication and other major bleeding [%]	TIA or stroke; hemorrhagic stroke [%]	Early device embolization [%]
WATCHMAN™ device						
Holmes et al. [25]	463	88	4.8	3.5	1.1; 0.2	0.6
Reddy et al. [61]	460	95	2.2	0.7	0.0	0.0
Reddy et al. [31]	150	95	1.3	2.0	0.7	1.3
Holmes et al. [27]	269	95	0.4	0.7	0.7	0.7
Boersma et al. [34]	1019	99	0.1	1.1	0.0 (0.3 between days 8 and 30)	0.2
Amplatzer™ devices						
Park et al. (ACP) [84]	143	96	3.5	n/a	2.1	1.4
Lam et al. (ACP) [78]	20	95	0.0	0.0	n/a	0.0
Urena et al. (ACP) [30]	52	98	0.0	3.8	1.9	1.9
Gloekler et al. (ACP and Amulet™) [76]	100	96	6.0	0.0	0.0	5.0
Tzikas et al. (ACP) [33]	1047	97	1.2	1.2	0.9	0.8
Abualsaud et al. (ACP and Amulet™) [77]	59	98	0.0	n/a	0.0	0.0
Berti et al. (ACP and Amulet™) [64]	110	96	2.7	0.9	0.9	0.0

Table 1. Implantation success and procedural safety; n/a = not applicable; TIA = transitory ischemic attack.

data usually refer to events within the first 7 days following the procedure. No procedure-related death occurring during the first week and only one procedure-related death (0.1%) within 30 days after the WATCHMAN™ device implantation was recently reported from the large multicenter observational EWOLUTION registry [34], a low rate, which also could be recently observed in a multicenter observational registry for the ACP [33]. The implantation success (≥ 95%) was highly satisfactory most recently. Comparing the periprocedural safety, the first and second generation Amplatzer™ devices appear equal [76, 77]. Not only for the procedural success but also for the reduction of overall complications, a learning curve over time was obvious [33, 60, 61].

2.5. Medium- and long-term outcome

As mentioned in the beginning, the WATCHMAN™ device was shown to be superior (posterior probability 96.0%) for the combined outcome of stroke, systemic embolism and cardiovascular death compared to a warfarin treatment in a long-term follow-up to the PROTECT-AF trial with a 2:1 randomization for the device implantation [26]. After a mean follow-up of 3.8 years (2621 patient-years) the primary annual event rate was 2.3% in the device versus 3.8% in the warfarin group (rate ratio 0.60; 95% credible interval 0.41–1.05) [26]. In the initial PROTECT-AF trial with a follow-up of 1065 patient-years, only the noninferiority could be demonstrated (posterior probability >99.9%) [25]. The primary annual event rate in the device group was 3.0 versus 4.9% in the warfarin group (rate ratio 0.62; 95% credible interval 0.35–1.25). The study is limited by a high dropout rate in the control groups as well as by collecting a per se OAC eligible collective with a low stroke risk ($CHADS_2$ score 2.2 ± 1.2).

Under the conditions of an equal study protocol but of a higher $CHADS_2$ score of 2.6 ± 1.0 the PREVIAL trial failed to reach noninferiority for the primary efficacy outcome within 18 months [27]. Only for the stroke and systemic embolization rate >7 days after randomization noninferiority could be stated. But the key message of this trial was the lower rate of safety events compared to PROTECT-AF despite a high proportion of untrained operators (25%) and a more inclusive definition of safety events compared to PROTECT-AF event rates were still lower (annual rates of 4.2 versus 8.7%, respectively; $p = 0.004$).

With a total of 5931 patient-years, a meta-analysis of the PROTECT-AF trial, the PREVAIL trial and the subsequent registries confirmed noninferiority for the predefined combined primary efficacy endpoint compared to warfarin treatment [79]. Annual event rates were 2.7 and 3.5%, respectively (hazard ratio 0.79; 95% credible interval 0.53–1.20 ; p=0.22). Worthy of note, only after subtracting the procedure-related strokes from the total number of strokes, the event rates in the device and the warfarin group were no longer significantly different (hazard ratio 1.56; 95% credible interval 0.78–3.09; $p = 0.21$). Reflecting a bleeding benefit, hemorrhagic stroke was significantly less frequent in the device group (0.15%; 95% credible interval 0.07–0.40) compared to the warfarin group (0.61%; 95% credible interval 0.55–1.70) (hazard ratio 0.22; 95% credible interval 0.08–0.61; $p = 0.004$).

The largest data set for the ACP was published by Tzikas et al. (prospective collection of the data and retrospective analyzation). He reports, after 1349 patient-years of follow-up, an annual systemic thromboembolism rate of 2.3% [33]. In terms of safety, an annual rate of major bleeding of 2.1% was registered. Based on a mean CHA_2DS_2-VASc score of 4.5 ±

1.6 and a mean HAS-BLED score 3.1 ± 1.2, this meant a risk reduction of 59% for systemic thromboembolism and 61% for major bleeding respectively, compared to the rates predicted by the scores.

Postinterventional DAPT was mainly proven effective and safe by the prospective observational studies of Reddy et al. (WATCHMAN™) [31] and Urena et al. (ACP) [30]. Annual event rates for all-cause stroke and systemic thromboembolism were 2.3 and 3.4%, respectively. Reddy et al. found an annual rate for hemorrhagic stroke of 0.6%. Urena et al. observed an annual major bleedings rate of 3.4%. Thus, these outcome measures were completely comparable to the event rates in the RCTs including OAC eligible patients. The mean/median CHA_2DS_2-VASc scores of 4.4 ± 1.7 and 5 (4–6), respectively, thereby correspond to a high-risk collective.

Concerning alternatives to vitamin K antagonists and DAPT following LAAC, two recently published studies reported data for the strategy of a single antiplatelet therapy after LAAC. After a total of 265 patient-years an annual stroke rate of 2.3% was observed by Korsholm et al. under a single ASA therapy [40]. The mean CHA_2DS_2-VASc score was 4.4 ± 1.6 and the mean HAS-BLED score was 4.1 ± 1.1. Jalal et al. [39] reported an annual stroke/TIA rate of 4.0% and an annual major bleeding rate of 1.3% after 75 patient-years of follow-up under ASA or clopidogrel monotherapy. The mean CHA_2DS_2-VASc score was 4.4 ± 1.3 and the mean HAS-BLED score 3.4 ± 0.9. Here again, the rates are in good accordance with the ones reported in the earlier mentioned RCTs. Initial retrospective data comparing NOAC to warfarin for 6 weeks following LAAC showed comparable rates for device-related thrombus, composite of thromboembolism or device-related thrombosis and postprocedural bleeding events [65].

In summary, LAAC with different devices was proven to be effective and safe or, in the long run, even superior to long-term warfarin treatment in respect to all-cause and cardiovascular mortality when it is combined with a 45-day warfarin intake following procedure. Moreover, LAAC could be shown to be more effective and less costly relative to warfarin and NOACs in recent analyses [80, 81]. LAAC was dominant over NOACs by year 5 and warfarin by year 10 [80].

2.6. Perspectives

On this basis, meanwhile, the LAAC procedure has found its status in clinical practice. Due to the inherent character of complications regarding any interventional cardiac procedure, it is unlikely that complication rates will further strongly decrease and, therefore, an individualized and risk-tailored approach in patient selection is a crucial step prior to the patient's transfer to the catheterization laboratory. It is hoped that further studies will focus on the identification of patients who will derive the most benefit from an interventional approach and will help to better characterize the term "contraindication for long-term OAC" [82].

As more and more patients will be implanted which are even ineligible for a short-term OAC treatment, the alternatives, i.e., DAPT and single antiplatelet agents following LAAC, have to be further evaluated. In this context, the knowledge of the optimal duration of DAPT and about the possibility of discontinuing any antithrombotic medication will help to treat certain very high-risk patients based on reliable data.

Unsolved questions derived from the postprocedural practice are the relevance of paradevice leaks especially ≥ 5 mm revealed during follow-up imaging procedures and the related need for action. Moreover, the value of CT angiography for device surveillance is not conclusively clarified yet.

But the most important would be to thoroughly compare LAAC to different NOACs as these substances currently are clearly recommended in AF patients without contraindications by the European guidelines [3]. Initial data show that the interventional approach does not need to be hidden away [83].

Author details

Christian Fastner*, Michael Behnes, Uzair Ansari, Ibrahim El-Battrawy and Martin Borggrefe

*Address all correspondence to: christian.fastner@umm.de

First Department of Medicine, University Medical Center Mannheim, University of Heidelberg, Mannheim, Germany

References

[1] Go, A.S., et al., *Prevalence of diagnosed atrial fibrillation in adults: national implications for rhythm management and stroke prevention: the AnTicoagulation and Risk Factors in Atrial Fibrillation (ATRIA) Study*. JAMA, 2001. **285**(18): pp. 2370-2375.

[2] Haim, M., et al., *Prospective national study of the prevalence, incidence, management and outcome of a large contemporary cohort of patients with incident non-valvular atrial fibrillation*. J Am Heart Assoc, 2015. **4**(1): p. e001486.

[3] Kirchhof, P., et al., *2016 ESC Guidelines for the management of atrial fibrillation developed in collaboration with EACTS*. Eur Heart J, 2016. **37**(38): pp. 2893-2962.

[4] Calenda, B.W., et al., *Stroke risk assessment in atrial fibrillation: risk factors and markers of atrial myopathy*. Nat Rev Cardiol, 2016. **13**(9): pp. 549-559.

[5] Lim, H.S., et al., *Effect of atrial fibrillation on atrial thrombogenesis in humans: impact of rate and rhythm*. J Am Coll Cardiol, 2013. **61**(8): p. 852-860.

[6] Watson, T., E. Shantsila, and G.Y. Lip, *Mechanisms of thrombogenesis in atrial fibrillation: Virchow's triad revisited*. Lancet, 2009. **373**(9658): pp. 155-166.

[7] Al-Saady, N.M., O.A. Obel, and A.J. Camm, *Left atrial appendage: structure, function, and role in thromboembolism*. Heart, 1999. **82**(5): pp. 547-554.

[8] Lupercio, F., et al., *Left atrial appendage morphology assessment for risk stratification of embolic stroke in patients with atrial fibrillation: A meta-analysis*. Heart Rhythm, 2016. **13**(7): pp. 1402-1409.

[9] Kimura, T., et al., *Anatomical characteristics of the left atrial appendage in cardiogenic stroke with low CHADS2 scores*. Heart Rhythm, 2013. **10**(6): pp. 921-925.

[10] Di Biase, L., et al., *Does the left atrial appendage morphology correlate with the risk of stroke in patients with atrial fibrillation? Results from a multicenter study*. J Am Coll Cardiol, 2012. **60**(6): pp. 531-538.

[11] Blackshear, J.L. and J.A. Odell, *Appendage obliteration to reduce stroke in cardiac surgical patients with atrial fibrillation*. Ann Thorac Surg, 1996. **61**(2): pp. 755-759.

[12] Hart, R.G., et al., *Antithrombotic therapy to prevent stroke in patients with atrial fibrillation: a meta-analysis*. Ann Intern Med, 1999. **131**(7): pp. 492-501.

[13] Kakkar, A.K., et al., *Risk profiles and antithrombotic treatment of patients newly diagnosed with atrial fibrillation at risk of stroke: perspectives from the international, observational, prospective GARFIELD registry*. PLoS One, 2013. **8**(5): p. e63479.

[14] Waldo, A.L., et al., *Hospitalized patients with atrial fibrillation and a high risk of stroke are not being provided with adequate anticoagulation*. J Am Coll Cardiol, 2005. **46**(9): pp. 1729-1736.

[15] Pisters, R., et al., *A novel user-friendly score (HAS-BLED) to assess 1-year risk of major bleeding in patients with atrial fibrillation: the Euro Heart Survey*. Chest, 2010. **138**(5): pp. 1093-1100.

[16] Investigators, A.W.G.o.t.A., et al., *Clopidogrel plus aspirin versus oral anticoagulation for atrial fibrillation in the Atrial fibrillation Clopidogrel Trial with Irbesartan for prevention of Vascular Events (ACTIVE W): a randomised controlled trial*. Lancet, 2006. **367**(9526): pp. 1903-1912.

[17] Connolly, S.J., et al., *Dabigatran versus warfarin in patients with atrial fibrillation*. N Engl J Med, 2009. **361**(12): pp. 1139-1151.

[18] Patel, M.R., et al., *Rivaroxaban versus warfarin in nonvalvular atrial fibrillation*. N Engl J Med, 2011. **365**(10): pp. 883-191.

[19] Granger, C.B., et al., *Apixaban versus warfarin in patients with atrial fibrillation*. N Engl J Med, 2011. **365**(11): pp. 981-992.

[20] Giugliano, R.P., et al., *Edoxaban versus warfarin in patients with atrial fibrillation*. N Engl J Med, 2013. **369**(22): pp. 2093-2104.

[21] Ruff, C.T., et al., *Comparison of the efficacy and safety of new oral anticoagulants with warfarin in patients with atrial fibrillation: a meta-analysis of randomised trials*. Lancet, 2014. **383**(9921): pp. 955-962.

[22] Alamneh, E.A., L. Chalmers, and L.R. Bereznicki, *Suboptimal use of oral anticoagulants in atrial fibrillation: has the introduction of direct oral anticoagulants improved prescribing practices?* Am J Cardiovasc Drugs, 2016. **16**(3): pp. 183-200.

[23] Tsai, Y.C., et al., *Surgical left atrial appendage occlusion during cardiac surgery for patients with atrial fibrillation: a meta-analysis*. Eur J Cardiothorac Surg, 2015. **47**(5): pp. 847-854.

[24] Chatterjee, S., et al., *Safety and procedural success of left atrial appendage exclusion with the lariat device: a systematic review of published reports and analytic review of the FDA MAUDE database.* JAMA Intern Med, 2015. **175**(7): pp. 1104-1109.

[25] Holmes, D.R., et al., *Percutaneous closure of the left atrial appendage versus warfarin therapy for prevention of stroke in patients with atrial fibrillation: a randomised non-inferiority trial.* Lancet, 2009. **374**(9689): pp. 534-542.

[26] Reddy, V.Y., et al., *Percutaneous left atrial appendage closure vs warfarin for atrial fibrillation: a randomized clinical trial.* JAMA, 2014. **312**(19): pp. 1988-1998.

[27] Holmes, D.R., Jr., et al., *Prospective randomized evaluation of the Watchman Left Atrial Appendage Closure device in patients with atrial fibrillation versus long-term warfarin therapy: the PREVAIL trial.* J Am Coll Cardiol, 2014. **64**(1): pp. 1-12.

[28] Kuramatsu, J.B., et al., *Anticoagulant reversal, blood pressure levels, and anticoagulant resumption in patients with anticoagulation-related intracerebral hemorrhage.* JAMA, 2015. **313**(8): pp. 824-836.

[29] Meier, B., et al., *EHRA/EAPCI expert consensus statement on catheter-based left atrial appendage occlusion.* Europace, 2014. **16**(10): pp. 1397-1416.

[30] Urena, M., et al., *Percutaneous left atrial appendage closure with the AMPLATZER cardiac plug device in patients with nonvalvular atrial fibrillation and contraindications to anticoagulation therapy.* J Am Coll Cardiol, 2013. **62**(2): pp. 96-102.

[31] Reddy, V.Y., et al., *Left atrial appendage closure with the Watchman device in patients with a contraindication for oral anticoagulation: the ASAP study (ASA Plavix Feasibility Study With Watchman Left Atrial Appendage Closure Technology).* J Am Coll Cardiol, 2013. **61**(25): pp. 2551-2556.

[32] Mehran, R., et al., *Standardized bleeding definitions for cardiovascular clinical trials: a consensus report from the Bleeding Academic Research Consortium.* Circulation, 2011. **123**(23): pp. 2736-2747.

[33] Tzikas, A., et al., *Left atrial appendage occlusion for stroke prevention in atrial fibrillation: multicentre experience with the AMPLATZER Cardiac Plug.* EuroIntervention, 2016. **11**(10): pp. 1170-1179.

[34] Boersma, L.V., et al., *Implant success and safety of left atrial appendage closure with the WATCHMAN device: peri-procedural outcomes from the EWOLUTION registry.* Eur Heart J, 2016. **37**(31): pp. 2465-2474.

[35] Ruiz-Garcia, J. and R. Moreno, *Percutaneous closure of left atrial appendage: device-indicated antiplatelet therapy may also lead to fatal bleeding. A call for evidence-based antiplatelet regimen.* J Thromb Thrombolysis, 2014. **37**(3): pp. 359-361.

[36] Llull, L., et al., *Intracranial hemorrhage during dual antiplatelet therapy after percutaneous left atrial appendage closure.* Cerebrovasc Dis, 2014. **38**(1): pp. 73-74.

[37] Rodriguez-Gabella, T., et al., *Single antiplatelet therapy following left atrial appendage closure in patients with contraindication to anticoagulation*. J Am Coll Cardiol, 2016. **68**(17): pp. 1920-1921.

[38] Renou, P., et al., *Left atrial appendage closure in patients with atrial fibrillation and previous intracerebral hemorrhage*. J Stroke Cerebrovasc Dis, 2016 26(3): pp. 545-551.

[39] Jalal, Z., et al., *Percutaneous left atrial appendage closure followed by single antiplatelet therapy: short- and mid-term outcomes*. Arch Cardiovasc Dis, 2017. [Epub ahead of print].

[40] Korsholm, K., et al., *Transcatheter left atrial appendage occlusion in patients with atrial fibrillation and a high bleeding risk using aspirin alone for post-implant antithrombotic therapy*. EuroIntervention, 2016. [Epub ahead of print].

[41] Connolly, S.J., et al., *Apixaban in patients with atrial fibrillation*. N Engl J Med, 2011. **364**(9): pp. 806-817.

[42] Zimmerman, D., et al., *Systematic review and meta-analysis of incidence, prevalence and outcomes of atrial fibrillation in patients on dialysis*. Nephrol Dial Transplant, 2012. **27**(10): pp. 3816-3822.

[43] Olesen, J.B., et al., *Stroke and bleeding in atrial fibrillation with chronic kidney disease*. N Engl J Med, 2012. **367**(7): pp. 625-635.

[44] Chan, K.E., et al., *Dabigatran and rivaroxaban use in atrial fibrillation patients on hemodialysis*. Circulation, 2015. **131**(11): pp. 972-979.

[45] Bonde, A.N., et al., *Net clinical benefit of antithrombotic therapy in patients with atrial fibrillation and chronic kidney disease: a nationwide observational cohort study*. J Am Coll Cardiol, 2014. **64**(23): pp. 2471-2482.

[46] Shah, M., et al., *Warfarin use and the risk for stroke and bleeding in patients with atrial fibrillation undergoing dialysis*. Circulation, 2014. **129**(11): pp. 1196-1203.

[47] Kefer, J., et al., *Impact of chronic kidney disease on left atrial appendage occlusion for stroke prevention in patients with atrial fibrillation*. Int J Cardiol, 2016. **207**: pp. 335-340.

[48] Mahajan, R., et al., *Importance of the underlying substrate in determining thrombus location in atrial fibrillation: implications for left atrial appendage closure*. Heart, 2012. **98**(15): pp. 1120-1126.

[49] Yosefy, C., et al., *A new method for direct three-dimensional measurement of left atrial appendage dimensions during transesophageal echocardiography*. Echocardiography, 2016. **33**(1): pp. 69-76.

[50] Nucifora, G., et al., *Evaluation of the left atrial appendage with real-time 3-dimensional transesophageal echocardiography: implications for catheter-based left atrial appendage closure*. Circ Cardiovasc Imaging, 2011. **4**(5): pp. 514-523.

[51] Donal, E., et al., *The left atrial appendage, a small, blind-ended structure: a review of its echocardiographic evaluation and its clinical role*. Chest, 2005. **128**(3): pp. 1853-1862.

[52] Jung, P.H., et al., *Contrast enhanced transesophageal echocardiography in patients with atrial fibrillation referred to electrical cardioversion improves atrial thrombus detection and may reduce associated thromboembolic events*. Cardiovasc Ultrasound, 2013. **11**(1): p. 1.

[53] Saw, J., et al., *Comparing measurements of CT Angiography, TEE, and fluoroscopy of the left atrial appendage for percutaneous closure*. J Cardiovasc Electrophysiol, 2016. **27**(4): pp. 414-422.

[54] Krishnaswamy, A., et al., *Planning left atrial appendage occlusion using cardiac multidetector computed tomography*. Int J Cardiol, 2012. **158**(2): pp. 313-317.

[55] Romero, J., et al., *Detection of left atrial appendage thrombus by cardiac computed tomography in patients with atrial fibrillation: a meta-analysis*. Circ Cardiovasc Imaging, 2013. **6**(2): pp. 185-194.

[56] Bai, W., et al., *Assessment of the left atrial appendage structure and morphology: comparison of real-time three-dimensional transesophageal echocardiography and computed tomography*. Int J Cardiovasc Imaging, 2016 [Epub ahead of print].

[57] Rajwani, A., et al., *CT sizing for left atrial appendage closure is associated with favourable outcomes for procedural safety*. Eur Heart J Cardiovasc Imaging, 2016 [Epub ahead of print].

[58] Miwa, Y., et al., *Resolution of a warfarin and dabigatran-resistant left atrial appendage thrombus with apixaban*. J Arrhythm, 2016. **32**(3): pp. 233-235.

[59] Masson, J.B., et al., *Transcatheter left atrial appendage closure using intracardiac echocardiographic guidance from the left atrium*. Can J Cardiol, 2015. **31**(12): pp. 1497 e7-1497 e14.

[60] Ledwoch, J., et al., *Learning curve assessment for percutaneous left atrial appendage closure with the WATCHMAN occluder*. J Interv Cardiol, 2016. **29**(4): pp. 393-399.

[61] Reddy, V.Y., et al., *Safety of percutaneous left atrial appendage closure: results from the Watchman Left Atrial Appendage System for Embolic Protection in Patients with AF (PROTECT AF) clinical trial and the Continued Access Registry*. Circulation, 2011. **123**(4): pp. 417-424.

[62] Freixa, X., et al., *The chicken-wing morphology: an anatomical challenge for left atrial appendage occlusion*. J Interv Cardiol, 2013. **26**(5): pp. 509-514.

[63] Badheka, A.O., et al., *Utilization and adverse outcomes of percutaneous left atrial appendage closure for stroke prevention in atrial fibrillation in the United States: influence of hospital volume*. Circ Arrhythm Electrophysiol, 2015. **8**(1): pp. 42-48.

[64] Berti, S., et al., *Left atrial appendage occlusion in high-risk patients with non-valvular atrial fibrillation*. Heart, 2016. **102**(24): pp. 1969-1973.

[65] Enomoto, Y., et al., *Use of non-warfarin oral anticoagulants instead of warfarin during left atrial appendage closure with the Watchman device*. Heart Rhythm, 2017. **14**(1): pp. 19-24.

[66] Bosche, L.I., et al., *Initial experience with novel oral anticoagulants during the first 45 Days after left atrial appendage closure with the Watchman device*. Clin Cardiol, 2015. **38**(12): pp. 720-724.

[67] Viles-Gonzalez, J.F., et al., *The clinical impact of incomplete left atrial appendage closure with the Watchman Device in patients with atrial fibrillation: a PROTECT AF (Percutaneous Closure of the Left Atrial Appendage Versus Warfarin Therapy for Prevention of Stroke in Patients With Atrial Fibrillation) substudy*. J Am Coll Cardiol, 2012. **59**(10): pp. 923-929.

[68] Hornung, M., et al., *Catheter-based closure of residual leaks after percutaneous occlusion of the left atrial appendage*. Catheter Cardiovasc Interv, 2016. **87**(7): pp. 1324-1330.

[69] Main, M.L., et al., *Assessment of device-related thrombus and associated clinical outcomes with the WATCHMAN left atrial appendage closure device for embolic protection in patients with atrial fibrillation (from the PROTECT-AF Trial)*. Am J Cardiol, 2016. **117**(7): pp. 1127-1134.

[70] Plicht, B., et al., *Risk factors for thrombus formation on the Amplatzer Cardiac Plug after left atrial appendage occlusion*. JACC Cardiovasc Interv, 2013. **6**(6): pp. 606-613.

[71] Aminian, A., et al., *Embolization of left atrial appendage closure devices: a systematic review of cases reported with the watchman device and the amplatzer cardiac plug*. Catheter Cardiovasc Interv, 2015. **86**(1): pp. 128-135.

[72] Behnes, M., et al., *--LAA Occluder View for post-implantation Evaluation (LOVE)--standardized imaging proposal evaluating implanted left atrial appendage occlusion devices by cardiac computed tomography*. BMC Med Imaging, 2016. **16**: p. 25.

[73] Saw, J., et al., *Cardiac CT angiography for device surveillance after endovascular left atrial appendage closure*. Eur Heart J Cardiovasc Imaging, 2015. **16**(11): pp. 1198-1206.

[74] Jaguszewski, M., et al., *Cardiac CT and echocardiographic evaluation of peri-device flow after percutaneous left atrial appendage closure using the AMPLATZER cardiac plug device*. Catheter Cardiovasc Interv, 2015. **85**(2): pp. 306-12.

[75] Fastner, C., et al., *Veno-venous double lasso pull-and-push technique for transseptal retrieval of an embolized Watchman occluder*. Cardiovasc Revasc Med, 2016. **17**(3): pp. 206-208.

[76] Gloekler, S., et al., *Early results of first versus second generation Amplatzer occluders for left atrial appendage closure in patients with atrial fibrillation*. Clin Res Cardiol, 2015. **104**(8): pp. 656-665.

[77] Abualsaud, A., et al., *Side-by-Side comparison of LAA occlusion performance with the amplatzer cardiac plug and amplatzer amulet*. J Invasive Cardiol, 2016. **28**(1): pp. 34-38.

[78] Lam, Y.Y., et al., *Left atrial appendage closure with AMPLATZER cardiac plug for stroke prevention in atrial fibrillation: initial Asia-Pacific experience*. Catheter Cardiovasc Interv, 2012. **79**(5): pp. 794-800.

[79] Holmes, D.R., Jr., et al., *Left atrial appendage closure as an alternative to warfarin for stroke prevention in atrial fibrillation: a patient-level meta-analysis*. J Am Coll Cardiol, 2015. **65**(24): pp. 2614-2623.

[80] Reddy, V.Y., et al., *Time to cost-effectiveness following stroke reduction strategies in AF: Warfarin Versus NOACs Versus LAA closure*. J Am Coll Cardiol, 2015. **66**(24): pp. 2728-2739.

[81] Reddy, V., et al., *TCT-617 Cost effectiveness following treatment initiation of stroke reduction strategies in non-valvular atrial fibrillation: Warfarin vs NOACs vs left atrial appendage closure.* J Am Coll Cardiol, 2016. **68**(18S): pp. B251-B252.

[82] Tzikas, A., et al., *Percutaneous left atrial appendage occlusion: the Munich consensus document on definitions, endpoints and data collection requirements for clinical studies.* EuroIntervention, 2016. **12**(1): pp. 103-111.

[83] Sahay, S., et al., *Efficacy and safety of left atrial appendage closure versus medical treatment in atrial fibrillation: a network meta-analysis from randomised trials.* Heart, 2017. **103**(2): pp. 139-147.

[84] Park, J.W., et al., *Left atrial appendage closure with Amplatzer cardiac plug in atrial fibrillation: initial European experience.* Catheter Cardiovasc Interv, 2011. **77**(5): p. 700-6.

Section 8

Heart Team Concept

Chapter 13

Collaboration between Interventional Cardiologists and Cardiac Surgeons in the Era of Heart Team Approach

Takashi Murashita

Additional information is available at the end of the chapter

http://dx.doi.org/10.5772/67788

Abstract

Along with the rapid evolution of transcatheter interventions, interventional cardiologists are playing more and more important role in the care of cardiovascular disease. The consequence of rapid change in the landscape has been fostering new and improved relationships between interventional cardiologists and cardiac surgeons and the formulation of Heart Team to facilitate patient management. A hybrid strategy is a combination of tools available only in the catheterization laboratory with those available only in the operative room in order to gain maximum profit from both of them. In the current era, the continuous development in transcatheter procedures along with the adoption of minimally invasive surgical approaches makes hybrid strategy an attractive alternative to conventional surgical or transcatheter techniques for any given set of cardiovascular diseases. In the areas of coronary revascularization, valve repair or replacement, and ablation for atrial fibrillation, hybrid approaches have shown great benefit especially in high-risk cases. With the technological evolutions in the treatment of cardiovascular disease, the Heart Team approach utilizing the expertise of all relevant specialties will be more and more invaluable in facilitating optimal patient selection, procedural planning, complication management, postprocedural care, and patient outcomes.

Keywords: interventional cardiologist, cardiac surgeon, hybrid, heart team

1. Introduction

A hybrid approach combines the treatments traditionally available only in the catheterization laboratory with those traditionally available only in the operative room in order to obtain maximum benefit from both procedures. The continuous evolution of transcatheter technology along with the adoption of minimally invasive surgical approaches make hybrid procedures an attractive alternative to conventional surgical or interventional techniques for a wide variety of cardiovascular diseases [1–3]. Angelini et al. reported the first case series of hybrid coronary artery revascularization in 1996 [4]. Since then, along with technological advancement, hybrid procedures are currently applied not only for coronary artery disease, but also for valvular heart disease, arrhythmia, congenital heart disease, aortic diseases, and peripheral vascular disease.

As a result of rapid evolution of transcatheter techniques, interventional cardiologists are playing a central role in the management of cardiovascular diseases. For a success of hybrid approach, a formulation of Heart Team combined with good collaboration between interventional cardiologists and cardiac surgeons is encouraged to facilitate patient management. The indications and patient selection for hybrid procedures need to be well discussed in Heart Team.

2. Hybrid coronary revascularization (HCR)

2.1. Rationale of HCR

Despite the increasing use of percutaneous coronary intervention (PCI) for coronary artery disease during the past decade [5], coronary artery bypass grafting (CABG) remains the gold standard for multivessel coronary artery disease or left main disease [6]. A number of major trials such as SYNTAX [7], ASCERT [8], and FREEDOM [9] reported superior long-term survival rates of CABG compared with PCI.

The main factor of the superiority of CABG over PCI is the use of left internal mammary artery (LIMA) to left anterior descending (LAD) artery [10, 11]. The excellent long-term patency of LIMA to LAD graft has been established [12–14], whereas the long-term outcomes of other conduits such as saphenous vein graft and radial artery have been reported to be poorer than those of LIMA. The patency rates of saphenous vein grafts were 71–87% at 1-year after surgery in previous studies [15–17], and up to 50% at 10-years [15–19].

On the other hand, newer generation of drug-eluted stents are associated with fewer restenosis and repeat revascularization compared to conventional bare metal stents [20], and are associated with similar or even better long-term patency rates than saphenous vein grafts [11, 17, 21–23]. Thus, the combination of LIMA-LAD bypass and PCI using new generation of drug-eluting stents to non-LAD lesions takes the advantage of both procedures. The rationale of HCR is to combine the survival benefit and high patency rates of LIMA graft with the lower restenosis rates of new generation drug-eluting stents for non-LAD lesions [11, 24, 25].

2.2. Indications of HCR

HCR is applicable in patients having multivessel coronary artery disease with CABG-suitable LAD disease and PCI-suitable non-LAD disease [1, 11, 26–28]. HCR takes the most advantage in patients with comorbidities such as diabetes mellitus, obesity, chronic kidney disease, chronic occlusive pulmonary disease, and advanced age [11, 28], because these comorbidities are known to increase the risk of conventional CABG.

http://dx.doi.org/10.5772/67788

On the other hand, there is a couple of situations where HCR is not suitable, such as left subclavian artery stenosis, nonusable LIMA graft due to prior radiation to the left chest, intramyocardial LAD, previous stent to the target lesions, and extensive calcification on LAD [27, 29].

American guidelines for HCR demonstrate that HCR is reasonable in patients with one or more of the following: limitations to traditional CABG, such as heavily calcified proximal aorta or poor target vessels for CABG but amenable to PCI; lack of suitable graft conduits; unfavorable LAD for PCI such as excessive vessel tortuosity or chronic total occlusion with Class IIa recommendation with level of evidence of B. Also, HCR may be reasonable as an alternative to multivessel PCI or CABG in an attempt to improve the overall risk-benefit ratio of the procedures with Class IIb recommendation with level of evidence of C [3].

2.3. Techniques of HCR

Several techniques have been reported for achieving minimally invasive CABG [1]. Thoracoscopic endoscopic CABG; LIMA graft is harvested with the use of thoracoscopy through a port-access approach. The LIMA-to-LAD anastomosis is then performed by hand on the beating heart using specially designed stabilizers and retractors [2]. Robotically assisted CABG; LIMA graft is harvested with an assistance of robot followed by a hand-sewn LIMA-to-LAD anastomosis on the beating heart [3]. Totally endoscopic CABG, LIMA harvest and the anastomosis are performed endoscopically with the robot. The anastomosis can be performed on the beating heart or on cardiopulmonary bypass on an arrested heart.

HCR can be performed either as a one-staged or a two-staged procedure. A two-staged procedure is defined as a PCI and CABG performed separately by hours or days. A one-staged HCR is defined as PCI and CABG performed in a hybrid-operating room in one operative setting. The advantages of one-staged HCR include complete revascularization with minimal patient discomfort, intraoperative confirmation of LIMA-to-LAD anastomosis, and easy conversion to conventional CABG if needed [29]. However, bleeding concerns due to dual antiplatelet therapy and incomplete heparin reversal, as well as acute stent thrombosis possibility are disadvantages of one-staged HCR [11].

In a two-staged approach, there is a concern of adverse coronary events between the procedures because patients are incompletely revascularized. When PCI is preceded, CABG needs to be performed under the effect of dual antiplatelet therapy, which leads to significant bleeding risk. On the other hand, when CABG is preceded, PCI can be performed under the protection of the LIMA-to-LAD graft and the ability to verify the patency of the LIMA-to-LAD graft while avoiding the risk of bleeding due to dual antiplatelet therapy. Therefore, CABG-first strategy for two-staged HCR is preferable.

2.4. Outcomes of HCR

The surgical outcomes of previous studies regarding HCR are summarized in **Table 1**. The 30-day mortality after HCR ranged from 0 to 2.4%. LIMA patency is reported to be over 90%. The event-free survival rate ranged from 83 to 100%, whereas the incidence of major adverse cardiac and cerebrovascular events (MACCEs) ranged from 0 to 12.2%. However, the sample size of each study was relatively small.

Study	Year	Number of pts	Follow-up (months)	30-day mortality (%)	MACCE (%)	Event-free survival (%)
Angelini et al. [4]	1996	6	–	0	–	89
Leacche et al. [25]	2013	80	1	–	2.5	91
Rab et al. [53]	2012	22	38.8 ± 22	0	0	95
Lewis et al. [54]	1999	14	1.44	0	–	93
Isomura et al. [55]	2000	37	24	1.4	–	92
Presbitero et al. [56]	2001	42	18	2.4	12.2	83
Lee et al. [57]	2004	6	12	0	0	–
Repossini et al. [58]	2013	166	64.6 ± 12.0	1.2	12	83 (at 5 years)
Gilard et al. [59]	2007	70	33	1.4	–	97
Kon et al. [60]	2008	15	12	0	–	93
Vassiliades et al. [61]	2006	47	7	0	–	90
Bonatti et al. [62]	2008	5	6	0	–	100

Note: MACCE; major adverse cardiac and cerebrovascular events.

Table 1. Outcomes of hybrid coronary revascularization.

Zhu et al. performed a meta-analysis to compare the short-term outcomes of HCR with those of CABG for multivessel coronary artery disease. They found that HCR was noninferior to CABG in terms of the incidence of death, myocardial infarction, stroke, and renal failure, whereas HCR was associated with less blood transfusion and shorter length of stay in hospital [30]. Halkos et al. compared the outcomes of 147 HCR cases with matched off-pump CABG cases. They reported 5-year survival rate and the incidence of MACCE were similar between HCR and off-pump CABG, whereas the need for repeated revascularization was higher in HCR group [31].

3. Transcatheter treatment for aortic valve disease

For the treatment of severe symptomatic aortic stenosis, surgical aortic valve replacement has been the gold standard. The advent and rapidly widespread adoption of transcatheter aortic valve replacement (TAVR) has now resulted in it becoming the option for patients who would have been considered inoperable or prohibitively high surgical risk [32]. Excellent mid-term

http://dx.doi.org/10.5772/67788

and long-term outcomes after TAVR have been reported [33, 34], and indications of TAVR are expanding to severe aortic valve regurgitation associated with moderate aortic valve stenosis and valve-in-valve procedures for surgical bioprosthetic valve failure.

TAVR procedures are now shifting to percutaneous approach and even general anesthesia is not mandatory. The percutaneous transfemoral route is the preferred approach in the majority of the cases due to its associated advantages [35]. Although some centers reported that transapical and transfemoral approach resulted in the similar outcomes [36], transapical approach is usually associated with poorer outcomes than transfemoral approach [37]. Interventional cardiologists possess the required skills for transfemoral TAVR including the handling of guidewires, catheters, and image selection. They can even take care of technical complications associated with TAVR, such as coronary obstruction and conduction disturbance by performing PCI or implanting pacemaker. Although interventional cardiologists can take a lead in TAVR procedures, surgeons still play an important role in managing life-threatening complications such as aortic root rupture, cardiac tamponade, and vascular complications. Those complications cannot be managed percutaneously and surgical interventions are the only viable rescue option. Furthermore, surgeons have the skill to ensure procedural success in patients whom transfemoral approach is not applicable. For the success of transapical and transaortic TAVR procedures, surgeons play a crucial role and they should be familiar with individual cases and technical aspects.

Postprocedural care and rehabilitation are undoubtedly important in optimizing functional status and clinical outcomes [38]. Cardiologists can take the leading role in this area by virtue of familiarity with all aspects of general cardiology issues such as heart failure and arrhythmia in the management of these complex patients.

In conclusion, a good collaboration between interventional cardiologists and cardiac surgeons and formulation of a Heart Team is essential for the success of TAVR. The decision making for patients selection and surgical approach, the actual performance of procedure in the operating room, and postoperative care should be performed by a Heart Team approach [39].

4. Transcatheter treatment for mitral valve disease

4.1. Transcatheter mitral valve repair

The prevalence of mitral regurgitation is higher than other valvular heart diseases [40, 41]. Surgical mitral repair remains the gold standard for patients with primary mitral regurgitation. However, there are a growing number of patients with mitral regurgitation underserved by surgical therapy due to prohibitive surgical risks. The recent development of transcatheter mitral valve technique provides an additional therapeutic option for some high-risk and inoperable patients [42, 43]. The optimal way to adjudicate innovative surgical and interventional mitral therapies is through a robust collaboration within a well-functioning Heart Team which includes not only cardiac surgeons and interventional cardiologists but also imaging specialists.

The current leader in the field of transcatheter mitral repair device is the MitraClip (Abbott Vascular, Santa Clara, CA). This device is delivered in an antegrade transseptal approach across the atrial septum from the femoral vein to achieve an edge-to-edge direct leaflet approximation (**Figure 1**). More than 30,000 patients worldwide have been treated with this procedure to date. In the United States, a Society of Thoracic Surgeons (STS)/American College of Cardiology database analysis of the first 564 cases performed through August 2014 showed the average patient age was 83 years, with a median STS predicted risk of mortality for mitral valve repair and replacement of 7.9 and 10.0%, respectively. The majority of the patients had prohibitive surgical risks such as severe frailty, prior cardiac surgery, and end-stage heart failure. The procedural success rate was 91.8% with a 30-day operative mortality of 5.8% [43].

The randomized EVEREST II trial showed that the need for surgery for residual mitral regurgitation was significantly higher in patients who received MitraClip compared with those who underwent surgery at 1 year and 5 years; however, the MitraClip procedure was associated with superior safety and similar improvements in clinical outcomes [44, 45]. Currently, guidelines state that MitraClip can be considered in patients with severe primary mitral regurgitation who meet the echocardiographic criteria of eligibility, and are judged inoperable or at prohibitive surgical risk by a Heart Team [32, 46]. Further studies are needed to apply this technique to intermediate- or low-risk patients.

In conclusion, the MitraClip procedure has proven reasonable safety and efficacy in high-risk patients and is already considered as an established part of the mitral valve program in high-volume centers. A multidisciplinary Heart Team approach will play a crucial role for careful patient selection and clinical application of the transcatheter interventions as a part of a successful and multimodal mitral valve program [47].

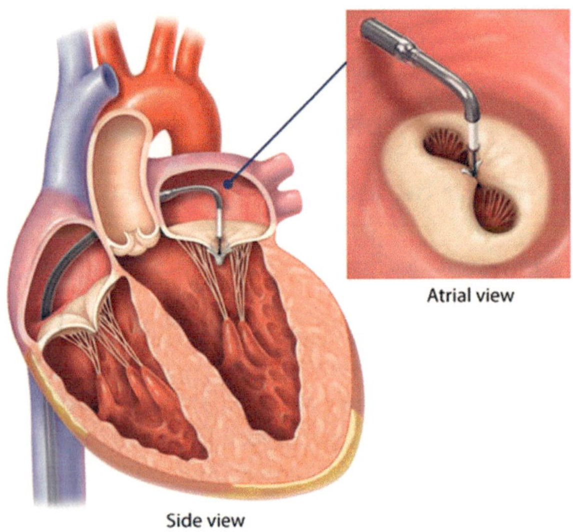

Figure 1. MitraClip (Abbott Vascular, Santa Clara, CA) is a percutaneous mitral valve repair using anterior-posterior edge-to-edge direct leaflet approximation.

4.2. Transcatheter mitral valve replacement

Unlike transcatheter mitral valve repair, the challenges of deploying and anchoring a functional prosthetic device into the mitral valve annulus amid the intact subvalvular apparatus is more complex. As of January 2016, the total human experience with transcatheter mitral valve replacement implantation surpassed 50 cases, with half of those performed in the United States [43]. The preliminary outcomes have been promising so far.

The Tendyne device (Abbott Vascular, Santa Clara, CA) is a potentially fully retrievable trileaflet porcine pericardial valve with an impermeable nitinol skirt which has a prominent cuff positioned to rest on the intertrigonal aortomitral curtain [48] (**Figure 2**). The Tendyne is an intraannular valve that does not specifically capture the leaflets, and thus the primary clinical target is patients with functional mitral regurgitation. The first US use of Tendyne device was in April 2015. Currently, multiple experienced centers have been chosen for the Food and Drug Administration (FDA) clinical trial for high risk patients inoperable for conventional mitral valve replacement. Several other devices for transcatheter mitral valve replacement are also in the stage of clinical investigation.

Despite continuing innovation, current transcatheter mitral valve replacement delivery systems remain large and the majority require a transapical retrograde approach to the mitral valve. Therefore, the collaboration between interventional cardiologists and surgeons is needed as with the transapical TAVR procedure.

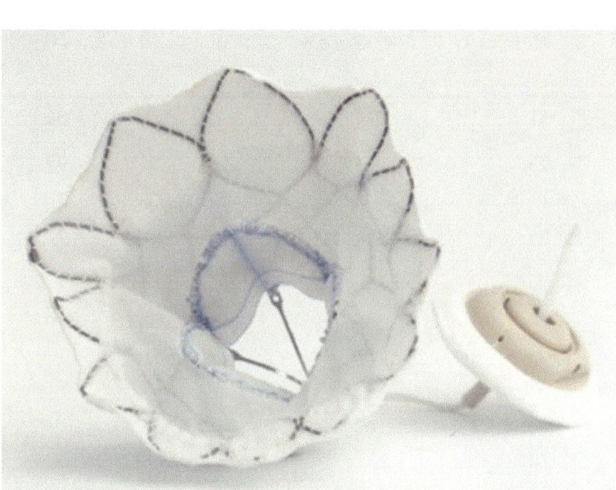

Figure 2. Tendyne (Abbott Vascular, Santa Clara, CA) is a transapically delivered porcine pericardial valve for transcatheter mitral valve replacement.

5. Hybrid approach for atrial fibrillation

Nowadays the majority of ablations for symptomatic atrial fibrillation are catheter-cased. In the United States from 2000 to 2010, over 93,000 catheter ablations were performed for atrial fibrillation [49]. However, the outcomes of catheter ablation for patients with significant valve disease and long-standing persistent atrial fibrillation remain poor [50]. For patients who have valvular heart disease or patients who are refractory to antiarrhythmic drugs or catheter ablation, surgical ablation called Cox-Maze procedure is recommended [51].

The hybrid approach for atrial fibrillation represents a collaborative between cardiac surgeons and cardiologists utilizing the strengths of both techniques in order to achieve outcomes that maximize the success rates and minimize the procedural complications. There are several potential advantages to a hybrid approach [50]. From a surgical standpoint, direct visualization allows surgeons to perform aggressive ablation at sites which may be challenging for catheter ablation due to risk of injuring esophagus or phrenic nerves, and also allows surgeons to confirm of transmurality of ablation. Moreover, the ability to exclude the left atrial appendage serves to potentially eliminate need for anticoagulation. On the other hand, catheter ablation allows more complex mapping of the left atrium for either complex fractionated atrial electrograms or rotors.

Hybrid procedures incorporate both an epicardial surgical ablation and endocardial catheter ablation [52]. The procedure can be done in either one-staged or two-staged fashion. The outcomes of hybrid approach for atrial fibrillation in previous studies are shown in **Table 2.** While all procedures were done through minimally invasive approach, the approach varied with right,

Study	Year	Number of pts	Follow-up (months)	Mortality (%)	Success rate off AA drugs (%)	Success rate on AA drugs (%)
Mahapatra et al. [63]	2011	15	20.7 ± 4.5	0	86.7	93.3
Krul et al. [64]	2011	31	12	0	86	–
Pison et al. [65]	2012	26	12	0	92	–
Muneretto et al. [66]	2012	36	30	0	77.7	91.6
Gersak et al. [67]	2012	50	24	4	87	–
La Meir et al. [68]	2013	35	12	0	91.4	–
Gehi et al. [69]	2013	101	12	2	60.7	73.3
Bisleri et al. [70]	2013	45	28 ± 1.7	0	88.9	–
Gersak et al. [71]	2014	73	12	0	52	80
Bulava et al. [72]	2015	50	12	0	84	94

Note: AA, antiarrhythmic.

Table 2. Outcomes of hybrid approach for atrial fibrillation.

and bilateral thoracoscopic approaches as well as subxiphoid and laparoscopic access. Overall, hybrid ablation procedures are associated with low mortality which is up to 4%. High success rates are reported noting sinus rhythm off antiarrhythmic drugs in about 87% of cases and in about 92% when antiarrhythmic drugs are added.

In conclusion, for the success of the hybrid ablation for atrial fibrillation, a creation of a collaborative team between cardiac surgeons and electrophysiologists is crucial. This collaboration will permit important advances in improving the outcomes of procedure especially in challenging patients.

6. Conclusions

Nowadays, the cases of patients who suffer from cardiovascular disease are more and more complex. Along with the technological advancement, patients who used to be thought inoperable can be treated by a new technology with a reasonable risk. Interventional cardiologists tend to be more invasive in their field, whereas cardiac surgeons tend to seek for minimally invasive approach. There are advantages and disadvantages in both surgery and interventions. The rational for hybrid procedures is to achieve the best outcome by combining the strengths of both surgery and interventional procedures. The key point for the success of hybrid procedures is the collaboration between interventional cardiologists and cardiac surgeons. In the current era, patient selection and indications for each procedure must be well discussed in a well-functioning Heart Team.

Author details

Takashi Murashita

Address all correspondence to: tmurashita@gmail.com

Heart and Vascular Institute, West Virginia University, Morgantown, WV, USA

References

[1] Byrne JG, Leacche M, Vaughan DE, Zhao DX. Hybrid cardiovascular procedures. JACC Cardiovasc Interv. 2008;1(5):459-68.

[2] Leacche M, Umakanthan R, Zhao DX, Byrne JG. Surgical update: hybrid procedures, do they have a role? Circ Cardiovasc Interv. 2010;3(5):511-8.

[3] Papakonstantinou NA, Baikoussis NG, Dedeilias P, Argiriou M, Charitos C. Cardiac surgery or interventional cardiology? Why not both? Let's go hybrid. J Cardiol. 2017; 69(1):46-56.

[4] Angelini GD, Wilde P, Salerno TA, Bosco G, Calafiore AM. Integrated left small thoracotomy and angioplasty for multivessel coronary artery revascularisation. Lancet 1996; 347(9003):787-8.

[5] Epstein AJ, Polsky D, Yang F, Yang L, Groeneveld PW. Coronary revascularization trends in the United States, 2001-2008. JAMA. 2011;305(17):1769-76.

[6] Serruys PW, Morice MC, Kappetein AP, Colombo A, Holmes DR, Mack MJ, et al. Percutaneous coronary intervention versus coronary-artery bypass grafting for severe coronary artery disease. N Engl J Med 2009;360(10):961-72.

[7] Mohr FW, Morice MC, Kappetein AP, Feldman TE, Ståhle E, Colombo A, et al. Coronary artery bypass graft surgery versus percutaneous coronary intervention in patients with three-vessel disease and left main coronary disease: 5-year follow-up of the randomised, clinical SYNTAX trial. Lancet. 2013;381(9867):629-38.

[8] Weintraub WS, Grau-Sepulveda MV, Weiss JM, O'Brien SM, Peterson ED, Kolm P, et al. Comparative effectiveness of revascularization strategies. N Engl J Med 2012;366(16): 1467-76.

[9] Farkouh ME, Domanski M, Sleeper LA, Siami FS, Dangas G, Mack M, et al. Strategies for multivessel revascularization in patients with diabetes. N Engl J Med. 2012; 367(25):2375-84.

[10] Wrigley BJ, Dubey G, Spyt T, Gershlick AH. Hybrid revascularisation in multivessel coronary artery disease: could a combination of CABG and PCI be the best option in selected patients? EuroIntervention. 2013;8(11):1335-41.

[11] Harskamp RE, Zheng Z, Alexander JH, Williams JB, Xian Y, Halkos ME, et al. Status quo of hybrid coronary revascularization for multi-vessel coronary artery disease. Ann Thorac Surg. 2013;96(6):2268-77.

[12] Shah PJ, Durairaj M, Gordon I, Fuller J, Rosalion A, Seevanayagam S, et al. Factors affecting patency of internal thoracic artery graft: clinical and angiographic study in 1434 symptomatic patients operated between 1982 and 2002. Eur J Cardiothorac Surg. 2004; 26(1):118-24.

[13] Cameron A, Davis KB, Green G, Schaff HV. Coronary bypass surgery with internal-thoracic-artery grafts—effects on survival over a 15-year period. N Engl J Med. 1996; 334 (4):216-9.

[14] Loop FD, Lytle BW, Cosgrove DM, Stewart RW, Goormastic M, Williams GW, et al. Influence of the internal-mammary-artery graft on 10-year survival and other cardiac events. N Engl J Med. 1986;314(1):1-6.

[15] Alexander JH, Hafley G, Harrington RA, Peterson ED, Ferguson TB, Jr., Lorenz TJ, et al. Efficacy and safety of edifoligide, an E2F transcription factor decoy, for prevention of vein graft failure following coronary artery bypass graft surgery: PREVENT IV: a randomized controlled trial. JAMA 2005;294(19):2446-54.

[16] Harskamp RE, Lopes RD, Baisden CE, de Winter RJ, Alexander JH. Saphenous vein graft failure after coronary artery bypass surgery: pathophysiology, management, and future directions. Ann Surg. 2013;257(5):824-33.

[17] Puskas JD, Williams WH, Mahoney EM, Huber PR, Block PC, Duke PG, et al. Off-pump vs conventional coronary artery bypass grafting: early and 1-year graft patency, cost, and quality-of-life outcomes: a randomized trial. JAMA. 2004;291(15):1841-49.

[18] Tatoulis J, Buxton BF, Fuller JA. Patencies of 2127 arterial to coronary conduits over 15 years. Ann Thorac Surg. 2004;77(1):93-101.

[19] Goldman S, Zadina K, Moritz T, Ovitt T, Sethi G, Copeland JG, et al. Long-term patency of saphenous vein and left internal mammary artery grafts after coronary artery bypass surgery: results from a Department of Veterans Affairs Cooperative Study. J Am Coll Cardiol. 2004;44(11):2149-56.

[20] Stettler C, Wandel S, Allemann S, Kastrati A, Morice MC, Schömig A, et al. Outcomes associated with drug-eluting and bare-metal stents: a collaborative network meta-analysis. Lancet 2007;370(9591):937-48.

[21] Yeung AC, Leon MB, Jain A, Tolleson TR, Spriggs DJ, Mc Laurin BT, et al. Clinical evaluation of the resolute zotarolimus-eluting coronary stent system in the treatment of de novo lesions in native coronary arteries: the Resolute US clinical trial. J Am Coll Cardiol. 2011;57(17):1778-83.

[22] Weisz G, Leon MB, Holmes DR, Jr., Kereiakes DJ, Popma JJ, Teirstein PS, et al. Five-year follow-up after sirolimus-eluting stent implantation results of the SIRIUS (Sirolimus-Eluting Stent in De-Novo Native Coronary Lesions) Trial. J Am Coll Cardiol. 2009; 53(17):1488-97.

[23] Alfonso F, Pérez-Vizcayno MJ, Hernandez R, Fernandez C, Escaned J, Bañuelos C, et al. Sirolimus-eluting stents versus bare-metal stents in patients with in-stent restenosis: results of a pooled analysis of two randomized studies. Catheter Cardiovasc Interv. 2008;72(4):459-67.

[24] Mauri L, Orav EJ, Kuntz RE. Late loss in lumen diameter and binary restenosis for drug-eluting stent comparison. Circulation. 2005;111(25):3435-42.

[25] Leacche M, Byrne JG, Solenkova NS, Reagan B, Mohamed TI, Fredi JL, et al. Comparison of 30-day outcomes of coronary artery bypass grafting surgery verus hybrid coronary revascularization stratified by SYNTAX and euroSCORE. J Thorac Cardiovasc Surg. 2013; 145(4):1004-12.

[26] Harskamp RE, Brennan JM, Xian Y, Halkos ME, Puskas JD, Thourani VH, et al. Practice patterns and clinical outcomes after hybrid coronary revascularization in the United States: an analysis from the society of thoracic surgeons adult cardiac database. Circulation. 2014;130(11):872-79.

[27] Green KD, Lynch DR, Jr., Chen TP, Zhao D. Combining PCI and CABG: the role of hybrid revascularization. Curr Cardiol Rep. 2013;15(4):351.

[28] Kappetein AP, Head SJ. CABG, stents, or hybrid procedures for left main disease? EuroIntervention. 2015;11:Suppl V:V111-4.

[29] Verhaegh AJ, Accord RE, van Garsse L, Maessen JG. Hybrid coronary revascularization as a safe, feasible, and viable alternative to conventional coronary artery bypass grafting: what is the current evidence? Minim Invasive Surg. 2013;142616.

[30] Zhu P, Zhou P, Sun Y, Guo Y, Mai M, Zheng S. Hybrid coronary revascularization versus coronary artery bypass grafting for multivessel coronary artery disease: systematic review and meta-analysis. J Cardiothorac Surg. 2015;10:63.

[31] Halkos ME, Vassiliades TA, Douglas JS, Morris DC, Rab ST, Liberman HA, et al. Hybrid coronary revascularization versus off-pump coronary artery bypass grafting for the treatment of multivessel coronary artery disease. Ann Thorac Surg. 2011;92(5):1695-701.

[32] Joint Task Force on the Management of Valvular Heart Disease of the European Society of Cardiology (ESC), European Association for Cardio-Thoracic Surgery (EACTS), Vahanian A, Alfieri O, Andreotti F, Antunes MJ, et al. Guidelines on the management of valvular heart disease (version 2012). Eur Heart J. 2012;33(19):2451-96.

[33] Mack MJ, Leon MB, Smith CR, Miller DC, Moses JW, Tuzcu EM, et al. 5-year outcomes of transcatheter aortic valve replacement or surgical aortic valve replacement for high surgical risk patients with aortic stenosis (PARTNER 1): a randomised controlled trial. Lancet. 2015;385(9986):2477-84.

[34] Kapadia SR, Leon MB, Makkar RR, Tuzcu EM, Svensson LG, Kodali S, et al. 5-year outcomes of transcatheter aortic valve replacement compared with standard treatment for patients with inoperable aortic stenosis (PARTNER 1): a randomised controlled trial. Lancet. 2015;385(9986):2485-91.

[35] Stortecky S, O'Sullivan CJ, Buellesfeld L, Windecker S, Wenaweser P. Transcatheter aortic valve implantation: the transfemoral access route is the default access. EuroIntervention. 2013;9 Suppl:S14-8.

[36] Murashita T, Greason KL, Pochettino A, Sandhu GS, Nkomo VT, Bresnahan JF, et al. Clinical outcomes after transapical and transfemoral transcatheter aortic valve insertion: an evolving experience. Ann Thorac Surg. 2016;102(1):56-61.

[37] Blackstone EH, Suri RM, Rajeswaran J, Babaliaros V, Douglas PS, Fearon WF, et al. Propensity-matched comparisons of clinical outcomes after transapical or transfemoral transcatheter aortic valve replacement: a placement of aortic transcatheter valves (PARTNER)-I trial substudy. Circulation. 2015;131(22):1989-2000.

[38] Zanettini R, Gatto G, Mori I, Pozzoni MB, Pelenghi S, Martinelli L, et al. Cardiac rehabilitation and mid-term follow-up after transcatheter aortic valve implantation. J Geriatr Cardiol. 2014;11(4):279-85.

[39] Colombo A RN. Transcatheter valve interventions: playground for cardiologists or cardiac surgeons? The cardiologist's view. EuroIntervention. 2015;11(SupplW):W20-2.

[40] Nkomo VT, Gardin JM, Skelton TN, Gottdiener JS, Scott CG, Enriquez-Sarano M. Burden of valvular heart diseases: a population-based study. Lancet. 2006;368(9540):1005-11.

[41] Lloyd-Jones D, Adams RJ, Brown TM, Carnethon M, Dai S, De Simone G, et al. Heart disease and stroke statistics-2010 update: a report from the American Heart Association. Circulation. 2010;121(7):e46-215.

[42] Maisano F, Alfieri O, Banai S, Buchbinder M, Colombo A, Falk V, et al. The future of transcatheter mitral valve interventions: competitive or complementary role of repair vs. replacement? Eur Heart J. 2015;36(26):1651-9.

[43] Badhwar V, Thourani VH, Ailawadi G, Mack M. Transcatheter mitral valve therapy: the event horizon. J Thorac Cardiovasc Surg. 2016;152(2):330-6.

[44] Feldman T, Foster E, Glower DD, Kar S, Rinaldi MJ, Fail PS, et al. Percutaneous repair or surgery for mitral regurgitation. N Engl J Med. 2011;364(15):1395-406.

[45] Feldman T, Kar S, Elmariah S, Smart SC, Trento A, Siegel RJ, et al. Randomized comparison of percutaneous repair and surgery for mitral regurgitation: 5-Year Results of EVEREST II. J Am Coll Cardiol. 2015;66(25):2844-54.

[46] Nishimura RA, Otto CM, Bonow RO, A. CB, Erwin JP, 3rd., Guyton RA, et al. 2014 AHA/ACC Guideline for the management of patients with valvular heart disease: a report of the American College of Cardiology/American Heart Association Task Force on Practice Guidelines. Circulation. 2014;129(23):e521-643.

[47] Nielsen SL. Current status of transcatheter mitral valve repair therapies—From surgical concepts towards future directions. Scand Cardiovasc J. 2016;50(5-6):367-76.

[48] Perpetua EM, Reisman M. The tendyne transcatheter mitral valve implantation system. EuroIntervention. 2015;11(Suppl W):W78-9.

[49] Deshmukh A, Patel NJ, Pant S, Shah N, Chothani A, Mehta K, et al. In-hospital complications associated with catheter ablation of atrial fibrillation in the United States between 2000 and 2010: analysis of 93 801 procedures. Circulation 2013;128(19):2104-12.

[50] Driver K, Mangrum JM. Hybrid approaches in atrial fibrillation ablation: why, where and who? J Thorac Dis. 2015;7(2):159-64.

[51] Badhwar V, Rankin JS, Damiano RJ, Jr., Gillinov AM, Bakaeen FG, Edgerton JR, et al. The society of thoracic surgeons 2017 clinical practice guidelines for the surgical treatment of atrial fibrillation. Ann Thorac Surg. 2017;103(1):239-41.

[52] Wang PJ. Hybrid epicardial and endocardial ablation of atrial fibrillation: is ablation on two sides of the atrial wall better than one? J Am Heart Assoc. 2015;4(3):e001893.

[53] Rab ST, Douglas JS, Jr., Lyons E, Puskas JD, Bansal D, Halkos ME, et al. Hybrid coronary revascularization for the treatment of left main coronary stenosis: a feasibility study. Catheter Cardiovasc Interv. 2012;80(2):238-44.

[54] Lewis BS, Porat E, Halon DA, Ammar R, Flugelman MY, Khader N, et al. Same-day combined coronary angioplasty and minimally invasive coronary surgery. Am J Cardiol. 1999;84(10):1246-47.

[55] Isomura T, Suma H, Horii T, Sato T, Kobashi T, Kanemitsu H. Minimally invasive coronary artery revascularization: off-pump bypass grafting and the hybrid procedure. Ann Thorac Surg. 2000;70(6):2017-22.

[56] Presbitero P, Nicolini F, Maiello L, Franciosi G, Carcagni A, Milone F, et al. "Hybrid" percutaneous and surgical coronary revascularization: selection criteria from a single-center experience. Ital Heart J. 2001;2(5):363-8.

[57] Lee MS, Wilentz JR, Makkar RR, Singh V, Nero T, Swistel D, et al. Hybrid revascularization using percutaneous coronary intervention and robotically assisted minimally invasive direct coronary artery bypass surgery. J Invasive Cardiol. 2004;16(8):419-25.

[58] Repossini A, Tespili M, Saino A, Kotelnikov I, Moggi A, Di Bacco L, et al. Hybrid revascularization in multivessel coronary artery disease. Eur J Cardiothorac Surg. 2013;44(2):288-93.

[59] Gilard M, Bezon E, Cornily JC, Mansourati J, Mondine P, Barra JA, et al. Same-day combined percutaneous coronary intervention and coronary artery surgery. Cardiology 2007;108(4):363-7.

[60] Kon ZN, Brown EN, Tran R, Joshi A, Reicher B, Grant MC, et al. Simultaneous hybrid coronary revascularization reduces postoperative morbidity compared with results from conventional off-pump coronary artery bypass. J Thorac Cardiovasc Surg. 2008; 135(2):367-75.

[61] Vassiliades TA, Jr., Douglas JS, Morris DC, Block PC, Ghazzal Z, Rab ST, et al. Integrated coronary revascularization with drug-eluting stents: immediate and seven-month outcome. J Thorac Cardiovasc Surg. 2006;131(5):956-62.

[62] Bonatti J, Schachner T, Bonaros N, Jonetzko P, Ohlinger A, Ruetzler E, et al. Simultaneous hybrid coronary revascularization using totally endoscopic left internal mammary artery bypass grafting and placement of rapamycin eluting stents in the same interventional session. The COMBINATION pilot study. Cardiology. 2008;110(2):92-95.

[63] Mahapatra S, LaPar DJ, Kamath S, Payne J, Bilchick KC, Mangrum JM, et al. Initial experience of sequential surgical epicardial-catheter endocardial ablation for persistent and long-standing persistent atrial fibrillation with long-term follow-up. Ann Thorac Surg. 2011;91(6):1890-98.

[64] Krul SP, Driessen AH, van Boven WJ, Linnenbank AC, Geuzebroek GS, Jackman WM, et al. Thoracoscopic video-assisted pulmonary vein antrum isolation, ganglionated plexus ablation, and periprocedural confirmation of ablation lesions: first results of a hybrid surgical-electrophysiological approach for atrial fibrillation. Circ Arrhythm Electrophysiol. 2011;4(3):262-70.

http://dx.doi.org/10.5772/67788

[65] Pison L, La Meir M, van Opstal J, Blaauw Y, Maessen J, Crijns HJ. Hybrid thoracoscopic surgical and transvenous catheter ablation of atrial fibrillation. J Am Coll Cardiol. 2012;60(1):54-61.

[66] Muneretto C, Bisleri G, Bontempi L, Curnis A. Durable staged hybrid ablation with thoracoscopic and percutaneous approach for treatment of long-standing atrial fibrillation: a 30-month assessment with continuous monitoring. J Thorac Cardiovasc Surg 2012;144(6):1460-65.

[67] Gersak B, Pernat A, Robic B, Sinkovec M. Low rate of atrial fibrillation recurrence verified by implantable loop recorder monitoring following a convergent epicardial and endocardial ablation of atrial fibrillation. J Cardiovasc Electrophysiol 2012;23(10):1059-66.

[68] La Meir M, Gelsomino S, Lucà F, Pison L, Parise O, Colella A, et al. Minimally invasive surgical treatment of lone atrial fibrillation: early results of hybrid versus standard minimally invasive approach employing radiofrequency sources. Int J Cardiol. 2013;167(4):1469-75.

[69] Gehi AK, Mounsey JP, Pursell I, Landers M, Boyce K, Chung EH, et al. Hybrid epicardial-endocardial ablation using a pericardioscopic technique for the treatment of atrial fibrillation. Heart Rhythm. 2013;10(1):22-8.

[70] Bisleri G, Rosati F, Bontempi L, Curnis A, Muneretto C. Hybrid approach for the treatment of long-standing persistent atrial fibrillation: electrophysiological findings and clinical results. Eur J Cardiothorac Surg. 2013;44(5):919-23.

[71] Geršak B, Zembala MO, Müller D, Folliguet T, Jan M, Kowalski O, et al. European experience of the convergent atrial fibrillation procedure: multicenter outcomes in consecutive patients. J Thorac Cardiovasc Surg. 2014;147(4):1411-6.

[72] Bulava A, Mokracek A, Hanis J, Kurfirst V, Eisenberger M, Pesl L. Sequential hybrid procedure for persistent atrial fibrillation. J Am Heart Assoc. 2015;4(3):e001754.